Patient Compliance
in
Medical Practice and Clinical Trials

Other Raven Press Books by Bert Spilker

Guide to Clinical Studies and Developing Protocols
(Raven Press, 1984)

Guide to Clinical Interpretation of Data
(Raven Press, 1986)

Guide to Planning and Managing Multiple Clinical Studies
(Raven Press, 1987)

Multinational Drug Companies: Issues in Drug Discovery and Development (Raven Press, 1989)

Presentation of Clinical Data (with John Schoenfelder, Raven Press, 1990)

Quality of Life Assessments in Clinical Trials (Editor, Raven Press, 1990)

Data Collection Forms in Clinical Trials (with John Schoenfelder, Raven Press, 1991)

Patient Compliance
in
Medical Practice and Clinical Trials

Editors

Joyce A. Cramer, B.S.
Project Director, Epilepsy Research
Epilepsy Center
Department of Veterans Affairs Medical Center
West Haven, Connecticut; and
Department of Neurology
Yale University School of Medicine
New Haven, Connecticut

Bert Spilker, Ph.D., M.D.
Director, Project Coordination, Burroughs Wellcome Company
Research Triangle Park, North Carolina
Adjunct Professor of Pharmacology and Clinical Professor of Medicine
University of North Carolina
Clinical Professor of Pharmacy
University of North Carolina School of Pharmacy
Chapel Hill, North Carolina

RAVEN PRESS   NEW YORK

Raven Press Ltd., 1185 Avenue of the Americas, New York, New York 10036

Made in the United States of America

Library of Congress Cataloging-in-Publication Data

Patient compliance in medical practice and clinical trials / editors,
  Joyce A. Cramer, Bert Spilker.
      p.   cm.
  Includes bibliographical references.
  Includes indexes.
  ISBN 0-88167-735-3
  1. Patient compliance. 2. Medical personnel and patient.
 I. Cramer, Joyce A. II. Spilker, Bert.
  [DNLM: 1. Patient Compliance. 610.69/6]
  R727.43.P38 1991
  610.69′6—dc20
  DNLM/DLC
  for Library of Congress   90-9013
                                                      CIP

9 8 7 6 5 4 3 2 1

*to all health care providers
who are encouraging patients
to take their medication
as prescribed*

Preface

As the 1990s unfold, the topic of compliance deserves fresh attention. The results of patient failure to comply with prescribed regimens affect every aspect of medical care. The purpose of this book is to identify the issues, to document the scope of the problem, and to suggest means of enhancing patient compliance in both medical practice and clinical trials. Improving patient compliance would decrease the total cost of health care worldwide, besides providing improved health for patients.

Topics are clustered in this volume to address the following questions:

1. What is noncompliance? How does it affect physician recommendations for safe and effective dosing and also the design of clinical trials?
2. Does the degree of compliance differ among special populations, and if so, how is this manifested?
3. What happens to patients when doses are missed? How can compliance be monitored?
4. How can the issue of partial compliance be handled in clinical trials?
5. What is the impact of partial compliance on health care and research?

Organized into five sections, the book opens with an overview of the issues at both the micro and macro levels. Other chapters in the first section set the stage for further discussion by presenting information on diminished and inconsistent compliance, communicating risk and benefit information to the patient, evaluating the magnitude of unfilled prescriptions, and designing clinical trials to evaluate and enhance compliance. Section II discusses the special compliance problems that are associated with pediatric, adolescent, and geriatric patient populations. The methods used to assess patient medication habits for specific diseases are discussed in Section III. These chapters illustrate that the clinical implications of partial compliance vary. Examples of state-of-the-art continuous electronic observation of patient dosing habits are described for a variety of patient populations and for a wide selection of electronic devices. Section IV addresses analytical aspects of compliance monitoring. Understanding the scope and impact of missed doses as precisely as possible is essential in clinical trials. Practicing clinicians should be aware of these problems in order to appreciate better how data from clinical trials should be interpreted. Perspectives on health care and research are covered in the fifth section. The use of information is described in terms of health belief models. Concerns of the Food and Drug Administration are presented in terms of how compliance data are used toward understanding the safety and effectiveness of new medicines. Practical suggestions and a series of checklists are offered on how to enhance compliance in medical practice and clinical trials.

This book is written for practicing physicians and health care personnel who recognize the possibility and occurrence of noncompliance by their patients but remain unable to reliably guess "who, when, and how much." Professional specialists in every therapeutic area are aware of compliance problems that have confronted them and usually take some comfort that theirs are not the only patient populations that do not completely listen to their physicians. Clinical researchers are increasingly aware that partial compliance has become a major concern in the interpretation of their data from clinical trials. Epidemiologists, behavioral scientists, and virtually all physicians will discover the many opportunities for important research that may and should be conducted on compliance issues.

Although this book is designed to be read as an integrated treatise on patient compliance, chapters may be read in any order or used as sources of information on specific topics. The editors hope that many readers will be stimulated to engage in new research that will advance the concepts discussed in this book.

Joyce A. Cramer
Bert Spilker

Acknowledgments

The Drug Information Association sponsored a conference in September 1989 (organized by JAC) on "The Impact of Partial Compliance in Clinical Trials." Several of the chapters in this book developed from presentations given at that conference. The willingness of the Drug Information Association to allow publication of this book is greatly appreciated.

A special note of gratitude is made by JAC to Richard H. Mattson, M.D., a skilled and caring physician, a creative and insightful researcher, and a dedicated teacher. His encouragement and support of independent investigations of pharmacologic and clinical issues in epilepsy led to initial explorations of the association between compliance and seizure control.

Incalculable appreciation to Marvin B. Cramer for generously and enthusiastically discussing various concepts about compliance, with JAC.

Contents

Contributors

Shaheda Ahmed, MD *Stanford University Medical Center, Department of Medicine, Stanford, CA 94305-5475*

Julie M. Backes, PharmD *Kaiser Foundation Health Plan Pharmacy, Fairfield, CA 94533*

Martha U. Barnard, RN, PhD *University of Kansas Medical Center, Department of Pediatrics, Kansas City, KA 66103*

Ivan Barofsky, PhD *Johns Hopkins School of Medicine, Francis Scott Key Medical Center, Division of Digestive Diseases, Baltimore, MD 21224*

Carol Barton, RN, MS *Stanford University Medical Center, Department of Medicine, Stanford, CA 94305-5475*

Delphine Bonduelle, MD *Stanford University Medical Center, Department of Medicine, Stanford, CA 94305-5475*

Joseph F. Collins, ScD *Cooperative Studies Program Coordinating Center, Department of Veterans Affairs Medical Center, Perry Point, MD 21902*

Joyce A. Cramer, BS *Epilepsy Center, Department of Veterans Affairs Medical Center, West Haven, CT 06516 and Yale University School of Medicine, Department of Neurology, New Haven, CT 06510*

Barbara A. Cromer, MD *The Ohio State University College of Medicine, Department of Adolescent Medicine, Children's Hospital, Columbus, OH 43205-2696*

Bengt Dahlström, PhD *Professional Medical Consultants AB, Glunten, S-751 83, Uppsala, Sweden*

J. Dickins *Division of Bioengineering, Clinical Research Centre, Northwick Park Hospital, Harrow, Middlesex, HA1 3UJ, United Kingdom*

R. John Dobbs, MD *Therapeutics in the Elderly, Research Group, Northwick Park Hospital, Harrow, Middlesex, HA1 3UJ, United Kingdom*

Sylvia M. Dobbs, MD *Therapeutics in the Elderly, Research Group, Northwick Park Hospital, Harrow, Middlesex, HA1 3UJ, United Kingdom*

Walter Dorus, MD *Department of Veterans Affairs, Edward Hines Jr. Hospital, Hines, IL 60141 and Department of Psychiatry, Loyola University of Chicago, Maywood, IL 60153*

Seth A. Eisen, MD, MSC *Washington University Medical Service, St. Louis Veterans Affairs Medical Center, St. Louis, MO 63106*

Sven-Åke Eckernäs, PhD, MD *Professional Medical Consultants AB, Glunten, S-751 83, Uppsala, Sweden*

Frederick W. Engstrom, MD *Park Nicollet Medical Center, Mental Health Department, Minneapolis, MN 55416*

Alvan R. Feinstein, MD *Yale University School of Medicine, Clinical Epidemiology Unit, New Haven, CT 06510 and Cooperative Studies Program Coordinating Center, Veterans Administration Medical Center, West Haven, CT 06516*

Marsha D. Fretwell, MD *Brown University Program in Medicine and Department of Medicine, Roger Williams General Hospital, Providence, RI 02910*

Rhonda B. Friedman, ScD *SysteMetrics/McGraw-Hill, Washington, DC 20008*

Russell E. Glasgow, PhD *Oregon Research Institute, Eugene, OR 97401*

Mae E. Gordon, PhD *Washington University School of Medicine, Department of Opthalmology and Visual Sciences and Division of Biostatistics, St. Louis, MO 63110*

Lawrence W. Green, DrPH *Henry J. Kaiser Family Foundation, Menlo Park, CA 94025*

Joerg Hasford, MD *Biometric Center for Therapeutic Studies, D-8000 München 2, West Germany*

Frank L. Hurley, PhD *Biometric Research Institute, Inc., Arlington, VA 22209*

Peter Barton Hutt JD *Covington and Burling, Washington, DC 20044*

Michael A. Kass, MD *Washington University School of Medicine, Department of Opthalmology and Visual Sciences, St. Louis, MO 63110*

Russell Katz, MD *Division of Neuropharmacological Drug Products, Office of Drug Evaluation I, Food and Drug Administration, Rockville, MD 20857*

Ronald L. Krall, MD *Pharmaceutical Products Division, Abbott Laboratories, Abbott Park, IL 60064-3500*

Wolfgang H.-H. Kruse, MD *University of Heidelberg, Krankenhaus Bethanien, Rohrbacher Str. 149, 6900 Heidelberg-1, Federal Republic of Germany*

E. Paul Larrat, MS, MBA *University of Rhode Island, College of Pharmacy, Providence, RI 02910*

Louis Lasagna, MD *Tufts University, Sackler School of Graduate Biomedical Sciences, Center for the Study of Drug Development, Boston, MA 02111*

Ilo E. Leppik, MD *Minnesota Comprehensive Epilepsy Program and University of Minnesota, Minneapolis, MN 55416*

Richard A. Levy, PhD *National Pharmaceutical Council, Reston, VA 22091*

Richard H. Mattson, MD *Epilepsy Center, Department of Veterans Affairs Medical Center, West Haven, CT 06516 and Department of Neurology, Yale University School of Medicine, New Haven, CT 06510*

Helen Mawhinney, MD, FRCP *Allergy Research Foundation, Los Angeles, CA 90025*

Louis A. Morris, PhD   *Food and Drug Administration, Rockville, MD 20857*

Patricia Dolan Mullen, DrPH   *University of Texas Health Science Center, Center for Health Promotion Research and Development, Houston, TX 77225*

Norma J. Owens, PharmD   *University of Rhode Island, College of Pharmacy, Providence, RI 02910*

Linda S. Potter, DPH   *Family Health International, Research Triangle Park, NC 27709*

Jeffrey L. Probstfield, MD   *National Heart, Lung, Blood Institute, Clinical Trials Branch, Bethesda, MD 20892*

Michael A. Rapoff, PhD   *University of Kansas Medical Center, Department of Pediatrics, Kansas City, KS 66103*

Peter Rudd, MD   *Stanford University Medical Center, Department of Medicine, Stanford, CA 94305-5475*

Jerome J. Schentag, PharmD   *State University of New York at Buffalo School of Pharmacy, and Clinical Pharmacokinetics Laboratory, Millard Fillmore Hospital, Buffalo, NY 14209-1194*

Sheldon L. Spector, MD   *Allergy Research Foundation, Los Angeles, CA 90025*

Bert Spilker, PhD, MD   *Department of Project Coordination, Burroughs Wellcome Company, Research Triangle Park, NC 27709*

John Urquhart, MD   *Aprex Corporation, Fremont, CA 94539 and University of Limburg, Department of Pharmaco-Epidemiology, 6200 Maastricht, The Netherlands*

Valerie Zachary, RN   *Stanford University Medical Center, Department of Medicine, Stanford, CA 94305-5475*

PART I

Introduction to the Topic of Patient Compliance

*Patient Compliance in Medical
Practice and Clinical Trials*
edited by J.A. Cramer and B. Spilker
Raven Press, Ltd., New York © 1991

1

Overview of Methods to Measure and Enhance Patient Compliance

Joyce A. Cramer

*Epilepsy Center, Department of Veterans Affairs Medical Center, West Haven,
Connecticut 06516; and Department of Neurology, Yale University School of Medicine,
New Haven, Connecticut, 06510*

HISTORICAL BACKGROUND

An historical perspective of concern about medication compliance can be traced to before the time of Hippocrates. Physicians were able to learn about the therapeutic effectiveness of medicinal remedies by observing patient outcome and noting whether the patient had used the potions. Throughout the history of medicine, patients have often had to purchase and ingest the prescribed potions in hopes of regaining their health. Nevertheless, human nature has led many patients to select their own plan for medication dosing, sometimes saving the leftover portion for a possible future episode.

The plethora of medical remedies available in this last decade of the 20th century includes chemical, biological, physical, and spiritual treatments for an increasingly detailed list of ailments. Although the physician's expectation of patient compliance with a medical regimen is usually high for seriously ill patients, the evidence to support this claim is not substantial. No consequence of poor compliance is so severe that all patients uniformly adhere to their physician's advice. Even the threat of kidney rejection after a transplant operation does not assure compliance with immunosuppressant medication by all patients (1). Not only is it easy for some patients to deny the need for treatment of asymptomatic conditions such as hypertension and elevated lipid levels, but it is also easy for many patients to discontinue treatment for disorders as soon as the symptoms of the acute event have passed (e.g., infections). The scope of noncompliance ranges across all age groups and medical disciplines, many of which are reviewed in later chapters. This chapter introduces the issues pertaining to patient compliance and describes some of the simple, practical strategies that medical staff can use to improve patient's compliance with their therapeutic plan.

DEFINITIONS

The term *compliance* in a medical context is generally defined in this book as following the instructions of the health care provider. Modifications and additional definitions are provided within individual chapters. Feinstein (2) provided humorous reasons why synonyms are not "preferred substitutes for compliance. *Adherence* seems too sticky; *fidelity* has too many connotations; and *maintenance* suggests a repair crew. Although *adherence* has its adherents, compliance continues to be the most popular term"(2). The expectation exists that a patient who accepts a prescription from a physician not only will fill the prescription but also will take the medicine as indicated. Physicians also assume that their patients will call to discuss adverse events or lack of efficacy rather than adjust or discontinue the medicine without professional medical advice.

Compliance can be total, partial, nil, or erratic. Neither age, education, nor socioeconomic level makes a difference in how patients use therapeutic plans. Sufferers seek professional medical opinions about their problems and appropriate therapy whether prescribed by a medicine man, "barefoot doctor," or clinician. However, once alone with their conscience, individual patients may choose to use all, part, or none of the treatment. Treatment defaulting (i.e., partial compliance) can occur during any stage of treatment. No single therapeutic plan has been found to create optimum compliance with a prescribed regimen. In this chapter, a review of practical strategies provides simple constructs that may be used in either medical practice or clinical trials to help patients develop positive patterns of compliance with medication regimens.

MEASUREMENT OF COMPLIANCE

The easiest strategy to assess compliance is to ask the patient (3). As suggested by Sackett (4), a nonjudgmental discussion can provide a straightforward explanation of missed doses that explains treatment failure or dose reduction because of adverse reactions. Unfortunately, patients tend to tell physicians what they think the physician wants to hear. Incorrect reports of full compliance might not be helpful to their treatment plan, but indications of missed doses can be accepted.

Pill counts at the end of a week or month usually are used only in research programs in which leftover doses are measured as an approximate measure of compliance (5). It is difficult to ensure that all pills are brought to the clinic for counting, which usually invalidates this measure (3). In general outpatient practice, counting pills would not be suitable, but an inventory of pills in a box with compartments for each dose would identify missed doses for the patient. The presence of leftover pills in the evening notifies the patient of a missed dose, which (for some drugs) should be made up by taking the leftover pills at bedtime. The absence of the last dose indicates inadvertent double-dosing during the day.

Therapeutic drug monitoring using blood and urine tests is well-established as an accurate and reliable marker for many medications. Variable drug serum concentrations can indicate erratic compliance (6). However, drug serum concentrations are a reasonable method of evaluating compliance only for medicines with long half-lives. Levels of short-acting medications reflect only recent dosing, not doses missed more than several days before the test (7).

A variety of devices are now available for electronic monitoring of doses, self-testing, and outpatient notation of events. Table 1–1 lists types of units that use microprocessors to record the date and time the apparatus is used to dispense a dose

TABLE 1-1. *Microelectronic monitors*

Device/developer	Use	Reference

Unit Dose Monitor
  DVA Medical Center
  St. Louis, Missouri
	Records removal of tablets from blister pack	See Chapter 18, *this volume*; (29)

Eye Drop Monitor
  Univ. Washington
  St. Louis, Missouri
	Records inversion of bottle to dispense liquid medication	See Chapter 13, *this volume*

Nebulizer Chronolog
  Advanced Technology Products
  Lakewood, Colorado
	Records spray of aerosol medication	See Chapter 12, *this volume*; (30)

Pill Box Monitor
  Clinical Research Center
  Harrow, United Kingdom
	Records opening of box to remove tablets or capsules	See Chapter 11, *this volume*; (31)

Medication Event Monitoring System (MEMS)
  Aprex Corp.
  Fremont, California
	Records opening of bottle for removal of tablets or capsules	See Chapter 10, *this volume*; (32)

MEMS Reader Display-Printer (RDP)
  Aprex Corp.
  Fremont, California
	Dosing data retrieval, display and printout from MEMS units	Aprex Corp., Fremont, California

Pill Ring Monitor
  Aprex Corp.
  Fremont, California and
  Johnson & Johnson Co.
  New Brunswick, New Jersey
	Records removal of each oral contraceptive tablet	See Chapter 16, *this volume*

Glucometer
  Ames/Miles
  Elkhart, Indiana
	Records time of test and glucose level	Gonder-Frederick et al. (8)

Mini Doc
  Professional Medical Consultants—AB
  Uppsala, Sweden
	Interactive electronic diary for notation of events by patient	See Chapter 19, *this volume*

of medication or record test information. Although these devices cannot assure that the medication was used (e.g., appropriate number of tablets ingested), they can document the initiative of bottle opening or aerosol spray as a presumptive dose. Analyses can include number and time of missed doses, frequency of over- or underdosing, trends in noncompliance during a week or month, or missed doses several half-lives before blood sampling. Microelectronic monitors can be used to correlate missed doses with breakthrough seizures, asthma attacks, or other medical crises or to note problems with glucose control. Examples are given and discussed in later chapters. The purpose of electronic monitoring is not merely to prove noncompliance but to ascertain whether adverse events occur after missed or excessive doses. Proof of either correlation would allow appropriate change of dose, medicine, or the addition of a second medicine.

OVERVIEW OF STRATEGIES TO ENHANCE COMPLIANCE

Four major strategies to aid in complying with a medical regimen include education, dosing, clinic scheduling, and communication. These approaches are pertinent to all types of patients experiencing a variety of medical problems (Table 1-2). These issues were reviewed a decade ago in a book edited by Haynes et al. (9). The simple, practical methods described in that book remain valid and useful but can be supplemented with new technological developments described below and in Table 1–1. Throughout this book, numerous authors address concepts pertinent to these four topics.

1. *Education* develops patient understanding to enhance the patient's compliance with the physician's recommendations. A thorough explanation of the need for the medication or alternate therapy, as well as the selection of a specific medicine, gives the patient an important overview and perspective of the treatment plan. Verbal explanations often have to be repeated to a family because, although a patient may comprehend the details during the interview, he or she often forgets or is unable to reexplain instructions after leaving the office (10). Ley et al. (11) found that categorization of information by the medical staff is helpful to patients in remembering oral instructions. Unfortunately, more than half of the information is forgotten immediately after the visit (12,13). Medical staff should provide written instructions on dosing, what to do if symptoms such as a seizure or an asthma attack recur, a plan if adverse reactions occur, and a plan for follow-up. Written information is taken home and may be reread long after the office discussion is forgotten (11,14).

2. Planning a *dosing schedule* that fits into the individual patient's life-style should be considered for patients who are unused to taking pills, already take a number of other medications, or are unable to conveniently take medication at certain times of day. Dose frequency is more important in maintaining compliance than is the number of pills per dose (15). The simplest possible regimen (e.g., one pill at bedtime) achieves the highest compliance, but often it is impossible to recommend for medicines with short duration of action. A mutually acceptable schedule should be planned, even if it is less than the desired number of doses. Such an act of partnership with the patient alleviates guilt when the patient knows he or she cannot remember or cannot take time for a midafternoon dose, and avoids judgmental disappointment on the part of the physician. Norell (16) demonstrated improved

TABLE 1–2. *Practical strategies to improve compliance*

Communication from the health care provider to the patient
  • discuss the diagnosis and the treatment plan
  • discuss the treatment plan selected
  • discuss the timetable for follow-up
Education about treatment
  • provide pamphlets or video information
  • arrange for staff to help the patient and family understand the treatment and how to
    implement it
Dosing
  • reduce the number of medications
  • reduce the number of doses each day
  • provide a dose checklist
  • provide a pill box with daily compartments or an alarm reminder
Scheduling of clinic visits
  • schedule a specific appointment and minimize total visit time
  • provide information about or reimbursement for transportation or parking
  • increase the frequency of visits
  • designate a specific clinic staff person for contacts

compliance with glaucoma treatment when dosing plans were tailored to individual habits but were within the required 8-hr dosing intervals.

The patient who already takes several medications faces the problem of coordinating the dosing of all pills. Various drugs may have been prescribed by several different physicians, each of which requires special scheduling. The patient should not be given instructions to take one pill at 8 AM, 12 noon, and 5 PM while other doses are given at 9 AM, 3 PM, and 10 PM. A review of all medications should be made, redundant medicines eliminated, and the simplest schedule created. Patients taking multiple medications occasionally require a dose checklist to help them remember which pills are to be taken at what time (17). If a log sheet is prepared listing doses of all medications for a week or a month, the patient can make a check mark after taking each dose to avoid double-dosing or missed doses. The importance of omitting the missed earlier dose or taking it with the bedtime dose should be explained by the physician.

Some patients manage well with a simple pill box with a compartment for each day of the week in which a full day's dose can be inserted once a week (Pill Memo Ring, Bridgerland Products, Logan, Utah). The Dosett box (18), widely used in Europe, has compartments for four doses daily for 7 days. The box can be filled weekly by a health care provider to assist patients who take multiple medicines in frequent doses. The size of the box, however, makes it unwieldy for most ambulatory patients. Oral contraceptives are traditionally packaged in a small pill ring with 21 or 28 daily doses. The woman clearly sees the sequence of daily doses as an aid to remembering whether she took the current day's pill.

Development of cues to remind the patient to take a dose takes careful planning. For example, pills can be set next to a razor for a man who shaves every morning or near the coffee for those who eat breakfast (19). Inexpensive wristwatches with alarms and small electronic memories to record brief messages can be programmed to cue the time for a dose or remind the patient about special instructions for therapy. Small pill boxes with a clock and alarm system are convenient for carrying a few pills in a shirt pocket (e.g., Medi-MindeRx-II and Pill Box Timer, Criterion Watch Company, Woodside, New York). A pill bottle with a clock-alarm on the cap shows the exact time at which the previous dose was taken or when the bottle was last opened (Prescript Timecap, Wheaton Medical Technologies, Millville, New Jersey). The drawback to all alarm systems is that unless the patient hears the buzzer and takes the pills immediately, the cue is quickly forgotten.

3. *Clinic scheduling* for patient follow-up also is an important factor in long-term compliance. The first clue that a patient might be noncompliant is failure to attend a scheduled appointment. The physician will not have an opportunity to examine or counsel the patient long-term if he or she has not done so early in treatment, because the patient will not return for follow-up. One study of hypertensive patients demonstrated a 56% loss to follow-up within 3 months (20). Similarly, a study of newly treated epilepsy patients lost 18% of participants despite free care at veterans' clinics (21). Cramer et al. (22) found that young, healthy men were likely to drop out of the treatment program as a method of denial of the diagnosis and need to take medication.

Some patients may not return for follow-up because they are asymptomatic. The patient apparently believes that the scheduled visit is unnecessary if no perceived benefit is expected. If a follow-up visit is planned to be a short assessment to assure lack of adverse reaction with adequate efficacy, the health care provider should respect the patient's time by avoiding lengthy delays in seeing the patient. Special attempts to maintain the specific appointment schedule so patients are seen without much delay enhance the patient's willingness to return for examinations. Transportation to the clinic and parking are nuisance matters that affect attendance. Some research projects provide parking tokens to eliminate lengthy delays in finding parking spaces, which often takes longer than the entire clinic visit.

Once treatment is started and the patient is given a follow-up appointment, the purpose of each visit should be carefully explained because it might make a difference in the patient's intention to take the time away from work and efforts of transportation to return. The patient's perspective may be that no follow-up is needed if all is well. The physician should indicate clearly that he or she wants to see the patient in 1 month even if the patient is feeling fine, so that the patient can be examined for mild or subtle problems. Appointment reminder cards should be mailed 1 to 2 weeks before the visit if visits are several months apart. Computer-generated phone calls can be programmed to serve as voice reminders for appointments, need for medication refills, or other cues (e.g., Automatic Appointment Verification System, Comtel Broadcasting Corporation, Sheridan, Indiana). Finding that compliance is improved before a check-up (7), scheduling of frequent visits can effectively improve therapeutic outcome (e.g., blood pressure, seizure, or diabetes control).

Liaison with a specific clinic staff person helps the patient in many ways (23). The patient is reassured to know that someone is familiar with his or her problems and special needs and is able to provide assistance and information immediately without having to wait for the physician to call back. When noncompliance is detected, a strategy should be implemented to assist the patient in coordination with the therapeutic plan established by the physician (24). An individual compliance plan can be designed in 15 min by a trained clinical or research assistant, nurse, technician, or pharmacist.

4. *Communication* between the physician and patient is the primary strategy to enhance compliance with medical treatment. A dialogue including discussion of diagnosis and need for treatment, description of possible adverse reactions as well as therapeutic effects, duration of treatment, convenience of dosing, and need for follow-up are as important to patients as the writing of the prescription.

Lima et al. (25) suggested that the time and attention spent on orienting patients to their course of treatment probably was the key to successful compliance rather than any reminder devices. Stanaway et al. (26) reported a significant correlation between compliance and perceived benefit from medicines. Simply asking the patient whether he or she *can* and *will* adhere to the plan provides an opportunity for discussion of the patient's point of view. A negative answer requires immediate consideration of alternate plans.

No single, specific strategy will work to enhance compliance for all patients. Knowledge does not assure compliance, as demonstrated by decline in compliance after counseling is discontinued (27). Morris and Halperin (14) suggest a multifaceted educational and behavioral approach tailored to individual needs. Working in partnership with the patient, instead of using a didactic approach, physicians and other health care providers will have great influence on compliance (28).

The concepts described in this introductory chapter are reiterated with different perspectives throughout the book. The contexts of special populations and specific illnesses necessitate a review of the impact of partial compliance on target groups and provide an opportunity for each author to recommend strategies tailored for that population. The similarity of problems and the diversity of approaches poignantly explain the need for more research on the scope and impact of partial compliance in medical practice and clinical trials.

ACKNOWLEDGMENT

This work was supported by the Veterans Administration Medical Research Service. This chapter is adapted from a report previously published in *Epilepsy Research* (suppl 1): *Compliance in Epilepsy,* 1988;163–175, eds. D. Schmidt and I.E. Leppik, by permission of Elsevier Science Publishers BV, Amsterdam.

REFERENCES

1. Rovelli M, Palmeri D, Vossler E, Bartus S, Hull D, Schweizer R. Noncompliance in organ transplant recipients. *Transplant Proc* 1989;21:833–834.
2. Feinstein AR. On white coat effects and the electronic monitoring of compliance. *Arch Intern Med* 1990;150:1377–1378.
3. Fletcher SW, Pappius EM, Harper SJ. Measurement of medication compliance in a clinical setting. *Arch Intern Med* 1979;139:635–638.
4. Sackett DL. A compliance practicum for the busy practitioner. In: Haynes RB, Taylor DW, Sackett DL, eds. *Compliance in Health Care.* Baltimore, Maryland: Johns Hopkins University Press, 1979;286–294.
5. Pullar T, Kumar S, Tindall H, Feely M. Time to stop counting the tablets? *Clin Pharmacol Ther* 1989;46:163–168.
6. Leppik IE, Cloyd JC, Sawchuk RJ, Pepin SM. Compliance and variability of plasma phenytoin levels in epileptic patients. *Ther Drug Monit* 1979;1:475–483.
7. Cramer JA, Scheyer R, Mattson R. Compliance declines between clinic visits. *Arch Int Med* 1990;150:1509–1510.
8. Gonder-Frederick LA, Julian DM, Cox DJ, Clarke WL, Carter WR. Self-measurement of blood glucose accuracy of self-reported data and adherence to recommended regimen. *Diabetes Care* 1988;2:579–585.
9. Haynes RB, Taylor DW, Sackett DL, eds. *Compliance in Health Care.* Baltimore, Maryland: Johns Hopkins University Press, 1979.
10. Ley P. Primacy, rated importance, and the recall of medical statements. *J Health Soc Behav* 1972;13:311–317.
11. Ley P, Bradshaw PW, Eaves D, Walker CM. A method for increasing patients' recall of information presented by doctors. *Psychol Med* 1973;3:217–220.
12. Spelman LP. Communications in an outpatient setting. *Br J Soc Clin Psychol* 1965;4:114–116.
13. Joyce CRB, Caple G, Mason M. Quantitative study of doctor–patient communications. *Q J Med* 1969;38:183–194.
14. Morris LA, Halperin JA. Effects of written drug information on patient knowledge and compliance: a literature review. *Am J Public Health* 1979;69:47–52.
15. Haynes RB, Sackett DL, Taylor DW, Roberts RS, Johnson AL. Commentary—Manipulation of the therapeutic regimen to improve compliance: conceptions and misconceptions. *Clin Pharmacol Ther* 1977;22:125–130.
16. Norell SE. Improving medication compliance: a randomised clinical trial. *Br Med J* 1979;2:1031–1033.
17. Gabriel M, Gagnon JP, Bryan CK. Improved patient compliance through use of a daily drug reminder chart. *Am J Public Health* 1977;67:968–969.
18. Rehder TL, McCoy LK, Blackwell B, Whitehead W, Robinson A. Improving medication compliance by counseling and special prescription container. *Am J Hosp Pharm* 1980;37:379–385.
19. Schmidt JP. A behavioral approach to patient compliance. *Postgrad Med* 1979;65:219–224.

20. Wilbur JA, Barrow JG. Reducing elevated blood pressure. Experience found in a community. *Minn Med* 1969;52:1303–1305.
21. Mattson RH, Cramer JA, Collins JF. Comparison of carbamazepine, phenobarbital, phenytoin, and primidone in partial and secondary generalized tonic-clonic seizures. *N Engl J Med* 1985;313:145–151.
22. Cramer JA, Collins JF, Mattson RH. Can categorization of patient background problems be used to determine early termination in a clinical trial? *Controlled Clin Trials* 1988;9:47–63.
23. Spector R, McGrath P, Uretsky N, Newman R, Cohen P. Does intervention by a nurse improve medication compliance? *Arch Intern Med* 1978;138:36–40.
24. Russell ML. Behavioral aspects of the use of medical markers in clinical trials. *Controlled Clin Trials* 1984;5:526–534.
25. Lima J, Nazarian L, Charney E, Lahti C. Compliance with short-term antimicrobial therapy: some techniques that help. *Pediatrics* 1976;57:383–386.
26. Stanaway L, Lambie DG, Johnson RH. Non-compliance with anticonvulsant therapy as a cause of seizures. *NZ Med J* 1985;98:150–152.
27. McKenney JM, Slining JM, Henderson HR, Devins D, Barr M. The effect of clinical pharmacy services on patients with essential hypertension. *Circulation* 1973;48:1104–1111.
28. Gillum RF, Barsky AJ. Diagnosis and management of patient noncompliance. *JAMA* 1974;228:1563–1566.
29. Eisen SA, Hanpeter JA, Kreuger LW, Michael G. Monitoring medication compliance: description of new device. *J Compliance Health Care* 1987;2:131–142.
30. Spector SL, Kinsman R, Mawhinney H, et al. Compliance of patients with asthma with an experimental aerosolized medication: implications for controlled clinical trials. *J Allergy Clin Immunol* 1986;77:65–70.
31. Cheung R, Sullens CM, Seal D, et al. The paradox of using a 7 day antibacterial course to treat urinary tract infections in the community. *Br J Clin Pharmacol* 1988;26:391–398.
32. Cramer JA, Mattson RH, Prevey ML, Scheyer R, Ouellette V. How often is medication taken as prescribed? A novel assessment technique. *JAMA* 1989;261:3273–3277.

Patient Compliance in Medical
Practice and Clinical Trials
edited by J.A. Cramer and B. Spilker
Raven Press, Ltd., New York © 1991

2

Failure to Refill Prescriptions

Incidence, Reasons, and Remedies

Richard A. Levy

National Pharmaceutical Council, Reston, Virginia 22091

The failure of patients to refill prescriptions is a frequently overlooked aspect of the medication compliance problem. Refill compliance is especially important for patients with chronic diseases who must often obtain prescription refills throughout their lives. Surprisingly, little information is available on refill behavior, but it has been estimated that at least 30% of refillable prescriptions are not refilled. The high incidence of this specific type of patient noncompliance has important clinical implications and significant economic consequences. This chapter discusses the incidence of and reasons for refill noncompliance and suggests solutions to the problem based on education and communications technologies (1).

A 1987 survey conducted by the Schering Corporation showed that half (50%) of all patients reported receiving instructions to have their prescriptions refilled, but 32% of these patients failed to refill their prescriptions (2). Hammel (3) found that refill compliance declined each month in long-term antihypertensive therapy, and only 44% of prescriptions for medications were being dispensed after 6 months.

The refill compliance problem will probably worsen as the population ages and the incidence of chronic disease increases. Additionally, patients are being discharged from hospitals sooner and are being forced to assume more responsibility for their drug therapies at home. The important role of the patient in the treatment of his or her own chronic disease must now be more fully recognized.

WHY PATIENTS FAIL TO REFILL PRESCRIPTIONS

A 1985 survey of consumers conducted by The Upjohn Company showed that 14% of patients receiving a prescription during the preceding 12 months reported that they did not have the prescription filled (4). Figure 2–1 shows the reasons these patients gave for not filling their prescriptions. It is significant that in this survey a total of 72.7% of the patients with unfilled prescriptions stated that they either did not need the medication or did not want to take the medication.

The Upjohn study also determined that older patients represent an important focus for the refill problem. Persons older than 60 years of age were prescribed refills significantly more often (63%) than younger adults (26%)(4). This is not surprising, because older patients have a higher incidence of chronic diseases that require long-

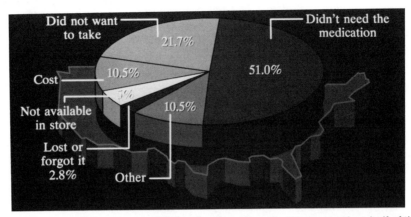

FIG. 2–1. Failure to fill. A survey by Upjohn Company revealed that more than half of the 14% of patients who failed to fill a prescription said they did so because they felt they did not need the medication. This chart shows the full set of reasons given by survey respondents. Source: Upjohn Survey, 1985.

term therapy. The study also showed a predominance of refills over new prescriptions in the elderly. These findings indicate the relative importance of assessing and improving refill behavior in this patient group. A 1982 survey by the American Association of Retired Persons (5) showed that approximately one of five (21%) consumers older than the age of 45 years has chosen, at one time, not to follow, from the outset, the physician's recommendations for taking a prescription (Fig. 2–2).

In both the American Association of Retired Persons and Upjohn surveys, the patient's decision not to take the medication was a major factor in refill noncompliance. The importance of the patient as a primary decision maker in ambulatory drug therapy is far greater than has been traditionally recognized.

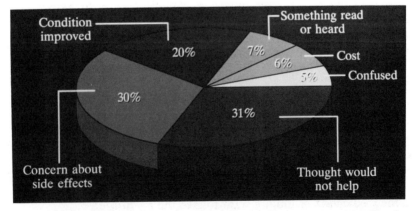

FIG. 2–2. Prescription resistance. Survey of 1,001 consumers conducted by American Association of Retired Persons reported the mix of reasons for noncompliance shown in this chart. Source: AARP (American Association of Retired Persons) survey of 1,001 consumers.

IMPROVING REFILL BEHAVIOR

A basic way to motivate patients to refill their prescriptions is to encourage physicians and pharmacists to stress the need for the medication to be taken on a regular basis. Patients must be told to obtain refills several days before the medication runs out. The Schering survey showed that only 20% of patients receive instructions on refills at the pharmacy (2). Patients should be given information on the importance, the timing, and the procedure for refilling the prescription each time it is dispensed.

Several innovative strategies using computer and telecommunications technologies have been developed to help patients remember to refill their prescriptions or to facilitate the refill process. These are discussed below.

Refill Reminders

Reminder systems, in the form of postcards or telephone reminders, have been shown to improve refill compliance. One study used computers linked to the pharmacy's patient profile system to generate refill reminder postcards for patients (6). The effect on refill compliance in patients taking chronic cardiovascular medication was assessed. Refill behavior in patients receiving these computer-generated postcard reminders was compared with a group receiving no reminders and a group receiving telephone call reminders. Refill compliance was monitored by a computerized patient profile system. Refill compliance improved significantly in patients receiving the postcard reminders and telephone call reminders. There was no significant difference in refill compliance between the postcard and the telephone call groups.

The efficacy of refill reminders has also been demonstrated in a study involving more than 1,000 type II diabetic patients having prescriptions for oral hypoglycemic agents (7). The use of refill reminders resulted in a refill compliance rate of 83%; the refill compliance rate in a control group of unreminded patients was only 57%. The combined use of refill reminders and special packaging resulted in a refill compliance rate of 92%.

The Schering survey noted that patients who have received such reminders appreciated the cards (2). Other studies, however, reported that some patients have reacted negatively (8). Some viewed the intervention as a sales technique, whereas others felt guilty about their lapse in compliance. Although physicians appear to be supportive of the general concept, problems could arise if the physician has changed the drug therapy and the patient receives an inappropriate reminder notice.

Refill reminder systems are currently not being extensively used in the United States. The Schering survey indicated that only one in 100 patients surveyed had received a refill reminder (2). The time required to prepare the reminder cards and the costs involved to mail them are the two primary reasons why pharmacists do not routinely send out refill reminder postcards and letters. Pharmaceutical companies marketing chronic medications could assist pharmacists by helping them develop, implement, and perhaps subsidize practical and effective refill reminder systems.

A 1988 survey by the California Pharmacists Association (9) identified 11 pharmacy computer companies currently offering equipment with refill reminder capabilities. A variety of features is available to pharmacists using these programs. Some programs simply print out a list of prescriptions due to be refilled on a given date or period of time. The patient's phone number may be included so the patient can be called. Other programs will print out a customized letter or note to be mailed to the patient in a computer-addressed envelope. One system will automatically telephone the patient and play a prerecorded message (see below). The patient is asked to use the touch-tone phone pad to indicate responses. The responses are stored and printed out, if desired.

Voice Mail

A relatively unexplored, but potentially effective tactic for reminding patients about refills is the use of prerecorded computer-generated messages transmitted over telephone lines. Although the elderly generally have negative attitudes toward new technology, the public is gradually becoming exposed to and accepting of prerecorded messages and other sophisticated uses of the telephone. Voice-synthesized messages and interactive programs are now commonplace and telecommunications technologies are becoming more "transparent." (Transparent technologies are "user friendly" devices, which, although complex, like the telephone can be easily used without any insight into how it works.)

For example, customers requesting telephone directory assistance are now presented with voice-synthesized phone numbers. Some banks now offer telephonic bill payment, in which customers use a touch-tone phone to access an interactive program. The telephone answering machine, with advanced features, has become an essential tool for small business and social life. Consumers are becoming familiar and comfortable with interactive programs when they call customer service numbers. These developments will facilitate the acceptance of telephone reminder systems.

An example of a telephone reminder system that is currently available is the "Med-Minder" program, marketed by the General Computer Corporation and endorsed by NARD (National Association of Retail Druggists). This computer-based automated system uses the pharmacy's patient profile data together with automatic telephone dialing and voice synthesizing or voice replication equipment. The patient is telephoned with a personalized reminder message containing the patient's name, the medicine name, the pharmacy name, and the suggested refill date. The system can also produce reports for the pharmacist or physician indicating which prescriptions were not filled. An interactive system is planned in which patients can use a touch-tone phone to signal if they intend to refill a prescription and when they will come to the pharmacy to pick it up.

Preliminary data suggests that telephone reminder systems can improve refill behavior. Using the Med-Minder system, 246 patients taking cardiovascular medications were followed during 6 months. Refills were obtained by 53% of patients who received no reminders and by 79% of those receiving telephone reminder messages (10). Similarly, Simkins and Wenzloff (6) have shown telephone reminders to improve refill compliance with cardiovascular medicines during a shorter (3 month) period. Additional studies are needed to better characterize the effectiveness of telephone refill reminders over longer periods and for different diseases, classes of medicines, and patient populations.

The potential uses of voice mail technology extend beyond reminding patients that refills are due. Elderly outpatients could be automatically called many times each day with preprogrammed reminders to assist them in adhering to complex medication regimens. Patients would signal compliance behavior using the telephone key pad. Public health messages could also be incorporated into these systems. For example, elderly persons could be informed or reminded about obtaining vaccinations for influenza or pneumonia. Phone calls have been shown to increase the rate of the elderly seeking influenza vaccination (11).

Voice mail may also have applications as an in-home emergency alert service for elderly persons. A cost benefit analysis conducted on such a system indicated a reduction in amount of time spent in the hospital and a reduction in medical costs for those who used it (12). The use of these additional voice mail applications along with refill reminders will enhance the use and cost-effectiveness of telephone refill reminder systems.

The acceptance of telephone and other types of refill reminder systems by the health care marketplace of the 1990s will depend on clear demonstrations of the cost-effectiveness of these systems in the commercial environments of pharmacy practice and managed care. Pharmacists must be convinced that these reminder systems will produce enough repeat business to justify their expense. The most likely market for these systems, however, is the managed care sector. If the use of refill reminders by these providers results in improved outcomes, the expense of operating these systems is likely to be greatly offset by large savings from reduced use of hospital or outpatient services.

Demonstrations of such savings should be of great interest to managed care providers. But to convince these providers, adequate studies are required showing that (a) reminders improve both compliance and clinical outcomes, (b) overall costs are reduced, and (c) the savings realized exceed the expense of operating the system.

Computerized Wrist Terminal

Because most people are accustomed to wearing a wristwatch, a "wrist terminal" signaling system can potentially be used to help patients remember to take medications on time and remember to refill prescriptions (13). Pharmacists could program and lease computer wrist terminals to patients. Several types of information could be programmed into the wrist terminal. An alarm could remind the patient to call for prescription refills. Another alarm could signal scheduled activities recurring each week, such as taking medications. At the appointed times during the day, the alarm would sound and the watch would display the name of the medication to be taken. A memo function could remind the patient about adverse reactions. It is also possible to enter information on whether the patient is a diabetic, heart patient, or contact lens wearer. Physician and pharmacy phone numbers could also be listed.

Once the pertinent information is entered on the terminal, the patient will carry a complete medicine profile on his or her wrist. The data can be stored on disks in the pharmacy and updated if the patient's medication schedule changes.

Although wrist terminals hold promise in improving compliance and refill behavior, they have not yet been tested in the real world and are not in general use (although Seiko briefly marketed such a device). Additionally, although new reminder technology is interesting, many patients give reasons other than forgetfulness for not having their prescriptions filled (4). Refill reminders will probably be of greatest value in those patients who cite forgetfulness as their primary reason for failing to fill a prescription.

Call-In Prescription Refill System

Another approach to improving refill behavior is the use of a telephone answering device that permits patients to order their refills 24 hr a day. The added convenience of such a system facilitates the ordering of refills and was shown to increase prescription volume by 16.9% in one outpatient pharmacy (14). This is a relatively inexpensive and cost-effective strategy for improving refill compliance.

Pharmaceutical Industry Strategies

Pharmaceutical manufacturers have made few product-specific attempts to improve refill behavior. However, one approach that has been taken is the development of medications that are more stable and require less frequent refills. A good example are the various nitroglycerin products. The original sublingual tablets were highly susceptible to moisture and heat. Potency was lost every time the container was opened. When the container was carried in a suit jacket or pocket, body heat caused the medication to evaporate. It was reported in 1987 that 17% of patients prescribed nitroglycerin were taking subpotent tablets and that some tablets contained no active medication (15).

Several years ago, a stabilized nitroglycerin sublingual tablet was marketed. More recently, a metered-dose aerosol form of nitroglycerin was developed. The product delivers the nitroglycerin in the form of spray droplets onto or under the tongue. Because this product is stable for 3 years, the manufacturer is able to offer patients 200 doses. This is in contrast to the stabilized tablets that are packaged with 100 doses. The older unstabilized tablets also come in bottles of 100, but patients are told to carry only a small number with them and to discard them after a few days.

These new stabilized products have strong clinical and marketing advantages over the older products because they have to be refilled less frequently. Research into the development of more stable dosage forms is a major approach pharmaceutical companies can take to help improve refill behavior.

CONCLUSIONS

Although technological solutions are now available to help improve the refill behavior of patients, many patients fail to refill their prescriptions because they decide they do not need the medication. The various manual and computerized systems must therefore be supported by educational and motivational programs.

Patients must be convinced that the medication will be of some benefit to them. They must also be told how to administer, manage, and store their medications correctly as well as why it is important to obtain refills at prescribed intervals. Once patients become more interested in taking their medications correctly, the various strategies to improve refill behavior will be more effective. In summary, patients must be educated—and convinced of the need—to refill their prescriptions at the appropriate intervals.

There are no well-designed studies on the incidence, patterns, and reasons for poor refill behavior. Most existing reports are consumer surveys and are subject to the methodological weaknesses inherent in this approach. A tremendous need exists to develop and implement remedial programs that will be cost-effective. As the population ages, the incidence of chronic disease will increase, and problems with refill behavior will become more widespread. It is astounding that the ethical drug industry in the United States has so little information on this vital subject and no overall strategy for improving refill behavior. Individual companies have a marketing opportunity to introduce products and services that will facilitate refill compliance.

SUMMARY

The high incidence of patient failure to refill prescriptions has important clinical implications and significant economic consequences. It has been estimated that at least one-third of refillable prescriptions are not refilled. When patients with chronic diseases do not refill their prescriptions on time, a suboptimal clinical response may occur.

Innovative strategies to improve refill behavior include postcard and telephone reminder systems. Some pharamaceutical manufacturers are addressing the problem by developing more stable products that can be packaged and prescribed in larger quantities, thus requiring less frequent refills.

These technological advances in improving refill behavior must be supported by educational and motivational programs. Commonly, patients fail to refill their prescriptions because they decide they do not need the medication. Thus, patients must be educated—and convinced of the need—to refill their prescriptions at the appropriate intervals.

REFERENCES

1. Levy RA, Smith DL. Staying the course: refill reminders can boost sales. *Pharmaceutical Executive* 1989;9:72–78.
2. *Schering Report IX: The Forgetful Patient: The High Cost of Improper Patient Compliance*. Kenilworth, New Jersey: Schering Laboratories, 1987.
3. Hammel RJ. Increased compliance means better health for patients, higher profits for you. *Am Druggist* 1981;184(4):98.
4. *1985 National Prescription Buyers Survey* conducted for The Upjohn Company by Market Facts, Inc., Kalamazoo, Michigan.
5. American Association of Retired Persons. *Prescription Drugs: A Survey of Consumer Use, Attitudes and Behavior.* Washington, DC, 1984.
6. Simkins CV, Wenzloff NJ. Evaluation of a computerized reminder system in the enhancement of patient medication refill compliance. *Drug Intell Clin Pharm* 1986;20:799–802.
7. Sclar, DA. Medication compliance: health policy and pharmacy economics. *Aust J Pharm* 1988;69:619–622.
8. Lachman BG. Increasing patient compliance through tracking systems. *California Pharmacist* 1987;35(3):54–58.
9. California Pharmacists Association. *A Pharmacist's Guide to Prescription Refill Reminder Systems.* Sacramento, California, 1988.
10. *Med-Minder Product Information,* Twinsburg, Ohio. General Computer Corporation, 1989.

11. McDowell I, Newell C, Rosser W. Comparison of three methods of recalling patients for influenza vaccination. *Can Med Assn J* 1986;135:991–997.
12. Ruchlin H, Morris J. Cost-benefit analysis of an emergency alarm and response system: a case study of a long-term care program. *Health Serv Res* 1981;16:65–80.
13. Allen LV Jr. Improving patient compliance: it's all in the wrist. *Comput Talk Pharmacist* January/February 1987:35–36.
14. Williams RF, Shepherd MD, Jowdy AW. Effect of a call-in prescription refill system on workload in an outpatient pharmacy. *Am J Hosp Pharm* 1983;40:1954–1956.
15. Curry SH, Mehta K, Shavlik TA, Felt R. Survey of sublingual nitroglycerine-tablet potency under conditions of patient use. *Intern Med Specialist* 1987;8:63–71.

*Patient Compliance in Medical
Practice and Clinical Trials*
edited by J.A. Cramer and B. Spilker
Raven Press, Ltd., New York © 1991

3

Interaction of Compliance and Patient Safety

Ronald L. Krall

Pharmaceutical Products Division, Abbott Laboratories, Abbott Park, Illinois 60064

Does poor compliance result in increased risk to patient health and safety? When failure to comply with a medication regimen represents a potential health hazard, do patients modify their drug-taking behavior accordingly? This chapter attempts to answer these two questions by drawing on selected data from the clinical trial literature.

EFFECT OF NONCOMPLIANCE ON PATIENT SAFETY

Does poor compliance result in increased risk to patient health? The evidence from two clinical trials and one epidemiologic study that evaluate this question suggests that it does. Patients who do not take medicines will not receive benefits from the medication, assuming that the medicines are effective. Patient health, therefore, will be adversely affected.

Lipid Research Clinics Coronary Primary Prevention Trial

This study examined the relation between serum cholesterol levels and risk of coronary heart disease in 3,806 asymptomatic middle-aged men (1). In this multicenter, randomized, double-blind study, patients received either cholestyramine or placebo for an average of 7.4 years. Compliance was measured in terms of packets of cholestyramine taken per day. As illustrated in Fig. 3–1, the number of packets consumed per day was proportional to reductions in serum cholesterol levels and in cardiac disease risk. Patients who were fully compliant, consuming five to six packets of cholestyramine per day, had the greatest reduction in cardiac disease risk and cholesterol levels. Those taking only two to five packets per day increased their risk of cardiac disease, compared with the fully compliant patients, by about 25%. The risk increased by 50% when compliance fell to less than two packets per day. This study illustrates that patient safety, defined as increased morbidity, can be affected by compliance.

Compliance in Organ Transplant Patients

In a study conducted at the University of Connecticut, Rovelli et al. (2) retrospectively reviewed the records of transplant patients and conducted a prospective study

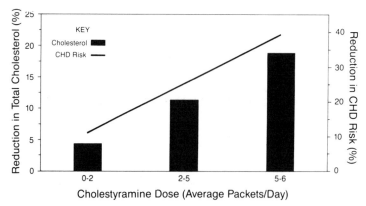

FIG. 3–1. Cholestyramine dose-response effect on total cholesterol and coronary heart disease (CHD) risk. (From ref. 1, with permission.)

of compliance and transplant outcome. Compliance with immunosuppressive medication was assessed during interviews (records of interviews for the retrospective study) with the patients and their families. In the retrospective study, 47 of 260 patients (18%) were noncompliant. Of those 47 patients, 43 (91%) experienced organ rejection or death, compared with 18% of the compliant patients. Of 182 patients in the prospective study, 30 (15%) were considered noncompliant. Of those, 11 (37%) experienced organ transplant rejection or death during the 3-year follow-up. In contrast, only two of 152 compliant patients (1%) in the prospective study experienced tissue rejection. Forty-nine percent of the total number of rejections in the retrospective study and 80% of the rejections in the prospective study were attributed to noncompliance. This transplant center has concluded that noncompliance with medication or other therapy is a major factor in tissue rejection, causing far more transplant failures than uncontrollable rejection in compliant patients.

Relative Risk of Coronary Heart Disease and Beta-Blocker Compliance

Psaty et al. (3) conducted a case-control study of the relative risk of coronary heart disease associated with poor compliance with beta-blockers in hypertensive patients with no prior history of ischemic heart disease. Using the Puget Sound health maintenance organization database, cases were selected from patients with treated hypertension and hospitalization or death from a first event of coronary heart disease between 1982 and 1984. The controls were a probability sample from the same database of patients who were also receiving antihypertensive therapy but were free of coronary heart disease. From pharmacy records of the Puget Sound Cooperative, patients who had stopped medication within 30 days of the coronary event (cases) or a randomly chosen date (controls) were identified using 80% compliance and the date of the last prescription, the number of doses prescribed, and the dosing instructions. The relative risk of coronary heart disease associated with recently stopping beta-blockers was 6.35 (95% confidence interval 1.67–24.21, $p = 0.0068$). There was no increase in relative risk associated with stopping diuretics (0.8, 95% confidence interval 0.35–1.82). The relative risk associated with stopping beta-blockers in-

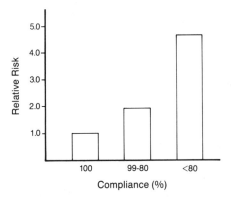

FIG. 3–2. Relative risk of coronary heart disease and compliance with beta-blockers. (From ref. 3, with permission.)

creased with decreasing compliance (Fig. 3–2). These data indicate that stopping the use of beta-blockers compromises their anticipated therapeutic benefit.

When studies do not assess risk or measure compliance, the link between poor compliance and increased risk to patient health may not be exposed. That link may exist, however, as the two following trials illustrate.

Compliance with Antiarrhythmic Therapy

Squire et al. (4) studied 98 consecutive patients receiving long-term oral antiarrhythmic therapy and attending an ambulatory cardiology clinic. Serum levels of the antiarrhythmic medicines procainamide and quinidine were measured in patients during a routine office visit and compared with medication dosages, dosing intervals, and time elapsed from the last dose. Of 98 patients, 75 (76.5%) had subtherapeutic serum drug levels as defined by the testing laboratory (Fig. 3–3). In most cases the levels were half or less than half of the minimum therapeutic level. These results could reflect inappropriate dosing schedules or inaccurate therapeutic ranges for the testing lab. However, among the 61 patients who claimed to have taken their last dose within 4 to 6 hr of the office visit, more than 10% had undetectable levels,

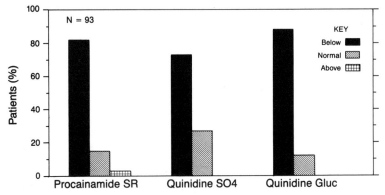

FIG. 3–3. Antiarryhthmic medicine levels: comparison with normal range. (From ref. 4, with permission.)

suggesting that noncompliance was the major cause of subtherapeutic levels. It is suspected that this degree of noncompliance would have resulted in significant morbidity.

Hypertension Treatment and Cardiac Risk

Alderman et al. (5) studied the relation between reductions in blood pressure and incidence of myocardial infarction in 1,765 patients with previously untreated mild-to-moderate hypertension. Patients were stratified into three groups based on the normal distribution of the change in diastolic blood pressure during an average of 4.2 years of treatment. The midpoint of the distribution was 12 mm Hg, and a range of 5 mm Hg was assigned to either side of the midpoint, establishing 7 to 17 mm Hg as the range of "moderate decline." Measurements above or below the moderate range were defined as "small" or "large" decreases in blood pressure. As shown in Fig. 3–4, the incidence of myocardial infarction was lowest in those patients with a moderate decrease in blood pressure and highest in the group with the smallest decrease in blood pressure. Surprisingly, the group with the largest decrease in blood pressure experienced a higher incidence of myocardial infarction than the moderate group, almost as high as the group with the smallest decline in blood pressure. This relation, known as the "J-shape" relation, persisted through various restratifications of the groups and after adjusting the analysis for potentially confounding risk factors (e.g., sex and smoking). The authors describe various explanations for these results, including physiological factors (e.g., a reduction in coronary blood flow caused by a large drop in blood pressure) or a difference between drug regimens. They do not, however, explore the possibility that compliance may have been a factor. It is conceivable that among the patient population were erratic users, who may have taken their medication immediately before their scheduled office visit but neglected the prescribed therapy between visits. This would result in a drop in blood pressure at the time of the measurement, but no consistent benefit in terms of reduced risk of myocardial infarction. The effect of erratic users would be greatest in the group with

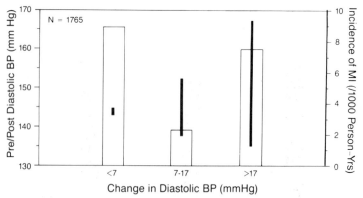

FIG. 3–4. Incidence of myocardial infarction (MI) by change in blood pressure (BP). *Solid bars* represent mean pretreatment (*top*) and during treatment (*bottom*) diastolic blood pressure in each group. (From ref. 5, with permission.)

the highest pretreatment blood pressure and would create the greatest disparity between blood pressure reduction and cardiac risk reduction.

PERCEPTIONS OF SAFETY: EFFECT ON COMPLIANCE

Many factors are thought to affect compliance. Younger patients and nonwhite patients have been reported to be more likely to be noncompliant (2). Mental disease and alcoholism (2), cost of medication (1,2), duration of therapy (2), and complexity of the medicine regimen (2) have been reported to influence compliance.

How do medicine and disease affect compliance? Theoretically, the perception that a medicine "works" should lead to improved compliance, whereas lack of drug efficacy might result in poorer compliance (Fig. 3–5). Adverse reactions that occur when treatment is stopped (e.g., the return of symptoms or the appearance of new ones) are likely to encourage improved compliance, whereas adverse experiences during treatment can be expected to lead to poor compliance. The extent to which these factors actually affect compliance is likely to be related to the patient's ability to perceive them. How apparent they are is a function of the nature of the consequence and how immediately and consistently it occurs.

Do treatment and disease affect compliance when failure to comply can be expected to create a threat to patient safety? In other words, when failure to comply presents a threat to patient safety, are patients more compliant? One way to answer this question is to compare compliance in two groups of patients receiving the same treatment but suffering from illnesses with differently perceived effects on health.

Two such illnesses are hypertension and angina. Both represent significant risks for cardiac morbidity. Stewart et al. (6), however, have shown that patients with angina perceive their health as compromised, whereas patients with hypertension perceive little impact on their health (Fig. 3–6). Based on the model above, in patients with hypertension, the inability to perceive the antihypertensive effect and the lack of noxious effects when the treatment is not taken remove a powerful stimulus for compliance. The only compliance-altering disease or treatment factors are ad-

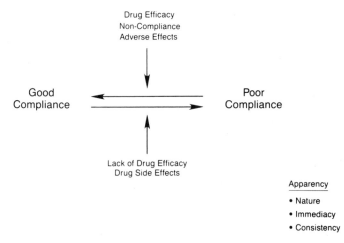

FIG. 3–5. Schematic of factors affecting patient compliance with drug therapy.

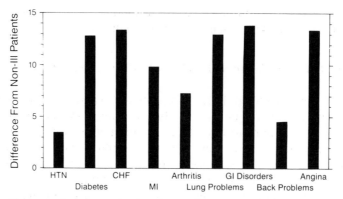

FIG. 3–6. Health perception scores in chronic conditions measured in the Medical Outcomes study. HTN, hypertension; CHF, congestive heart failure; MI, myocardial infarction; GI, gastrointestinal. (From ref. 6, with permission.)

verse reactions, cost, and regimen complexity, all of which stimulate poor compliance. In contrast, the disappearance of angina during treatment and its return when treatment is missed would be expected to be powerful influences encouraging compliance.

In two unpublished studies conducted by Lorex Pharmaceuticals, patients with hypertension or angina were treated with the same medicine. Both trials were double-blind, parallel-group, placebo-controlled studies with fixed-dose design. In the angina trial, medicine doses were 10, 20, and 40 mg, compared with 5, 10, and 20 mg in the hypertension trial. The duration of each trial was 4 weeks with visits every 2 weeks, although there was an opportunity for approximately 17 days of medication between visits. Noncompliance was defined as taking less than 80% of the allotted medication in the scheduled time. The results of these trials are illustrated in Fig. 3–7, with a much higher rate of noncompliance among the hypertension patients (5%) than among the angina patients (0.8%). These results support the hypothesis that the

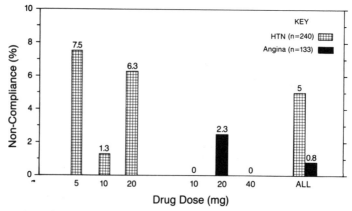

FIG. 3–7. Noncompliance in clinical trial patients. HTN, hypertension. (Data on file, Lorex Pharmaceuticals.)

perception of health and the apparency of the benefit of treatment affect drug-taking behavior.

CONCLUSION

The worst consequence of failing to comply with medication regimens is generally considered to be the loss of the intended effect. For many disorders, however, this loss of therapeutic benefit results in a significant threat to patient well-being. Even when illness represents a risk to patient health and well-being, many patients will only improve compliance if the treatment effect is apparent. Understanding the factors that affect compliance and using them to modify patient behavior can be expected to have an important impact on the efficacy of medicines and on patient safety.

REFERENCES

1. Lipid Research Clinics Program. The Lipid Research Clinics Coronary Primary Prevention Trial results. *JAMA* 1984;251:351–374.
2. Rovelli M, Palmeri D, Vossler E, Bartus S, Hull D, Schweizer R. Noncompliance in organ transplant recipients. *Transplant Proc* 1989;21:833–834.
3. Psaty BM, Koepsell TD, Wagner EH, LoGerfo JP, Inui TS. The relative risk of incident coronary heart disease associated with recently stopping the use of beta-blockers. *JAMA* 1990;263:1653–1657.
4. Squire A, Goldman ME, Kupersmith J, Stern EH, Fuster V, Schweitzer P. Long-term antiarrhythmic therapy: problem of low drug levels and patient noncompliance. *Am J Med* 1984;77:1035–1038.
5. Alderman MH, Ooi WL, Madhavan S, Cohen H. Treatment-induced blood pressure reduction and the risk of myocardial infarction. *JAMA* 1989;262:920–924.
6. Stewart AL, Greenfield S, Hays RD, et al. Functional status and well-being of patients with chronic conditions. Results from the medical outcomes study. *JAMA* 1989;262:907–913.

*Patient Compliance in Medical
Practice and Clinical Trials*
edited by J.A. Cramer and B. Spilker
Raven Press, Ltd., New York © 1991

4

Partial Compliance as a Source of Variance in Pharmacokinetics and Therapeutic Drug Monitoring

*Julie M. Backes and **Jerome J. Schentag

*Kaiser Foundation Health Plan Pharmacy, Fairfield, California 94533; and
**State University of New York at Buffalo School of Pharmacy, and Clinical
Pharmacokinetics Laboratory, Millard Fillmore Hospital, Buffalo, New York 14209*

The development of pharmacokinetics as a science during the past three decades has had a great impact on the current practice of medicine. The discipline has evolved through several processes. Techniques have been developed that measure the concentration of medicines in various body fluids; pharmacokinetic properties of various medicines in the body have been characterized; therapeutic ranges for plasma concentrations have been defined for a variety of medicines; and several physiologic and environmental factors that may affect pharmacokinetic parameters of certain medicines in the body have been identified.

The application of pharmacokinetic principles to the practice of medicine occurs in a variety of ways. Knowledge of pharmacokinetics is used in the research setting to develop medicines and drug formulations with desirable pharmacokinetic properties. In a clinical setting, clinicians have the capability of predicting patient-specific pharmacokinetic parameters and thus select an individualized dosage regimen for a patient. Obtaining appropriate drug plasma concentrations enables a practitioner to determine patient-specific pharmacokinetic parameters and adjust a patient's regimen accordingly. Pharmacokinetic principles can help achieve optimal therapeutic benefits and avoid unnecessary adverse drug reactions when used appropriately. This aids clinical monitoring and improves patient care.

Although beneficial, the application of this knowledge in both clinical and research settings is limited by several factors. One of these factors is patient compliance to a prescribed medication regimen. Because the concentration of some medicines in serum has a direct effect on efficacy, it follows that a decrease in serum drug concentration as a result of a missed dose may result in a diminished drug response. Although this is a simple concept, partial compliance can be a major issue in both clinical and research settings. Unfortunately, it is seldom recognized or considered.

Why should one be concerned with the effects of partial compliance on pharmacokinetics? One reason is the prevalence of noncompliance. A review of several studies assessing compliance indicated that the percentage of noncompliant patients may range from 20 to 82% (1). Second, the number of ambulatory patients with chronic diseases who are maintained on medicines requiring serum drug concentration monitoring is substantial. Pharmacokinetic monitoring is an integral part of management of ambulatory patients taking such medicines as theophylline, digoxin, lithium, anticonvulsants, antiarrhythmics, and antidepressants. In an ambulatory setting, practitioners rely heavily on serum drug concentrations to manage patients because it is difficult to monitor outpatients clinically for efficacy and toxicity. Weintraub et al. (2) analyzed the effects of factors such as renal function, age, dosage, and compliance on serum digoxin concentrations in outpatients. They found compliance to be the most important determinant of digoxin concentrations.

Finally, in a research setting, compliance may be a major factor affecting the apparent pharmacokinetics and efficacy of a medicine under study. In turn, clinical practices are once again based on the outcome of such studies. The overall number of patients receiving medicines requiring serum drug concentration monitoring is significant, and the fact that these patients do not always comply with their prescribed medication regimen creates major problems with both study and monitoring of these medicines.

METHODS OF ASSESSING COMPLIANCE

Several methods have been used in assessing rates of patient compliance. These include patient interviews, pill counts, measurement of medicines in blood and urine, and medication monitoring systems. Each method has specific limitations, and none is totally reliable. A review of studies that assessed patient compliance by interviews indicated that 25 to 50% of noncompliant patients can be identified by interviews but emphasized that a significant number of noncompliant patients cannot be identified by interviews (3). The accuracy of pill counts in monitoring compliance is dependent on the number of doses actually ingested by the patient versus the number of doses removed from the bottle. Measurement of drug concentrations in blood and urine has also been used in assessing compliance. This method also has limitations, which are discussed below. Recently, continuous monitoring devices have been used to measure patient compliance (4) (see Chapter 1, *this volume*). A limitation of these monitoring systems, however, is that device opening may not be associated with ingestion of a dose, or it may be associated with ingestion of more than one dose. This method of assessing compliance appears to be the most reliable in that it allows continuous monitoring of a patient's drug administration patterns. None of these methods when used alone is totally reliable but, if used together, may give a more accurate estimate of compliance.

ASSESSING COMPLIANCE BY PHARMACOKINETIC METHODS

Benefits

One beneficial aspect of using a serum drug concentration as an indication of compliance is the fact that it is a measurable form of data. Unlike patient interviews, which are subjective, drug concentrations are objective. Measurement of serum drug concentrations may be helpful in patients who are not responding to therapy despite maximization of their dosage regimen. In these situations, inability to detect the prescribed medicine in the patients' serum is an almost certain indication of erratic dosing or discontinuation of the medication. Livingston and Pruce (5) found the most important indication for monitoring anticonvulsant serum levels to be determination of whether a patient is taking medication appropriately. When a patient is suspected of erratic drug ingestion, serially obtained serum drug concentrations may be helpful. Large fluctuations in regular measurements may indicate irregular dosing, particularly if organ function is stable during the same period.

Limitations

Although beneficial, serum drug concentrations also have limitations when used to assess compliance. Serum drug concentrations obtained at intermittent office visits are isolated measurements that do not represent previous long-term compliance patterns but reflect only recent drug ingestion. They do not reveal the impact of events occurring between drug concentration determinations. The greatest limitation of using plasma concentrations in assessing compliance is the fact that so many other variables exist that may alter plasma concentrations. To appreciate these sources of variance, first consider the factors involved in measuring a serum drug concentration regardless of purpose. Often, the usefulness of a measurement is limited by several possible sources of error. For instance, time of drug ingestion in relation to sampling is an important consideration in evaluating a measured concentration. In an ambulatory setting, this information must be obtained from the patient and therefore is not always accurate. Other sources of variance include timing and technique of blood sampling, transport of blood to the lab, assay variance itself (usually small), and reporting of results to the practitioner. Not only are these elements possible sources of error, but one rarely knows if and where an error may have occurred. When assessing a drug concentration, one must consider the possibility of error in all steps involved in simply obtaining and processing a sample.

Once a sample has been obtained from the lab, the results must be interpreted. Oftentimes, the result is not what is expected, and it may be attributed to patient noncompliance. In this situation, other variables that may be responsible for altering the drug concentration must be considered. For instance, a low concentration may simply reflect an inadequate dose. A subtherapeutic level may also represent a non-steady state concentration in a patient receiving a medicine with a long half-life who has only been taking the medicine for a short time. It may also represent altered pharmacokinetics in a patient. Absorption of a medicine in a patient may be affected by the bioavailability of a particular dosage form or by physiologic factors such as gastric pH or may be incomplete as a result of a drug interaction. Recently, Kossoy et al. (6) reported four patients with low or variable serum theophylline concentrations, which they initially attributed to noncompliance. After closer evaluation, the patients were found to have altered theophylline absorption, which resulted in low theophylline concentrations. Metabolism of a medicine may be increased because of patient age, a drug interaction, or an environmental factor such as smoking. Each of these factors would result in low concentrations. Elimination of a medicine may be enhanced by a physiologic factor such as urinary pH. Any of these modifications in pharmacokinetic parameters could account for a "lower than expected" serum drug concentration. Likewise, a high serum drug concentration may be attributed to an excessive dose, altered pharmacokinetics, or "overcompliance."

IMPACT OF NONCOMPLIANCE ON PHARMACOKINETICS

Several different types of noncompliance exist. The drug concentrations used to assess compliance may be affected differently by different types of noncompliance. Practitioners should be aware of several possible patient scenarios that may occur in which patient noncompliance may affect pharmacokinetics. A patient may be "consistently" noncompliant (i.e., they may invariably eliminate a midday dose). This may result in a subtherapeutic plasma concentration, which would prompt a physician to increase the patient's dose. If the patient remains consistently noncompliant and continues to miss one daily dose, he or she may achieve a new serum concentration in the therapeutic range because the new dose now compensates precisely for his or her noncompliance. If, however, the patient suddenly becomes fully compliant with the prescribed dose, the plasma concentration may increase and approach toxicity. If the patient were receiving a medicine with nonlinear kinetics (e.g., phenytoin), a slight increase in prescribed dose in addition to a sudden increase in compliance may result in a dramatic increase in serum drug concentration and cause toxicity. As the reason for the sudden onset of toxicity seldom will be clear, the change in compliance is not usually considered as the cause of the problem.

Physician office visits may affect a patient's drug-taking behavior. A patient may begin taking medication more regularly shortly before an appointment with the physician. If they happen to be taking a medicine with a long half-life, a serum drug concentration may be low because it has not yet reached steady state. A subsequent increase in prescribed dose and continued increase in compliance could result in a steady-state serum concentration in the toxic range. A patient may attempt to compensate for previous noncompliance and become "overcompliant" by ingesting an excessive dose immediately before an appointment (7). Results of a serum drug concentration may be high, prompting the physician to decrease the dosage unnecessarily with a subsequent decrease in drug efficacy.

The most likely scenario is that a patient "becomes" compliant shortly before an office visit and achieves a therapeutic drug concentration because of this recent increase in compliance. However, because of previous partial compliance and a history of low serum drug concentrations, the medicine may appear to be ineffective. This may result in trials with several different therapeutic agents and many unnecessary changes in drug therapy, even though the problem originates with the patient and not the medicine. Review of these scenarios demonstrates that misinterpretation of patient pharmacokinetic parameters as a result of partial compliance may have significant consequences. These include the potential for toxicity and diminished response to drug therapy.

As previously mentioned, partial or irregular compliance may have a significant impact on studies determining patient-specific pharmacokinetics. Studies have assessed the value of monitoring serum phenytoin levels in outpatients with epilepsy. Low initial phenytoin concentrations were attributed to noncompliance or inadequate dosage (8,9). Increased medical staff support and supervision resulted in increases in subsequent phenytoin levels.

PHARMACOKINETIC METHODS VERSUS OTHER ASSESSMENTS OF COMPLIANCE

Several studies have been conducted that associate pharmacokinetics with compliance. These studies are summarized in Table 4–1. Measurement of medicines,

TABLE 4–1. Studies using pharmacokinetics to assess compliance

Objective	Reference	Patient diagnosis	Medicine	Pharmacokinetic method
Use and comparison of various methods of assessing noncompliance	10	Streptococcal pharyngitis	Penicillin	Urine assay
	11	Diabetes	Phenobarbital in oral hypoglycemic agents	Plasma phenobarbital
	12	Peptic ulcer disease	Sodium bromide in liquid antacids	Blood bromide levels
Use of pharmacokinetics to estimate compliance rates	13–15	Tuberculosis	Para-aminosalicylic acid and/or isoniazid	Urine assay
	16	Psychiatric patients	Chlorpromazine	Urine assay
	17	Psychiatric patients	Chlorpromazine, imipramine	Urine assay
	18	Epilepsy	Phenytoin	Serum concentrations
	19,20	Epilepsy	Phenytoin	Ratio of urinary hydroxyphenyl phenylhydantoin to creatinine
Evaluation of relation between noncompliance and drug response	21	Streptococcal pharyngitis	Penicillin	Urine assay
	22	Hypertension	Thiazides	Urine assay
	23,24	Depression	Antidepressants	Plasma concentrations
	25	Absence seizures	Ethosuximide	Plasma concentrations
Evaluation of pharmacokinetic variance as an indication of noncompliance	26	Epilepsy	Phenobarbital	Plasma concentrations
	27,28	Epilepsy	Phenytoin	Plasma concentrations
	29,30,31,32	Depression	Antidepressants	Plasma concentrations
	4	Epilepsy	Phenytoin	Plasma concentrations

their metabolites, and tracers in plasma and urine have been used as indicators of compliance. Detection of a medicine or tracer in the body as a means of identifying noncompliant patients has been compared with alternative methods such as pill counts and patient interviews. A study in patients with streptococcal pharyngitis treated with penicillin showed that negative urine assays for penicillin identified more noncompliant patients than both pill counts and patient interviews (10). A more recent study used detection of low-dose phenobarbital as an indicator of compliance (11). The phenobarbital was incorporated into oral hypoglycemic agents administered to diabetic patients. This pharmacologic indicator was also found to be superior to patient interviews and pill counts in identifying noncompliance. Roth et al. (12) assessed compliance in patients with peptic ulcer disease by adding a trace of sodium bromide to liquid antacid preparations. They found that "bottle counts" overestimated compliance by at least 20% when compared with the number of noncompliant patients identified by blood bromide level determinations. These studies suggest that measurement of medicines or tracers in the body is a more objective and sensitive indicator of noncompliance than pill counts or patient interviews. Although pharmacokinetic methods of assessing compliance are objective, they are limited by their inability to characterize chronic patterns of noncompliance. They cannot reveal drug-taking behavior between drug concentration determinations.

PHARMACOKINETICS IN ESTIMATING COMPLIANCE RATES

Investigators have used pharmacokinetic measurements to estimate compliance rates in patients taking a variety of medicines. The prevalence of noncompliance became an issue in the late 1950s as increasing numbers of tuberculosis patients were being treated on an outpatient basis. Investigators addressing this issue evaluated compliance by detecting the presence of para-aminosalicylic acid or isoniazid in the urine (13–15). The results of one study found that 50% of patients had negative urine assays and were therefore not taking medication as prescribed (13). Studies employing positive urine assays of antipsychotics as a criterion for compliance found rates of noncompliance in psychiatric patients to range from 10.7% (16) to 48% (17).

In a study of epileptic outpatients, investigators attempted to identify reasons for noncompliance (18). This study used plasma concentrations of phenytoin to classify patients as compliant or noncompliant. Compliance was indicated by two serial phenytoin levels within 10% of each other and an 80% clinic attendance record. The major metabolite of phenytoin found in the urine, hydroxyphenyl phenylhydantoin, has also been used to assess compliance as an alternative to serum phenytoin determinations (19,20). The ratio of the metabolite to the creatinine concentration in urine is used as an index of compliance because it remains fairly stable over time.

NONCOMPLIANCE AND DRUG EFFICACY

Patients who do not take medication as prescribed would be expected to have a decreased response to drug therapy. Several authors have shown a relation between noncompliance demonstrated by pharmacokinetic methods and diminished drug response. Compliance was studied in a group of patients with streptococcal pharyngitis treated with penicillin (21). Compliance was judged by pill counts and urine assays for penicillin. There were more negative urine assays for penicillin in patients who had positive culture on reexamination and were not responding to drug therapy.

Lowenthal et al. (22) studied the usefulness of obtaining urine assays for methyldopa and thiazides to identify noncompliant hypertensive patients. They found a relation between positive urine assays for thiazides and blood pressure control. Studies in patients treated with antidepressants have also found that patients who relapsed had subtherapeutic plasma concentrations, which were attributed to noncompliance (23,24). Sherwin et al. (25) found control of absence seizures to be associated with increases in therapeutic plasma ethosuximide levels as a result of increased compliance.

Although these studies associated low or absent plasma or urinary concentrations of medicine with decreased response to drug therapy, most, unfortunately, assume that the low levels are secondary to noncompliance. Using additional methods to assess compliance would have ruled out pharmacokinetic differences that may have altered plasma or urine concentrations.

PHARMACOKINETIC VARIANCE INDICATING NONCOMPLIANCE

As previously mentioned, variations in serially obtained plasma concentrations may reveal a patient with erratic drug administration. A study in epileptic outpatients used this concept to identify patients with unreliable intake of phenobarbital and phenytoin (26). Patients were classified as noncompliant if a difference of more than 20% existed between two phenobarbital blood levels obtained a month apart. By this criterion, 28% of patients in the group were considered noncompliant. Lund (27) also studied outpatients with epilepsy and found less variance in phenytoin blood levels in a group of patients with a daily dispenser versus a control group without the dispenser. Noncompliance was assumed to be the cause of variation in drug concentrations in these studies.

Leppik et al. (28) assessed the variability of serum phenytoin concentrations in supervised, "probably compliant," and noncompliant patients. Compliance status was determined by patient interviews and pill counts. Supervised and probably compliant patients had coefficients of variation of serially obtained serum phenytoin concentrations of less than 20%. These studies indicate that large intraindividual fluctuations in drug levels may be helpful in identifying noncompliant patients. However, this method may not identify patients who are consistently overcompliant or undercompliant. Fluctuations in plasma concentrations may also be caused by variables other than partial compliance, and a patient may be mistakenly considered noncompliant.

Several studies have evaluated compliance of patients on tricyclic antidepressants by measuring plasma concentrations of these medicines and their metabolites (29,30,31,32). Loo et al. (29) obtained tricyclic antidepressant levels on a monthly basis in 17 ambulatory patients with depression. They found small intrapatient fluctuations in plasma concentrations to be associated with good response, whereas large fluctuations were associated with poor response. They attributed the large fluctuations to erratic compliance.

The application of tricyclic antidepressant plasma level/dosage ratios has also been used to assess patient compliance (30). In these studies, patients with large fluctuations in level/dosage ratio values were considered erratically or partially compliant and had a decreased response to drug therapy (31,32).

A recent study conducted by Cramer et al. (4) incorporated a medication monitoring device to assess compliance in outpatients with epilepsy. The Medication

Event Monitor System records the date and time of vial opening, thus allowing for continuous monitoring of drug intake. This method was compared with both pill counts and serum drug concentrations in identifying noncompliant patients. A positive correlation was found between pill counts and compliance rates as determined by the monitoring device. The authors found no correlation between coefficients of variation of drug serum concentrations and compliance rates determined by the device. There was also no relation between pill counts and coefficients of variation. Serum drug concentrations were therefore unreliable in identifying noncompliant patients. Although the majority of serum drug concentrations obtained at office visits were in the therapeutic range, the Medication Event Monitor System revealed that seizure activity in some patients was associated with missed doses. These patients may have had intermittent subtherapeutic plasma concentrations secondary to erratic or partial compliance. Serum drug concentrations obtained at office visits, however, were unsuccessful in capturing these fluctuations. The authors emphasize the limitations inherent in serum drug concentration determinations as indicators of noncompliance. These results differ from previous studies using variance in serum drug concentrations to identify noncompliance (28). One possible consequence of studies that measure compliance using Medication Event Monitor System is that fluctuating serum concentrations on repeat sampling may not indicate partial compliance but may reflect pharmacokinetic variations.

SUMMARY

The impact of pharmacokinetics on medicine is growing as the knowledge of pharmacokinetic properties of medicines increases. Because pharmacokinetics is impacted by partial compliance, compliance in turn affects the practice of medicine and how patients are managed. The number of patients receiving medicines requiring pharmacokinetic monitoring who do not fully comply with their prescribed medication regimen is significant. Therefore, erratic compliance has an impact on patients in both clinical and research settings. Assaying of medicines, drug metabolites, and tracers in blood and urine is one of several methods used in analyzing patient compliance. Benefits of drug concentrations in assessing compliance include the objectiveness of the method and the ability to determine if a patient has discontinued his or her medication. Limitations include inability to disclose a patient's chronic drug administration behavior and the existence of several other variables that may affect pharmacokinetic values. Erratic or partial compliance may alter drug levels and make them difficult to interpret. Misinterpretation may result in drug toxicity or apparent drug failure.

Several studies have been conducted that have analyzed different aspects of pharmacokinetics and the role it plays in assessing noncompliance. Most studies have found drug level determinations to be a more sensitive indicator of noncompliance than pill counts or patient interviews. The absence of medicine in the body or fluctuations in drug concentrations have been used to indicate noncompliance. Several authors have used this method to estimate rates of compliance in different types of patients. Noncompliance determined by this method has also been associated with diminished response to drug therapy. A recent study using Medication Event Monitor System, however, found no correlation between coefficients of variation of serum drug concentrations and noncompliance (4). Thus, partial compliance is part of the variability in drug response but so is intrasubject variance in pharmacokinetics and perhaps drug absorption. Development of new medication monitoring devices offers exciting implications for future research. These devices will allow one to link patient compliance to pharmacodynamics and pharmacokinetics and allow one to better understand the interactions among these variables. Patient compliance can be determined by the monitoring device and pharmacodynamics by a measured physiologic response. Pharmacokinetics will then be determined by correctly interpreting the relation between actual dosage taken and the resulting measured serum concentration.

REFERENCES

1. Stewart RB, Cluff LE. A review of medication errors and compliance in ambulant patients. *Clin Pharmacol Ther* 1972;13:463–468.
2. Weintraub M, Au WY, Lasagna L. Compliance as a determinant of serum drug concentrations. *JAMA* 1973;224:481–485.
3. Norell SE. Methods in assessing drug compliance. *Acta Med Scand* 1983;suppl 683:35–40.
4. Cramer JA, Mattson RH, Prevey ML, Scheyer RD, Ouellette VL. How often is medication taken as prescribed? *JAMA* 1989;261:3273–3277.
5. Livingston S, Pruce I. Clinical response is more important than measurement of blood levels in managing epileptic patients. In: Lasagna L, ed. *Controversies in therapeutics*. Philadelphia: W. B. Saunders Company, 1980:118–130.
6. Kossoy AF, Hill M, Lin FL, Szefler SJ. Are theophylline levels a reliable indicator of compliance? *J Allergy Clin Immunol* 1989;84:60–65.
7. Cramer JA, Scheyer RD, Mattson RH. Compliance declines between clinic visits. *Arch Intern Med* 1990;150:(*in press*).
8. Gibberd FB, Dunne JF, Handley AJ, Hazleman BL. Supervision of epileptic patients taking phenytoin. *Br Med J* 1970;1:147–149.
9. Dawson KP, Jamieson A. Value of blood phenytoin estimation in management of childhood epilepsy. *Arch Dis Child* 1971;46:386–388.
10. Bergman AB, Werner RJ. Failure of children to receive penicillin by mouth. *N Engl J Med* 1963;268:1334–1338.
11. Pullar T, Birtwell AJ, Wiles PG, Hay A, Feely MP. Use of a pharmacologic indicator to compare compliance with tablets prescribed to be taken once, twice, or three times daily. *Clin Pharmacol Ther* 1988;44:540–545.
12. Roth HP, Caron HS, Hsi BP. Measuring intake of a prescribed medication. A bottle count and a tracer technique compared. *Clin Pharmacol Ther* 1970;11:228–237.
13. Dixon WM, Stradling P, Wootton IDP. Outpatient P.A.S. therapy. *Lancet* 1957;2:871–872.
14. Fox W. The problem of self-administration of drugs with particular reference to pulmonary tuberculosis. *Tubercle* 1958;39:269–274.
15. Berry D, Ross A, Huempfner H, Deuschle K. Self medication behavior as measured by urine chemical tests in domiciliary tuberculosis patients. *Am Rev Resp Dis* 1962;86:1–7.
16. Neve HK. Demonstration of largactil (chlorpromazine hydrochloride) in the urine. *J Ment Sci* 1958;104:488–490.
17. Willcox DRC, Gillan R, Hare EH. Do psychiatric outpatients take their drugs? *Br Med J* 1965;2:790–792.
18. Bryant SG, Ereshefsky L. Determinants of compliance in epileptic outpatients. *Drug Intell Clin Pharm* 1981;15:572–577.
19. Zysset T, Rudeberg A, Vassella F, Kupfer A, Bircher J. Phenytoin therapy for epileptic children: evaluation of salivary and plasma concentrations and of methods of assessing compliance. *Dev Med Child Neurol* 1981;23:66–75.
20. Rambeck B, May T. Urinary hydroxyphenytoin/creatinine ratios as an index of compliance in adult epileptic patients on phenytoin therapy. *Ther Drug Monit* 1984;6:164–172.
21. Leistyna JA, Macaulay JC. Therapy of streptococcal infections. Do pediatric patients receive prescribed oral medications? *Am J Dis Child* 1966;111:22–26.
22. Lowenthal DT, Briggs WA, Mutterperl R, Adelman B, Creditor MA. Patient compliance for antihypertensive medication: the usefulness of urine assays. *Curr Ther Res* 1976;13:405–409.
23. Sorensen PK, Hvidberg EF, Hansen CE, Baastrup PC. Therapeutic control of plasma concentrations and long term effects of nortriptyline in recurrent affective disorders. *Pharmacopsychiatry* 1976;9:178–182.

24. Coppen A, Ghose K, Montgomery S, Rama Rao VA, Bailey J, Jorgensen A. Continuation therapy with amitriptyline in depression. *Br J Psychiatry* 1978;133:28–33.
25. Sherwin AL, Preston RJ, Lechter M. Improved control of epilepsy by monitoring plasma ethosuximide. *Arch Neurol* 1973;28:178–181.
26. Driessen O, Hoppener R. Plasma levels of phenobarbital and phenytoin in epileptic outpatients. *Eur Neurol* 1977;15:135–142.
27. Lund M. Failure to observe dosage instructions in patients with epilepsy. *Acta Neurol Scand* 1973;49:295–306.
28. Leppik IE, Cloyd JC, Sawchuk RJ, Pepin SM. Compliance and variability of plasma phenytoin levels in epileptic patients. *Ther Drug Monit* 1979;1:475–483.
29. Loo H, Benyacoub AK, Rovei V, Altamura CA, Vadrof M, Morselli PL. Long term monitoring of tricyclic antidepressant plasma concentrations. *Br J Psychiatry* 1980;137:444–451.
30. Pollock BG, Perel JM. Tricyclic antidepressants: contemporary issues for therapeutic practice. *Can J Psychiatry* 1989;34:609–617.
31. Altamura AC, Mauri M. Plasma concentrations, information, and therapy adherence during long-term treatment with antidepressants. *Br J Clin Pharmacol* 1985;20:714–716.
32. Perel JM. Compliance during tricyclic antidepressant therapy: pharmacokinetic and analytical issues. *Clin Chem* 1988;34:881–887.

Patient Compliance in Medical Practice and Clinical Trials
edited by J.A. Cramer and B. Spilker
Raven Press, Ltd., New York © 1991

5

Methods of Assessing and Improving Patient Compliance in Clinical Trials

Bert Spilker

Department of Project Coordination, Burroughs Wellcome Company, Research Triangle Park, North Carolina 27709

IMPORTANCE OF ASSESSING COMPLIANCE

The term *compliance* is generally used in clinical trials to describe the adherence of patients to taking their medicines as prescribed. Patient compliance means a great deal more than merely "the patients took their drugs as directed." Several other types of compliance may be described. In addition, the compliance of several different groups of people (e.g., investigators, sponsors) involved with a clinical trial may be described.

Assessment of compliance often enables the determination of whether a negative clinical trial resulted from an inactive medicine or from a failure of patients to take their medicine. To assess the efficacy and safety of a medicine under various conditions, patients must take the medicine as prescribed. Negative results of a clinical trial could also relate to either a failure of an investigator to follow adequately (i.e., comply with) a protocol or from a failure of the medicine to work. Compliance of both patients and investigators should be measured and evaluated before the results of a clinical trial are interpreted. Compliance by investigators is only briefly discussed in this chapter.

POTENTIAL RAMIFICATIONS OF POOR PATIENT COMPLIANCE

Poor compliance that is undetected in a clinical trial may result in invalid results and in a medicine that is actually effective for certain populations (under certain conditions) being labeled as ineffective. A number of reasons for poor patient compliance are listed in Table 5–1. Positive data regarding a medicine's effectiveness obtained in compliant patients should not be extrapolated to noncompliant patients. The opposite situation of extrapolating ineffective data obtained in noncompliant patients to compliant patients may also be inappropriate. Data obtained in a mixed population of both compliant and noncompliant patients may not be appropriate to extrapolate to a single patient. Thus, dosage recommendations in package inserts that are based on patients with an average rate of compliance may be inappropriate for patients who take full doses and definitely will be inappropriate for noncompliant patients. Another ramification of poor patient compliance is that excess medicine

TABLE 5–1. *Selected reasons for poor patient compliance*

Disease-related
    Few symptoms present (e.g., mild hypertension)
    Terminal illness known to patient, particularly when accompanied by physical debilitation
Patient-related
    Forgetfulness
    Lack of complete belief in the value of the treatment
    Poor taste of the medicine
    Size of the medicine tablets or capsules
    Cost of therapy
    Adverse reactions
    Safety containers
    Mental illness
    Lack of understanding of terms used (e.g., take with meals may mean before, during, or after
      meals)
    Anger at or dissatisfaction with investigator or his or her staff
    Incomplete understanding of how to be compliant with the protocol
Clinical trial– or medical practice–related
    Number of pills required to ingest at each dosing
    Number of times a day the medicine must be taken
    Large number of medicines prescribed
    Medicine regimens that tend to be confusing or complex
    Requirements of protocol may be too painful, stressful, or demanding
    Long duration of therapy
Investigator-related
    Long time from referral to appointment
    Long time kept waiting
    Failure of physician to keep appointment
    Poor physician–patient relation[a]

[a]See Table 5–7.

from the clinical trial is available to patients after their participation is completed. This potential health hazard is aggravated by the already large number of partially consumed medicines available in most households.

When physicians observe that a medicine is ineffective and they are unaware of a patient's noncompliance, they often inappropriately increase the dose in an attempt to improve efficacy. This occurs both during clinical trials and treatment. Figure 3.12 in *Presentation of Clinical Data* (1) is an example of this phenomenon. Numerous studies have attempted to identify compliers and noncompliers based on personality traits and behavior (2,3), but the results of such studies are mixed and universal generalizations have not emerged. Some patient behaviors required for compliance are listed in Table 5–2.

TABLE 5–2. *Patient behavior required for compliance in an outpatient clinical practice*

Patient must
    Visit physician or clinic
    Answer questions about their medical history honestly
    Cooperate in testing, particularly where a voluntary effort is requested (e.g., forced expiratory
      volume in 1 sec)
    Allow required tests to be performed
    Purchase or obtain medicines prescribed
    Take medicines as prescribed in terms of doses and timing
    Adhere to appointment schedule
    Adhere to advice or requests regarding diet, exercise, relaxation, or other aspects of behavior

TYPES OF COMPLIANCE

For ease of discussion, the types of compliance in a clinical trial are categorized by their primary relation to patients, sponsors, or investigators. Compliance issues could also be described in terms of problems of omission (e.g., failure to take medicine, to file a regulatory document, or to report an adverse reaction) or commission (e.g., overdose, inappropriate self-medication, not adhering to protocol requirements by doing something differently).

Patient Compliance and Noncompliance

Patients must comply with the investigator's instructions by taking the recommended number of medicines at the correct times, coming to the clinic as directed, being cooperative and honest with the staff who are conducting the study, and adhering to all other aspects of the study (e.g., avoiding the forbidden concomitant medicines, following the recommended diet, following the prescribed exercise program). Additionally, in some clinical trials, patients must fill prescriptions. It is usually assumed that patients who ingest their medicine as prescribed are also compliant with other aspects of a protocol, but this is certainly not always the case.

Patients who are noncompliant with the protocol often withdraw from a clinical trial. If patients from different treatment groups withdraw from a clinical trial at variable rates, results may be affected, especially in longitudinal studies.

Although noncompliance is at the opposite end of a spectrum from compliance, both are relative concepts. In some clinical trials, patients may be (or must be) discontinued because of noncompliance. Although there are pros and cons to this practice, it should not be done during phase III clinical trials. If it is to be done during a phase II clinical trial, a standard of noncompliance should be defined before the trial starts that will be used as a basis for patient discontinuation. The standard may contain any one or more of the following concepts: (a) fewer than $X\%$ tablets used, based on pill counts or medication bottle openings; (b) tablets missed for Y days, based on patient history or medication bottle openings; (c) blood levels below Z; (d) poor attitude and cooperation with staff; (e) missing two or more consecutive clinic visits without an excellent excuse; (f) use of prohibited medicines; or (g) failure to cooperate in a specified manner. Several patterns of noncompliance are described by Urquhart (4).

Sponsor Compliance

Sponsors of clinical trials must adhere to regulatory compliance. This involves many steps and processes including producing an Investigational New Drug Application; submitting the protocol to the Food and Drug Administration; ensuring that the investigator has had the protocol approved by the ethics committee or Institutional Review Board; and adhering to Good Manufacturing Practices, Good Laboratory Practices, and Good Clinical Practices regulations. Other regulations affecting the sponsor's compliance with a protocol may also apply (e.g., reporting of adverse reactions).

Investigator Compliance in Clinical Trials and Medical Practice

Investigators must comply with numerous aspects of a clinical protocol. These include submitting the protocol to their ethics committee or Institutional Review Board and providing periodic updates and an end-of-clinical-trial report, adhering to agreements made through negotiations with sponsors (and vice versa), adhering to details of the protocol in treating patients, and adhering to administrative responsibilities (e.g., reporting adverse reactions, completing data collection forms).

In private medical practice, clinicians may not comply with the manufacturers' advice in the package labeling about using a medicine.

WHY AND HOW PATIENTS DO NOT COMPLY WITH CLINICAL TRIAL REQUIREMENTS

There are many reasons why patients may not comply with the requirements of a protocol. These may relate to the characteristics of the study design, study medicine, individual patient's personality, relations with study personnel, or other factors. Some of these reasons are listed in Table 5–1.

The quality of most outpatient studies is enhanced by incorporating a test or tests for compliance in the protocol. A compliance test with follow-up questioning of noncompliant patients may uncover a reason for diminished compliance that could be addressed in a protocol amendment (or new protocol). The revised protocol would enable data to be collected that would have a greater chance of meeting the objectives of the clinical trial.

Information on why protocol compliance was inadequate might assist in the interpretation of the data. A number of the ways in which patients fail to comply with a clinical trial are listed in Table 5–3. These illustrations of decreased compliance are

TABLE 5–3. *Selected ways in which patients fail to comply with a protocol[a]*

Noncompliance primarily related to the clinical trial medicine
    Patients do not fill their prescriptions for medicine
    Patients do not take the medicine as directed; patients take
        Too few doses per day but at the correct times
        Too few doses per day and at irregular times
        Irregular number of doses per day
        Correct number of doses per day, but at incorrect fixed times (i.e., in relation to meals or
          during too short a period)
        Too many doses on some days
        Irregular number of tablets per dose
        No doses on some days and a correct or incorrect pattern on other days
    Patients may prematurely discontinue the medicine (this is especially significant if antibiotics or
        some other classes of medicines are prematurely stopped)
    Patients place the medicine in their "cheek" (for inpatient studies) and then discard the dosage
        (or otherwise improperly ingest the medication)
Noncompliance unrelated to the clinical trial medicine
    Patients may not adhere to the clinic visit schedule, may not contact the clinic as directed (e.g.,
        for adverse reactions), or may fail to bring their medicines, diaries, or biological samples
        (e.g., urine) to the clinic
    Patients may not properly complete patient diaries or other materials
    Patients may not maintain a diet, exercise program, or other outpatient aspect of the clinical trial

[a]From ref. 25, with permission.

broadly divided into those related to the trial medicine and those related to other aspects of the trial.

DIRECT METHODS TO MEASURE AND EVALUATE PATIENT COMPLIANCE

Patient compliance with taking medicines may be assessed directly (i.e., proof of a certain degree of compliance) or indirectly. Indirect methods depend on patient reports or on data that could be modified, if desired, by the patient. A summary of these methods is given in Table 5–4.

Observation

Probably the most direct method to assess compliance is to observe patients taking their medication. This approach would be limited to a few inpatient trials or those outpatient trials in which patients are required to come to a clinic to receive medicine each time it is to be taken. Even in those situations, some patients are not compliant. For example, they may "cheek" their medicine or merely pretend to put it in their mouth. If this is suspected, it may be possible to assay blood or urine samples directly for the medicine, a metabolite, or an added marker.

Biological Markers

Markers are sometimes added as a means of determining compliance when assays are unavailable to measure the level of medicine or its metabolites present in a plasma or urine sample. Markers are also considered for clinical trials in which a placebo is used. The marker that is added must be (a) nontoxic at doses added, (b) stable in biological fluids, (c) easily detected by methods that are sensitive and spe-

TABLE 5–4. *Tests for compliance*

Direct methods
   Observation
   Measure the levels of a medicine or metabolite in biological fluids (e.g., blood, urine)
   Measure the presence of a biological marker attached to placebo or medicine
   Conduct unannounced spot checks on patients at their homes to obtain a biological fluid or sample
   Measure clinic attendance and count the number of missed and canceled appointments
   Screen urine or blood samples for medicines prohibited by protocol (e.g., caffeine and nicotine, if relevant)
Indirect methods
   Question the patient at the outset of a clinical trial
   Assess patients' compliance based on their clinical response
   Conduct pill counts of trial and possibly other medicines
   Use electronic counters
   Determine the number of prescriptions filled and also refilled at pharmacies (i.e., the total quantity of drug dispensed is calculated)
   Question the patient verbally or via questionnaire during treatment
   Use medication monitors (i.e., mechanical dispensers)
   Measure physiological markers
   Evaluate patient diaries for completeness and compliance with instructions
   Assess children's compliance through a school nurse or teacher

cific, and (d) biologically inert. It is also important that absorption and kinetic parameters are similar to those of the medicine it is combined with. Riboflavin may be added as a marker to both placebo and medicine. It is eliminated in the urine and fluoresces when exposed to ultraviolet light. If the medicine is excreted or eliminated via the urine, fluorescing agents may be used as markers and urine samples collected for evaluation. Biological markers include quinine, phenol red, sodium bromide, phenobarbital, and digoxin.

Levels in Biological Fluids

When medicines have a long half-life, arbitrarily defined as greater than 24 hr, their presence in a biological fluid does not confirm compliance, because recent doses may have been skipped. A medicine with a short half-life may be ingested by a patient shortly before going to a clinic, and thus its presence in blood or urine does not confirm compliance. In fact, the presence of a medicine, its metabolite, or a marker in blood or urine only confirms that one or a few doses have been taken within a limited period, whose length is determined by the half-life of the medicine, metabolite, or marker.

The interpretation of medicine levels in biological samples may be viewed in either qualitative or quantitative terms. In qualitative terms, the test result is scored as present or absent, and in quantitative terms, the precise level is measured and evaluated. In evaluating the quantitative levels of medicine and comparing different patients, it is important that each patient have ingested his or her most recent dose at the same time interval before the taking of the biological sample.

A problem may arise in interpreting blood level data if the clinical trial test medicine has a short half-life. For example, consider three patients who took their medicine at the same time on the day of their clinic visit: one patient had not taken the medicine since his or her last clinic visit, the second patient had only taken the medicine for the day preceding the present visit, and the third had taken all the prescribed medicine. The problem would be that all three patients might have the same blood level recorded on the day of the clinic visit, and the data would therefore be misleading in terms of measuring patient compliance.

Coefficient of Variation

Other obstacles to direct measurement of compliance include variations in a medicine's metabolism and dose–response relation. These issues also make single determinations of blood levels uncertain indicators of compliance. Leppik et al. (5) proposed a coefficient of variation as a method to overcome these problems in epileptic patients treated with phenytoin. A problem with this measurement is that if patients consistently take one-half or other fraction of their prescribed dose, they will have a low coefficient of variation, which implies a high degree of compliance. Another potential problem is that this method can only test medicine-taking events for a few half-lives before the time of sampling.

Other biological samples have been used to assess compliance in selected cases. These include secretion of a medicine into sweat (collected with absorbent pads), saliva samples, and breath samples.

Spot Checks on Patients

If it is believed that outpatients are compliant for a short period before their clinic visit but may not be compliant at other times, it is often possible to conduct spot checks on some or all patients in the clinical trial. Using this method, a member of the clinical team makes unannounced visits to patients at their homes sometime between clinic visits. This clinician or nurse collects a blood, urine, or other biological sample in which the amount of study medicine is measured. This method represents a potential invasion of privacy and must be carefully discussed with patients before their enrollment in the clinical trial. The agreement of patients to this procedure of spot checking should be part of the informed consent. This technique is only feasible if patients live relatively close to the clinical trial site and resources are available to visit patients and collect samples.

Clinic Attendance

If compliance is assessed in terms of clinic attendance, examining the records of clinic attendance is a direct method to assess patient compliance.

INDIRECT METHODS TO MEASURE AND EVALUATE PATIENT COMPLIANCE

Numerous indirect measures of patient compliance exist. The extrapolation of acceptable compliance from data gathered with some of these methods may be unwarranted.

Questioning the Patient at the Outset of a Clinical Trial

Patients may be asked at the outset of a clinical trial whether they intend to be compliant (e.g., ask patients if they are willing to take the medicine as directed). An affirmative response to this question should be one of the inclusion criteria in almost any clinical trial. Any patient answering "no" should not be enrolled or should be discontinued, except for extenuating circumstances (e.g., psychosis, parents to assure compliance).

Assessment Based on Clinical Response

The patient is assumed to be compliant if he or she improves on the active treatment or does not improve on placebo.

Pill Counts

The most commonly used measure of compliance apart from direct questioning is probably that of the pill count. The actual number of tablets or capsules in the drug container used by the patient is counted at each (or selected) clinic visits, and the expected number to be used is also determined. The ratio of actual pill use divided by expected pill use (times 100) gives a figure that may be referred to as percent compliance. Any drug refills obtained by the patient must be considered in calculating the actual number of pills used, and any changes in the dose prescribed must be considered in calculating the expected number of pills to be used. Care must be used in determining these figures, because patients often switch medicines between bottles (e.g., a "purse" bottle may be created by the patient), which could affect the numbers counted. Some protocols are written to exclude some of or all a patient's data from analysis if the patient's percent compliance falls below a defined level and to discontinue patients who are unable to offer a satisfactory explanation of their failure to comply adequately with the clinical trial.

If the patient does not bring his or her medications to the clinic or office visit, a definite plan should have been evolved to deal with the situation. The patient may be asked to count the number of pills at home and to telephone the information to the investigator, but this is not a wholly satisfactory method because it alerts the patient to the attention paid to pill counts and may make the patient feel that he or she is being watched too closely. In fact, all pill counts should be conducted out of the patient's sight. Another alternative is to omit performing the pill count in question and to give special attention to the pill count at the next visit. This option is reasonable if there are several pill counts scheduled during the clinical trial, but if the instance in question represented the only pill count in the trial, requesting the patient to return to the clinic the next day or having a member of the clinical trial team visit the patient's home should be considered. Mailing medicines to patients or to the trial site is not generally advocated except when absolutely necessary and under carefully controlled conditions.

The method of pill counting has been validated in some clinical trials (6), but other more recent publications have been highly critical of this approach (7,8). The value of pill counts undoubtedly depends on the particular clinical trial and group of patients enrolled. Pill counts cannot be assumed to be an accurate reflection of patient compliance. It is expected that the use of this method will decrease in the future.

Electronic Counters

Electronic counters in the tops of specially prepared medicine bottles have been developed that record the exact day, hour, and minute each time the bottle of medicine is opened or used (9–14). This method may demonstrate that patients open the container the correct number of times or either too few or too many. It also can demonstrate whether patients take their medicines at correct intervals. Despite the inability to know with certainty that patients have ingested the correct dose of medicine each time the bottle is opened, this is probably the best method to measure compliance in most outpatient trials. Selected advantages and disadvantages are listed in Table 5–5.

Pharmacy Refills

Pharmacy records demonstrate whether patients fill and refill their prescriptions at appropriate intervals. When this method is available, it may be valuable, because most patients do not purposely try to fool pharmacists. However, some patients

TABLE 5–5. *Selected advantages and disadvantages of assessing compliance with electronic medication counters*

Advantages
  Precise data are obtained
  Data are easily quantifiable and expressed
  Provides the most accurate compliance data possible in numerous situations (e.g., medicine has
    a very short or very long half-life)
Disadvantages
  Patients may purposely fool the system if they desire (e.g., open lid an excessively large or
    small number of times)
  Patients may inadvertently invalidate the data (e.g., put medicine in other containers, check
    contents frequently, remove extra medicine for later dosing)
  The approach is expensive and therefore often impractical for large clinical trials
  The approach is an indirect measure in that it does not assure ingestion of an appropriate
    number of tablets at the time the bottle is opened

stockpile medicines, especially those they obtain at no cost or low cost. Obtaining refills of medicine according to a set schedule does not ensure ingestion of those medicines on schedule.

Questioning the Patient During Treatment

Physicians question patients informally about whether the patient remembers to take their medicines as prescribed, and the physician believes the patient's compliance to be acceptable. The most simple and open approach to measuring compliance is to ask the patient a direct question such as "Are you taking all of your medicine?" or "Have you missed taking any of your medicine?" or, somewhat indirectly and possibly in a less threatening manner, "Are you having any difficulty remembering to take your medicine?"

Medication Monitors

Medicine bottles containing either the precise number of pills for a daily dose or a standard number of pills may be placed into a mechanical device, sometimes called a *medication monitor*. In inpatient studies, the patient may be advised to operate this machine to obtain medication but is not informed that the number of bottles is being monitored. The number of bottles of trial medicine dispensed to a patient may be easily determined, although it is a separate question whether all doses of the trial medicine dispensed were actually ingested.

Physiological Markers

In certain clinical trials, physiological markers provide an indication of the degree of patient compliance. A well-known example is that of measuring heart rate in patients receiving β-adrenergic receptor-blocking medicines. If the heart rate is not in the expected range and the patient is receiving a dose shown to decrease heart rate, this is indirect evidence of a lack of compliance, if there were no other reasonable explanations for the "elevated" heart rate.

Patient Diaries

Another means of estimating compliance is by evaluating patient diaries. Both the frequency (i.e., the number of times an entry was made compared with the number of times an entry should have been made) and the quality of the entries may be evaluated. The quality of the entry might be judged by whether the clinical trial medicine was taken as scheduled and whether all requested information was filled out (e.g., daily evaluations of the patient's pain).

Assessment Through a School Nurse

A child's container of medicine is collected from his or her school where it is kept, and the school nurse is questioned about the child's compliance.

Each of the indirect methods described may be misleading, and direct methods should also be used when possible to confirm findings. Numerous examples are referenced by Pearson (15). Under certain circumstances, each of the indirect methods may yield accurate data. The validity of results obtained by these measures depends on such factors as disease severity, degree of hope for improvement, and cultural and social factors in the population.

REASONS FOR POOR PATIENT COMPLIANCE

Number of Doses per Day

It has long been believed that compliance decreases with the number of doses required per day. This hypothesis was recently proven (16).

Disease Severity

Another factor that affects patient compliance is disease severity. This often affects patient's motivation to comply with a clinical trial. Patients with mild forms of a disease tend to comply less than patients with moderate and moderately severe disease. Patients with extremely severe or even terminal disease usually comply less than the moderate group (Fig. 5–1). This may be because those with severe disease are depressed and have lost hope or the physical ability to take care of themselves appropriately. The accuracy of this generalization depends, in part, on personality factors of the patient, as well as the patient's values, culture, religion, and previous experiences with the disease and medical establishment.

A patient's motivation often depends on the severity of his or her disease, how the disease affects his or her quality of life, and how he or she views the anticipated benefits (and costs) of the clinical trial. Another factor for assessing compliance in severely ill patients is how well they are physically able to comply with a clinical trial (e.g., to open childproof caps).

Other Reasons

Other reasons for poor patient compliance relate to requests made of them that they consider unfair, unclear, made with too-short notice, too expensive, too incon-

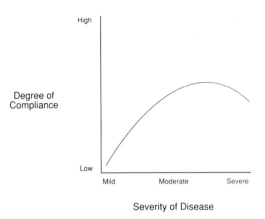

FIG. 5–1. Generalized relation between a patient's degree of compliance and severity of their disease.

venient, or made without discussion with them. Poor relationships with medical professionals is sometimes a major factor in compliance. Adverse reactions that the patient wishes to avoid are another problem. Sackett and Snow (17) reported that patients kept about 75% of clinic appointments they made for themselves but only about 50% of the appointments made for them.

The degree of noncompliance clearly varies enormously from trial to trial. Authors who have reviewed compliance data in the literature have documented noncompliance ranging from about 15 to 93% (18,19). Part of this variation may be explained by differences in definitions used, methods used to measure compliance, severity of disease, and the treatments used.

Compliance has been found to be unrelated to a patient's income, social class, occupation, or educational background (20).

WHEN SHOULD MEDICATION COMPLIANCE BE MEASURED?

Phase I

There is little need to measure compliance in most phase I acute safety or pharmacokinetic clinical trials. Medicines are often given directly to patients by staff who observe the ingestion or injection, and compliance is seldom an issue in single dose or short-term clinical trials. For chronic phase I clinical trials, compliance may be more of an issue.

Phase IIa

During pilot efficacy trials it may be extremely valuable to assess patient compliance, particularly if unexpectedly poor activity occurs. Patient interviews concerning compliance may be more valuable than merely assessing it in objective terms.

Phase IIb

It is almost always important to have an assessment of compliance during these clinical trials. The degree to which this factor should be evaluated must be judged for each clinical trial.

Phase III

The value of obtaining data on compliance greatly varies and must be judged for each clinical trial.

Phase IV

It is not generally possible to assess compliance during observational studies. Compliance is generally impossible to assess in retrospective phase IV studies and not practical in most prospective studies, but exceptions do occur.

HOW TO CHOOSE A METHOD TO EVALUATE PATIENT COMPLIANCE

To obtain accurate compliance data, the manner in which compliance is assessed may be more important than the specific methods used. Physicians or others who do not behave in an empathetic manner or who ask questions about compliance in a negative tone may not only obtain false data, but may encourage some patients to alter their degree of compliance with the clinical trial's requirements. Nonthreatening questions about the patient's compliance should be created and included in the protocol to help ensure that everyone associated with the clinical trial uses the same wording in eliciting information. A description of the empathetic tone to be used should also be included.

In some clinical trials it is so important that patients receive medicine that it should always be given by the staff. There is no question about patient compliance in these trials, although there could be questions about staff compliance. If patients are to medicate themselves, the relative importance of their compliance should determine which method(s) are chosen to evaluate it. The amount of resources available to evaluate compliance will determine whether it is possible to use medication bottles with electronic counters or whether it is necessary to rely on pill counts. The nature of the protocol will determine whether audits of pharmacy records can be used to measure refills. If that method is desirable but impractical to use, it may be possible to modify a protocol ahead of time to allow that method to be used.

Overall, a review of the pros and cons of each method for a particular clinical trial will indicate which methods should be used and how the methods should be modified to provide the best compliance data possible. One of the golden rules of measuring compliance is that a combination of methods is most effective, especially because most methods are extremely easy to implement (e.g., general probe, patient diary, pill count).

DESIGNING CLINICAL TRIALS TO MEASURE COMPLIANCE

Assessing compliance is rarely the primary objective in a clinical trial, but it is often one of the secondary ones. Compliance is rarely a major objective for inpatient trials because patients have less control over medicine intake, diet, and exercise as compared with patients in outpatient trials. Compliance may be the primary objective when a sponsor wants to determine whether compliance is enhanced by switching medicine regimens (e.g., comparing twice-a-day and four-times-a-day regimens, comparing capsules with suppositories).

If a clinical trial is designed primarily to evaluate compliance, it is critical to determine the basis for enrolling patients. Patients with the highest rates of compliance are those with the greatest motivation. Many of these patients can be identified in advance. If this is done and a select group of patients is chosen for the clinical trial, the representativeness of the groups must be assessed carefully, as well as the ability to extrapolate the trial's results to other patients.

Types of clinical trials that could be conducted to measure compliance include:

1. Cross-over or parallel trials with two formulations of the same medicine (e.g., uncoated tablet with a bitter taste and a film-coated tablet in which the bitter taste is masked)
2. Cross-over or parallel trials with two packages of the same medicine (e.g., blister pack and screw-top bottle, bottles with and without a child-resistant cap)
3. Cross-over or parallel trials with capsules (or tablets) of two different colors
4. Cross-over or parallel trials with capsules (or tablets) of two different sizes
5. Parallel trials with and without a patient package insert
6. Parallel trials with and without frequent encouragement of professional staff to comply with the medicine regimen
7. Cross-over or parallel trials with two (or more) dosing regimens (e.g., twice a day versus three times a day, drug holiday versus none)

Compliance Run-In Technique

If patient compliance during a clinical trial is deemed particularly important or even critical, a run-in period of X days or weeks may be included in the trial. Only patients with a satisfactory rate of compliance are then randomized to enter the true clinical trial. This approach is similar to that used to eliminate placebo responders from trials in which a large placebo effect is anticipated. Just as the "placebo run-in technique" is appropriate to use for phase II but not phase III clinical trials, the "compliance run-in technique" is also appropriate to use for phase II but not phase III clinical trials.

Electronic Monitors of Compliance

Electronic monitors of container openings have become more sophisticated in recent years and the Medication Event Monitor Systems (Aprex Corporation, Freemont, California) have been widely studied (14). The goal for Medication Event Monitor Systems is that it may help explain apparent failure of a regimen because of variable compliance. This goal is only an ideal, because this system is, at best, an indirect method of assessing compliance. One drawback of the system is that if each dose consists of two tablets, it is impossible to know the number of tablets actually taken. Other drawbacks of this system are that a patient may transfer some or all medicine to another container or may lay pills on a counter ahead of time. Table 5–5 summarizes selected advantages and disadvantages of electronic medication counters. A system under development for monitoring use of oral contraceptive pills has the advantage of using sensors to count the number of pills removed from a ring device for each dose (see Chapter 16, *this volume*). Nonetheless, for most outpatient trials, this method offers a more reliable measure of compliance than virtually all others. It may also be used to monitor use of rescue or concomitant medicine in addition to, or instead of, the clinical trial medications. An important issue is whether the additional validity of the data obtained is sufficient justification for the cost.

Cheung et al. (9,10) described a different electronic system of tracking compliance based on the principle used in the Medication Event Monitor Systems (i.e., each opening is recorded). Cheung et al. reported that their system overestimated compliance but to a lesser degree than did pill counts. Eyedrop monitors and nebulizer monitors based on the same principle are also available. These devices log the exact amount of liquid medicine dispensed (see Chapters 12 and 13, *this volume*).

METHODS TO IMPROVE COMPLIANCE

Improving Patient Compliance

Give the Medicine to Patients Directly

The best approach to assure total patient compliance is for the clinical trial staff to give the medicine(s) to patients. This is appropriate for depot injections and for medicines with long half-lives or if the patient lives within a reasonable distance of the clinic and can arrange to come for the medicine.

Demonstration and Practice of Techniques

For any medicine or therapy that involves techniques to self-administer the treatment that are not familiar to the patient, it is necessary to demonstrate the techniques and to have the patient practice. This approach is routinely followed when diabetic patients are first taught to inject themselves. Other methods that require practice are the use of inhalers and nasal insufflation. The compliance of patients who are uncomfortable or unfamiliar with a technique can be enhanced by practice with nonjudgmental professional staff.

Instructions

Another aspect of education that affects compliance relates to the nature of verbal instructions given patients. Simple instructions have a better chance of being understood and followed than do more complex or less clear instructions. Even for college graduates or those with advanced degrees, the Keep It Short and Simple rule applies. Asking patients to repeat what they are told helps ensure that the message transmitted is received accurately. Providing written instructions is a further tool that enhances the verbal message and assists patients' accurate recall of the verbal instructions. Details that cannot easily be remembered (e.g., dosing information, telephone numbers, names of contacts, instructions for completing patient diaries) may be provided on paper. In addition, some professional groups have prepared videos about taking medicines that can be shown to groups of patients in a clinic.

Clear labeling of medicine containers, as well as appropriate packaging, will enhance compliance in studies in which label instructions are unclear or packages are inconvenient to use (e.g., too large, too difficult to open).

TABLE 5–6. *Methods of improving compliance[a]*

Simplify the demands of the protocol on patients
Minimize the number and duration of unpleasant or painful tests
Maintain relatively frequent contact with patients, especially at emotionally or physically difficult periods for the patient; contact the patient before scheduled visits
Allow for flexible dosing regimens to deal with adverse reactions, toxicity, and unanticipated situations
Provide the patient with appropriate information on the clinical trial and strive for a positive physician–patient relation[b]
Avoid making the patient feel guilty about poor compliance and provide positive feedback to all patients
Establish a therapeutic goal in conjunction with the patient and assess the patient's progress toward that goal
Plan patient visits at a mutually convenient time and ensure that the patient has a minimal delay in waiting to see the physician or staff
Allow for and encourage patients to participate in their own care (e.g., with self-monitoring of their disease and treatment)
Involve the patient's spouse, family, or support group in the clinical trial

[a]This table does not include a number of methods described in the text or used in general medical practice, in which different factors must be considered and different techniques exist to improve compliance (e.g., switching patients to a different medicine or manipulating factors that are not permitted in most protocols).
[b]See Table 5–7.

Methods to enhance patient compliance are summarized in Table 5–6, have been reviewed elsewhere (20), and are listed below in a modified form. Few of these methods have been systematically assessed, and most represent a common sense approach.

1. *Ask Patients Why They Did Not Take Their Medicines.* Although the reasons offered may be only excuses and not necessarily true, they should be sought and taken seriously. Patients may be asked about compliance in a diary rather than in conversation. Patients may be noncompliant for reasons related to the clinical trial's outcome (e.g., cure obtained, no cure obtained, adverse reactions) or personal factors (e.g., forgetfulness, anger with staff, anger with demands of trial). A discussion about the topic may encourage patients to take their compliance more seriously and to improve their degree of compliance.

2. *Improve the Physician–Patient Interaction.* Many facets of this relationship have an important effect on a patient's compliance. A number of ways to enhance this relationship and patient compliance are listed in Table 5–7.

TABLE 5–7. *Selected methods to enhance compliance through improving the physician–patient relation*

Have patients see the same physician at each visit
Education physicians about the importance of being sympathetic and caring with patients
Provide positive feedback to patients about their performance
Interview patients about what aspects of a clinical trial they object to or what aspects interfere with their full compliance; discuss these situations and remedy them insofar as possible
Negotiate how the patient will take medicines if it is difficult to arrange a suitable schedule (e.g., take the medicine after school versus during school)
Prepare patients for expected adverse reactions so that they do not become upset and discontinue therapy when the reactions occur

3. *Creating Fear About Consequences of Noncompliance.* The impact on patient compliance through use of fear-arousing messages is uncertain. This method has (at best) only limited (if any) usefulness in clinical trials.

4. *Educating Patients About Their Disease.* The importance of educating interested patients about their disease is clear from an ethical perspective. But education's effect on compliance is not yet known and may not always be positive. There are reports of both enhanced compliance (21) and no effect (22) after educational interventions. Videotapes may be prepared to encourage patients to enroll in a trial as well as to adhere to assigned dosing schedules.

5. *Providing Written Instructions.* Written instructions have been found to be effective in increasing compliance for short-term therapy. For long-term therapy this approach does not necessarily elicit the same benefit. The instruction sheet should be reviewed with patients, not merely handed to them. Patients have been known to take all their pills for the entire day early in the morning because they are planning to be away from home; others take all their pills for a week at one time because they are afraid of forgetting to take them later.

6. *Using Special Medicine Packaging.* This is a valuable method of improving compliance in clinical trials. This improvement is achieved by reducing or eliminating confusion about dose schedules and by making medicines easier to remove from containers. This may involve using easy opening bottles or blister packs in which dates and times are printed on the foil.

7. *Tailoring Reminders to Patients.* Patients can be reminded about when to take their medicines through simple cues (e.g., notes put on a refrigerator or bathroom mirror, telephone calls from relatives or friends, alarms that ring at preset intervals). In long-term clinical trials as well as in private practice, a reminder to refill a prescription may be sent before the expected date of need. This must be carefully considered and, preferably, discussed with patients, because they may resent this method. Automatic telephone calls with computerized voice reminders represent a similar method that may annoy patients rather than improve their compliance.

8. *Allowing Patients to Schedule Their Own Appointments.* In some clinical trials it may be possible to do this, within limits; the method has been shown to work.

9. *Self-Monitoring.* Providing calendars or cards to be checked off may remind those patients who are noncompliant because of forgetfulness. This method will not improve the compliance of those who are noncompliant for other reasons.

10. *Rewards.* Patients may be given tokens for complying with medicine taking and other aspects of a clinical trial. Tokens may be exchanged for desired rewards (e.g., a trip to town). This approach is only appropriate for some selected patients (e.g., patients in institutions) and is primarily applicable to medical practice. The use of rewards in clinical trials is almost always inappropriate.

An additional approach is to simplify the therapeutic regimen. Although this is usually a possibility in medical practice, it has limited applicability in a clinical trial. Appointments should be scheduled at times that are convenient for the patient, and patients should be encouraged to participate in their own care, in clinical trials as well as in medical practice. Having a parent, friend, spouse, or other person (e.g., pharmacist) take an active role in ensuring medicine compliance has been shown to be effective, especially for patients who live alone or are known to be somewhat noncompliant.

A behaviorally oriented strategy (i.e., providing blood pressure measuring equipment to hypertensive patients known to be noncompliant) enhanced compliance (23), but several biases may have accounted for the improvements in compliance observed.

To dispel any doubts about the importance of trial design to compliance, imagine the following trial. Patients are required to take two huge (size zero) capsules six times per day, every 4 hr around the clock. Capsules are dispensed in childproof containers, and patients must complete their diaries three times a day. Every 3 days, for 6 weeks, patients must attend the clinic. In the clinic they undergo a rigorous 8-hr period of forms, tests, and blood draws and are questioned about adverse reactions every 20 min. This hypothetical scenario could be continued, but it makes the point that in many cases the compliance of both patients and investigators is a function of the clinical trial's design. Clearly, compliance could be improved by careful attention to the clinical trial's design, particularly by minimizing its complexity.

Assessing and Improving Investigator Compliance

Monitoring a clinical trial and evaluating the conduct of its investigators and staff is the best way to ensure that personnel are complying with the trial in the many ways required. Deviations should be discussed with the investigator, who should also be involved in planning modifications. Issues that are not readily resolved should be discussed with senior executives at the sponsoring institution. In some situations, creative solutions must be found. For example, one investigator was suspected of avoiding his responsibilities because he was not completing data collection forms. But when the situation was explored, he was found to be simply overworked. The solution reached was to have him hire an assistant for the duration of the clinical trial whose job included filling out the data collection forms.

Investigator compliance can also be assessed by evaluating audits conducted by sponsors or regulatory authorities. In private practice, the reports of adverse reactions reaching the manufacturer or published in the literature should indicate whether the medicine is being used correctly (i.e., as labeled). Physicians who are noncompliant with a medicine's labeling may observe a higher incidence or different nature of adverse reactions.

Activities by Sponsors to Enhance Compliance in a Clinical Trial

Sponsors may enhance compliance by writing a protocol in a logical sequence that makes sense to physicians and patients. Complex, unnatural, or unusual dosing regimens, tests, or other activities in a clinical trial will diminish compliance by both physicians and patients. For example, if 16 hr of tests are scheduled on a single day, if patients are awakened during the night to answer questions about adverse reactions, if patients are starved unnecessarily, or if they are otherwise harassed, patient noncompliance and dropouts will result.

The preparing and dispensing of medicine varies enormously between clinical trials and certainly affects compliance. A patient given a large glass jar containing a month's supply of medicine to take four times a day will comply less (on average) than one given four separate weekly blister packs in which each day's dose is labeled. Alternatively, a calendar pack (similar to the oral contraceptive packages) could be used to package the medicine for a whole month.

INTERPRETING DATA ON COMPLIANCE

Electronic monitors may help interpret clinical trial results. For example, an excess number of medicine bottle openings associated in time with adverse reactions may be related to an overdose, and too few bottle openings associated in time with adverse reactions may be related to an underdose and withdrawal effects or to re-emergence of disease symptoms.

In clinical trials with a test medicine and active control but no placebo, data may be analyzed separately for the groups of high versus the groups of low compliers. If efficacy is found to be greater in both groups of high compliers than in the comparable groups of low compliers, the validity of the clinical trial can probably be substantiated, and both treatments can be assessed as effective.

If compliance is less than expected, it may be necessary to examine the data and question patients to determine if the problem is primarily with the clinical trial design (e.g., too arduous), medicine (e.g., poor tasting), clinical response (e.g., improvement, lack of improvement), patient (e.g., personality, motivation to be in the trial), or some other factor.

In clinical trials with a placebo control, the relation of efficacy versus degree of compliance should be assessed for both the active medicine and placebo. These results allow the determination of the degree of patient compliance necessary to obtain full efficacy.

SHOULD NONCOMPLIANT PATIENTS BE DISCONTINUED FROM A CLINICAL TRIAL?

Yes, if it is a phase II clinical trial and if it is important to determine that a medicine is effective. Poor compliers may yield poor efficacy data, which will confound the results and lead to an incorrect conclusion about a medicine. If poor compliers are discontinued from a clinical trial, their data still *must* be included in the safety analyses. Their data should probably also be included in the efficacy analysis (under intention-to-treat principles) for the time they were in the clinical trial. Do not use "last observation carried forward" methods of statistics for patients discontinued for noncompliance because this could greatly bias and influence the outcome.

If the principle of eliminating poorly compliant patients from a clinical trial is accepted, it becomes necessary to establish a critical level of compliance and a method(s) for measuring it. The standard or cut-off level of compliance will depend on the disease and its severity and on the medicine's characteristics, value, and rate of use. Overall, the level that is considered reasonable must be established before the start of the clinical trial. The ultimate answer must involve clinical judgment and should be discussed by a group of appropriate individuals.

No, if a phase III clinical trial is involved, because the objective of phase III trials is to evaluate a medicine under conditions of essentially normal use. Eliminating patients who are poor compliers could skew results and result in the loss of important information.

A number of clinical trial reports have stated that a medicine is more effective with compliant patients than with noncompliant patients (24). This has also been observed with patients treated with placebo (see Table 5–8). These observations raise the question whether noncompliant patients differ from compliant patients in

TABLE 5–8. *Five-year mortality in patients given clofibrate or placebo according to cumulative compliance with protocol prescription[a]*

	Clofibrate		Placebo	
Compliance	N	% Mortality	N	% Mortality
Less than 80%	357	24.6 ± 2.3	882	28.2 ± 1.5
Greater than 80%	708	15.0 ± 1.3	1,813	15.1 ± 0.8
Total	1,065	18.2 ± 1.2	2,695	19.4 ± 0.8

[a]From ref. 26, with permission. The differences between the two groups of compliers was found to be statistically significant for both clofibrate and placebo.

substantial ways that affect mortality and suggest a number of subgroup analyses that may be conducted.

CONCLUSIONS

Compliance of a single patient or group is rarely an all-or-none phenomenon; instead it may be expressed as a percentage varying from 0 to 100. It should be measured in all well-controlled clinical trials, particularly during phase II. Before their initiation, clinical trials conducted during other phases should also be examined to determine the value of assessing compliance. Thought should be given while designing the protocol for a clinical trial to attaining as high a level of compliance as possible. The ideal method of measuring compliance is not yet available, but the use of multiple methods will yield reasonable data for most clinical trials. Where compliance is measured, data for overcompliers should be compared with data for undercompliers. The interpretation and extrapolation of data must consider these results. In phase II well-controlled clinical trials, efforts may be made to exclude noncompliers from entering, but this should not be done in phase III clinical trials. Data from noncompliant patients should not be omitted from most statistical analyses in a clinical trial.

The discussion in this chapter was based on the assumption that it is desirable to have as high a degree of patient compliance as possible. Although this assumption is not being questioned in most trials, partial compliance is usually sufficient to evaluate a medicine's efficacy. If compliance was poor, this fact should be apparent and can then be factored into the data analysis and interpretation of the results.

REFERENCES

1. Spilker B, Schoenfelder J. *Presentation of clinical data.* New York: Raven Press, 1990.
2. Davis MS. Variations in patients' compliance with doctors' advice: an empirical analysis of patterns of communication. *Am J Public Health* 1968;58:274–288.
3. Schwartz S, Griffin T. *Medical thinking: the psychology of medical judgment and decision making.* New York: Springer-Verlag, 1986.
4. Urquhart J. Noncompliance: the ultimate absorption barrier. In: Prescott LF, Nimmo WS, eds. *Novel drug delivery and its therapeutic application.* Chichester: John Wiley and Sons, 1989; 127–137.
5. Leppik IE, Cloyd JC, Sawchuk RJ, Pepin SM. Compliance and variability of plasma phenytoin levels in epileptic patients. *Ther Drug Monit* 1979;1:475–483.
6. Cromer BA, Steinberg K, Gardner L, Thornton D, Shannon B. Psychosocial determinants of compliance in adolescents with iron deficiency. *Am J Dis Child* 1989;143:55–58.

7. Rudd P, Byyny RL, Zachary V, et al. The natural history of medication compliance in a drug trial: limitations of pill counts. *Clin Pharmacol Ther* 1989;46:169–176.
8. Pullar T, Kumar S, Tindall H, Feely M. Time to stop counting tablets? *Clin Pharmacol Ther* 1989;46:163–168.
9. Cheung R, Sullens CM, Seal D, et al. The paradox of using a 7 day antibacterial course to treat urinary tract infections in the community. *Br J Clin Pharmacol* 1988;26:391–398.
10. Cheung R, Dickins J, Nicholson PW, et al. Compliance with anti-tuberculous therapy: a field trial of a pill-box with a concealed electronic recording device. *Eur J Clin Pharmacol* 1988;35:401–407.
11. Kass MA, Meltzer DW, Gordon M. A miniature compliance monitor for eyedrop medication. *Arch Ophthalmol* 1984;102:1550–1554.
12. Kass MA, Meltzer DW, Gordon M, Cooper D, Goldberg J. Compliance with topical pilocarpine treatment. *Am J Ophthalmol* 1986;101:515–523.
13. Spector SL, Kinsman R, Mawhinney H, et al. Compliance of patients with asthma with an experimental aerosolized medication: implications for controlled clinical trials. *J Allergy Clin Immunol* 1986;77:65–70.
14. Cramer JA, Mattson RH, Prevey ML, Scheyer RD, Ouellette VL. How often is medication taken as prescribed? A novel assessment technique. *JAMA* 1989;261:3273–3277.
15. Pearson RM. Who is taking their tablets? *Br Med J* 1982;285:757–758.
16. Pullar T, Birtwell AJ, Wiles PG, Hay A, Feely MP. Use of a pharmacologic indicator to compare compliance with tablets prescribed to be taken once, twice, or three times daily. *Clin Pharmacol Ther* 1988;44:540–545.
17. Sackett DL, Snow JC. The magnitude of compliance and noncompliance. In: Haynes RB, Taylor DW, Sackett DL, eds. *Compliance in health care.* Baltimore: Johns Hopkins University Press, 1979.
18. Blackwell B. The drug defaulter. *Clin Pharmacol Ther* 1972;13:841–848.
19. Greenberg RN. Overview of patient compliance with medication dosing: a literature review. *Clin Ther* 1984;6:592–599.
20. Peck CL, King NJ. Increasing patient compliance with prescriptions. *JAMA* 1982;248:2874–2877.
21. Norell SE. Improving medication compliance: a randomised clinical trial. *Br Med J* 1979;2:1031–1033.
22. Pye G, Christie M, Chamberlain JO, Moss SM, Hardcastle JD. A comparison of methods for increasing compliance within a general practitioner based screening project for colorectal cancer and the effect on practitioner workload. *J Epidemiol Community Health* 1988;42:66–71.
23. Haynes RB, Sackett DL, Gibson ES, et al. Improvement of medication compliance in uncontrolled hypertension. *Lancet* 1976;I:1265–1268.
24. Noseworthy JH. There are no alternatives to double-blind, controlled trials. *Neurology* 1988;38(suppl 2):76–79.
25. Spilker B. *Guide to clinical studies and developing protocols.* New York: Raven Press, 1984.
26. Coronary Drug Project Research Group. Influence of adherence to treatment and response of cholesterol on mortality in the coronary drug project. *N Engl J Med* 1980;303:1038–1041.

*Patient Compliance in Medical
Practice and Clinical Trials*
edited by J.A. Cramer and B. Spilker
Raven Press, Ltd., New York © 1991

6

Impact of Risk Communication on Accrual, Regimen, and Follow-up Compliance

*Louis A. Morris and **Ivan Barofsky

*Food and Drug Administration, Rockville, Maryland 20857; and **Johns Hopkins
School of Medicine, Francis Scott Key Medical Center, Division of Digestive Diseases,
Baltimore, Maryland 21224*

The clinical trial is in many ways an analogue of routine medical care. In both clinical trials and medical care, the patient must agree to enroll in a treatment program, adhere to a regimen, and return for follow-up treatments. These three aspects of clinical trial participation may be conceived as three different elements of patient compliance. As shown in Fig. 6–1, each of these three elements refers to qualitatively different behaviors on the part of physicians and patients.

Accrual compliance refers to the enrollment of patients in the clinical trial. Physicians must request that appropriate candidates enter the trial, and patients must decide they are willing to participate to meet the objectives of the trial. Starfield et al. (1) have shown that physician behavior in offering treatment options and soliciting patient agreement is critical to determining if patients initiate treatment.

Regimen compliance refers to the degree to which patients follow the prescribed regimen. Noncompliance rates ranging from 30 to 50% have been reported in the literature (2). Understanding the numerous factors that have been found to modify compliance rates requires conceptual models that examine how patients' knowledge and beliefs influence their health behavior.

Follow-up compliance refers to the extent to which patients return for treatment. In this instance, patients' experience with the treatment and their interpretation of this experience are critical in determining if patients stay in treatment or dropout. This is an issue both in medical practice and clinical trials.

RISK COMMUNICATION

The thesis of this chapter is that risk communication plays a critical role in determining each of these three compliance behaviors. The physicians' knowledge and perception of the risks of treatment and the manner and extent to which risks are communicated to and understood by patients helps determine all three types of compliance.

The risks of medical treatments are communicated in a number of ways. As Kraus and Slovic (3) have shown, risks are perceived and evaluated along two independent dimensions. First, the risks of treatment are assessed by an analysis of the "dread-

Type of Compliance	Accrual	Regimen	Follow-up
Illustrative Behavior	Enters Trial	Takes Medicine	Keeps App'ts
Measure of Compliance	Refusal	Non-Adher-ence	Drop Out

FIG. 6–1. Compliance processes.

edness" of the perceived outcomes. Second, risks are evaluated by how confident the participants in the communication process feel that the treatment has been fully evaluated and that the risks of treatment are known (at least to expert scientists). Thus, risks are communicated by both the disclosure of hazards the patient undertakes by using a particular therapy and by the "transmission of confidence" (i.e., the feelings of certainty or uncertainty communicated to those who prescribe and use the treatment).

ACCRUAL COMPLIANCE

Patients generally perceive both societal and personal benefits from participating in clinical trials (4,5). However, some patients may actively or passively refuse to participate in a study. A certain percentage of eligible patients actively refuse to enter clinical trials. Barofsky and Sugarbaker (6) found that 14% of eligible patients refused to enroll in a cancer study. In a study of nocturnal oxygen therapy, Williams et al. (7) found that of 1,043 patients who had passed an initial screening, 12% refused, and an additional 2% were judged "uncooperative" or "unreliable."

Assessment of the perceived risks compared with the perceived benefits appears to describe the general process underlying the decision to participate in a clinical trial (8). Although active resistance to treatment may be a function of risk-avoidance, passive resistance may be a function of the lack of perceived benefits of trial participation. Alternatively, passive accrual noncompliance may be attributed to the unwillingness of patients to refuse directly the request of health professionals.

Passive resistance to clinical trial participation can be manifested by the failure to return to initiate the study. DeVries et al. (9) tracked participation rates in phase I and II drug studies across a range of products. After informed consent was obtained but before the initial physical examination, 15% of the patients cancelled or failed to appear, accounting for one-third of the total recruitment losses during the course of the study. A follow-up telephone survey of these candidates indicated that the most frequent reasons given for failure to attend the physical screening was job conflict, failure to remember, and family problems. Thus, conflict between clinical trial entry and other life events may interfere with patient participation. The patient may provide a logical justification for not attending the entry session if the clinical trial is not perceived as important enough or if the patient simply wants to provide a situationally acceptable excuse for not participating.

These three studies illustrate that a notable proportion of a patient sample may be noncompliant with the accrual phase of a clinical trial. The impact of such attrition on the representativeness of a patient sample should not be underestimated. Accrual noncompliance occurs before exposure to the treatment under study. Thus, the patient's decision not to participate must be based on information that permits an assessment of the benefits and risks of treatment.

Informed Consent and Accrual Compliance

The primary method of communicating the risks and benefits of treatment to the patient is the informed consent procedure. Informed consent is designed to assure that the patient's right to be fully informed about a clinical trial is not infringed. Further, given the diversity of situational factors and values underlying patients' ability and willingness to participate in a trial, a certain percentage of patients would be expected (actively or passively) to refuse to participate in a trial. To understand how the informed consent process influences recruitment, the physician's disclosure of risks and how the patient's understanding of those risks influences participation rates must be examined.

Physician Perceptions

The physician's willingness to disclose the risks and uncertainty the patient faces when entering a clinical trial is a major factor influencing accrual compliance. Taylor et al. (10) examined the problems physicians had recruiting patients for a clinical trial of surgery for breast cancer. Ninety-four institutions had enrolled as participants in the study, and the expected accrual rate was 75 patients per month. However, the actual accrual rate was only 12 patients per month. To understand the reasons for the lack of patient recruitment, the authors conducted a survey of the physicians who served as principal investigators at the 94 institutions.

The most frequently endorsed reason for not entering patients in the trial was concern expressed about the physician–patient relationship (noted by 73% of the respondents). Slightly more than one-third (38%) said they had trouble with informed consent, about one-fourth (23%) disliked open discussions of uncertainty, and 18% said they had a conflict with their dual roles of clinician and scientist. Only 9% said they had practical difficulties with the informed consent procedure, and only 8% said they felt personally responsible if the treatments were unequal.

Perceived Impact on Accrual and Regimen Compliance

As a follow-up to the study described above (10), Taylor and Kelner (11) surveyed 170 oncologists in eight countries. Included in the survey were questions about how the informed consent process influenced accrual and regimen compliance. Results from the 68 United States physicians indicated differing views about the influence of informed consent on accrual and regimen compliance.

Most physicians believed that informed consent had a direct impact on recruitment for clinical trials. About three-quarters (78%) said that informed consent sometimes made placing patients in the protocol difficult. A significant number (41%) said they would enroll more patients in protocols if informed consent restrictions were eliminated.

However, there were considerable differences in views about the relation between informed consent and regimen compliance. About half (51%) of the physicians stated that informed consent never led to greater regimen compliance, 30% stated it sometimes increased regimen compliance, and the remaining 19% felt it always increased regimen compliance.

Other responses in the survey suggest that the difficulty with accrual compliance stemmed with physicians' discomfort with their dual role as an investigator and a clinician. Although most physician-investigators believed that the risk disclosure on the informed consent sheet was helpful to patients (71% signified sometimes or always), most also admitted that the disclosure made them uncomfortable (94% signified always or sometimes).

Most physicians believed that obtaining informed consent changed the physician–patient relation (76% signified sometimes or always). In addition, 91% endorsed the concept that admitting uncertainty about which treatment is best had a negative effect on the relation.

In summary, Taylor and Kelner found that although many physicians acknowledged benefits of informed consent in increasing the disclosure of risks to patients, they also perceived many negative influences. The disclosure of risks and uncertainty (especially as it related to the choice of the "best" treatment) was particularly difficult for physicians.

Patient Perceptions About Communications of Risk

The studies of Taylor et al. indicated that physicians' beliefs about the risk communication process (i.e., the informed consent process), influences accrual noncompliance. From patients' perspective, risk communication appears to be a more welcomed aspect of the accrual process. Evidence for this comes from a survey performed for the President's Commission for the Study of Ethical Problems in Medicine and in Biomedical and Behavioral Research (12). Views about risk disclosure were solicited from 805 primary care physicians and a random sample of 1,251 members of the general public. Figure 6–2 displays results from several questions about risk disclosure in which physicians were asked about the risks they routinely disclose to patients, and the public was asked if they would want to know about these risks.

For the likely adverse reactions of treatment, a slightly higher proportion of physicians (95%) than the public (88%) signified the likelihood/desire for risk disclosure. Similarly, if the probability of dying was one chance in 100, slightly more physicians (81%) than the public (75%) signified a likelihood/desire for disclosure. However, when the probability of death from the treatment was one chance in 1,000, only half (52%) of the physicians said they were likely to disclose risks to patients. Although there was some reduction, there was only an 11% decline (to 64%) in the public's desire to know. When the outcome was switched from 1/1,000 chance of death to a 1/1,000 chance of disability, the percentage of physicians stating that they routinely disclose risks was reduced to 43% (down 11% from the level set for death), but for patients, there was an equally strong percentage stating their desire for risk disclosure (65%).

Therefore, as risk outcomes and probabilities change, physicians tend to moderate their disclosure of risks. However, patients' desire for risk information does not vary

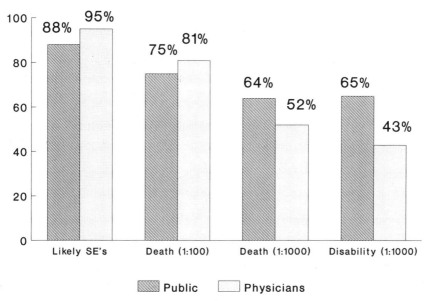

FIG. 6–2. Disclosure/desire for risk information.

to the same degree. It is evident that patients want to know more about the nonfatal and lower probability risks of treatment than physicians are willing to disclose. To explain the difference between physicians and patients, Morris (13) suggested consideration of differences in (a) the value system used by physicians and patients, as well as (b) the decision-making process used to evaluate willingness to undertake treatment.

The invariance of patients' desire for risk information across morbidity outcomes may be motivated by differences in values between patients and physicians. Quality of life research (14) suggested that when disability is compared with death, physicians view death as a more dreaded outcome. However, for patients, certain forms of disability are perceived as worse than death.

The invariance in patients' desire for risk information across estimates of the probability of occurrence, however, may be due to differences in how decisions are made about treatment acceptabilities. Jeffery (15) suggested that much of the difference in peoples reaction to hazards comes from contrasting perspectives about personal risk-taking (i.e., the individual perspective) compared with the perspective of individuals who communicate risk information (i.e., the population perspective). Although physicians may focus on probabilities of various outcomes to make a choice about which treatment option to select, patients may be more concerned about assessing their ability to cope with the worse-case outcome should it occur. Studies in decision making after genetic counseling indicate that probability information is not particularly useful to patients (16). Regardless of how rare the event, if it occurs, patienntsand their families must cope with its effects. Thus, patients tended to envision their ability to cope with the outcomes rather than to use the probability information to weigh options.

It can be speculated that patients' willingness to participate in a clinical trial may be due to their assessment of the perceived severity of the risks, as opposed to the probability that the risks will occur. Patients may be less willing to discount totally extremely small probabilities. However, the vividness and disruption of the disease is omnipresent for patients. It may be further speculated that patients' perspectives about the perceived severity of the risks of therapy must be evaluated in comparison to the risks of the disease. Patients' reactions to acquired immune deficiency syndrome treatments suggests that when faced with a fatal disease, patients may become assertive about obtaining all possible treatments. Coping with the risks of the disease, rather than making optimal choices about the best available treatment, dominates patient responses to acquired immune deficiency syndrome therapy.

With most disease entities, patients tend to be more passive participants to therapeutic decision making. Even if patients are passive and do not communicate reservations about undergoing treatment within the confines of a clinical trial, however, the informed consent process forces the physician personally to confront the risks of treatment each time a patient is approached for enrollment. This may foster physicians' projections of their own reservations about participating in clinical trials (17), increasing the physician's resistance to patient enrollment. Physician projections may be particularly important, as several studies suggest that from one-fourth to one-third of the patients who participate in clinical trials lack a basic understanding of the trial, do not comprehend that the randomization process rather than the physician selects their treatment, or even realize that they are participating in a clinical trial (18–20).

REGIMEN COMPLIANCE

Although it would be assumed that the patient, motivated to maintain or achieve a healthier state, would follow the physician's instructions, large numbers of patients fail to follow the proposed treatment regimen. It is often assumed that patients fail to follow prescribed regimens because they do not understand instructions or do not have the physical or cognitive skills to do what is expected. It has also been postulated that barriers such as adverse reactions or complex regimens cause noncompliance. However, Conrad's (21) study of patients with epilepsy demonstrated that for many patients, noncompliance is motivated by deeper meanings. In this study, patients failed to take their medication because they wanted to exert control over their illness. They resented being dependent on a medication and wished to express independence.

It must be assumed that a certain percentage of patients have strong reasons to avoid following their physician's instructions. For these patients, not following the physician's orders is a coping strategy that helps them adapt to or master their illness. Merely providing instructions to these patients will not necessarily promote the desired behavior. These patients must be persuaded that the behavior suggested is important, that their current coping strategy is inappropriate, and that there may be severe consequences for failing to follow the physician's orders. Finding meaningful persuasive arguments to convince patients about the necessity of doing what the physician suggests is an important element in promoting healthier behavior. Communicating the risks of treatment may be an important factor underlying patient compliance with their regimen.

Reasons Underlying Regimen Noncompliance

Several conceptual models have been advanced to explain reasons for lack of regimen compliance (22). Communication, health belief, and self-regulatory models provide a framework for understanding the conditions leading to noncompliance. Each of these models posits the importance of perceptions and appraisal of threatening events and their impact. In general, the most effective health messages are those that increase the perceived value of health goals (avoiding or ameliorating illness) or the perceived likelihood that a prescribed behavior will reduce threats to health or achieve a desired goal.

The Health Belief Model organizes the relevant beliefs that patients hold about their illness or its treatment into four categories: beliefs about the severity of illness, patient susceptibility to illness, benefits from taking the prescribed action, and barriers to taking action (23). In a recent review of 46 studies of the Health Belief Model, Janz and Becker (24) found that beliefs about barriers to undertaking the prescribed behavior (89%) were most often predictive of compliance, followed by beliefs about susceptibility to the disease (81%), beliefs about benefits of the recommended action (78%), and lastly, beliefs about the severity of the disease (65%).

Given this construct and set of findings, it is no wonder that physicians may be more inclined to focus on risks of the illness as opposed to the risks of treatment. Problem-solving activities to overcome barriers to regimen compliance are also necessary to provide patients with better skills to maintain compliance with the regimen. Furthermore, the benefits of treatment rather than their risks are more likely to be communicated.

Limiting Treatment

However, by their very nature, any intervention powerful enough to cure, treat, or prevent disease will also have negative effects. At times, compliance with treatment may necessitate limiting use. Certain treatments may have severe negative consequences if overused. Physicians and, occasionally, societal institutions are inclined to convey risks of these treatments more straightforwardly to persuade patients to limit use of the treatment. For example, a strong case can be made for convincing people to limit medication subject to abuse or addiction. Medicines that may be used illicitly (e.g., pain killers, antidepressants, and steroids) are often viewed as dangerous if used outside of an approved medical context.

The persuasive impact of risk messages, however, is problematic. Providing patients with threatening, sometimes fear-inducing information can be effective but often is ineffective. Leventhal and Cameron (22) concluded that the persuasive impact of threatening messages is short-lived and does not necessarily lead to behavior change. In a recent review of the mass media communications literature, Job (25) concluded that five conditions were necessary before fear operates as an effective persuasive device: (a) fear onset needs to precede the desired behavior, (b) the fear-producing event needs to be perceived as a likely occurrence, (c) the specific desired behavior needs to be effectively communicated, (d) the level of fear produced should be controlled (offset) by the desired behavior, and (e) fear offset should reinforce the desired behavior, confirming its effectiveness.

Job's analysis suggests that messages intended to reduce the use of a treatment will only be successful if several conditions are met. First, patients must believe that their action (stopping the treatment) will alleviate the threat. For example, if patients taking oral estrogens believe that they have used the product for such a long time that their risk of getting cancer will not be reduced by stopping the therapy, there is no incentive to stop using estrogens. Second, the level of fear produced by prolonging the treatment must be adjusted to match the fear of the disease. For the estrogen patient, the fear of the embarrassing and discomforting symptoms of menopause immediately returning must be reduced or the fear of cancer caused by estrogens must be increased if the patient is to be persuaded to stop the regimen. Third, any external event that increases the salience of cancer increases the persuasive impact of the therapy reduction message. If a friend gets cancer or if a vivid story appears on television, the threat of the disease becomes increased. Similarly, if a vivid event occurs involving the negative elements of the disease or symptoms under treatment, the fear level produced by the therapy may not be great enough to arouse motivations to stop treatment. Finally, reinforcements need to follow the suggested behavior. If the estrogen patient is shown that the feared symptoms of menopause do not return or if the level of discomfort is not as great as expected, the positive behavior may be reinforced and continued.

In summary, regimen compliance is a complex function of many cognitive, motivational, and behavioral elements. Knowledge about the risks of disease or of therapy overuse must be one of the factors that patients evaluate to make decisions and commitments to follow the physicians' advice. In this instance, risk information is essential to maintaining a clear treatment goal for the patient.

FOLLOW-UP COMPLIANCE

Once patients have initiated treatment, they must continue to maintain the regimen, periodically returning for follow-up visits. Long-term compliance necessitates a different range of behaviors during which patients must learn to live with their illness and their therapies. Experience with treatments, particularly the adverse reactions of treatment, can drastically modify compliance.

Providing risk and adverse reaction information has been viewed as a barrier to follow-up compliance. Loftus and Fries (26) suggested that providing patients with risk information can be "hazardous to their health" because of placebo-induced adverse reactions. Many physicians view suggestion-induced adverse reactions as occurring often in their practice (27). Indeed, in a classic report by Pogge (28), 23% of patients given placebos reported the occurrence of adverse reactions.

However, in sick patients, symptoms frequently occur that may or may not be due to taking medication. Even healthy patients report spontaneous symptoms that could be considered adverse reactions if they were taking medication. Reidenberg and Lowenthal (29) interrogated healthy patients not in treatment and found that 81% reported some symptoms that, had they been taking some treatment, might have been considered an adverse reaction.

Risk Communication and Adverse Reactions

In an effort to discern how the knowledge that a pill has been taken influences the reporting of adverse reactions, Shapiro et al. (30) gave patients a placebo tablet and asked them to report the occurrence of new symptoms after waiting in a quiet room for an hour. A second (control) group of patients was not given the placebo but asked to report on how their symptoms varied spontaneously after an hour. There was no statistical difference in the percentage of patients who reported adverse reactions in the placebo (61%) and control (64%) conditions. However, those who received the placebo were more likely to label their symptoms as primarily somatic (e.g., headache, burning eyes, stomach pain), whereas those in the control condition labeled their symptoms as primarily cognitive or affective (e.g., crying, upset, feeling sorry for self). Thus, patients expect medicines to produce physical changes and label observed bodily state changes as such.

The suggestion that a medicine causes adverse reactions influences how observed reactions are labeled, whether as drug reactions or caused by some other cause. In a study by Cartwright and Smith (31), only 6% of the patients reported no symptoms after the ingestion of medication. Evidently, patients are likely to use the knowledge that they have taken a medication as an explanation of observed bodily events.

To provide a direct test of how risk information influences the occurrence and reporting of adverse reactions, Morris and Kanouse (32) provided a group of hypertensive patients with explicit information in the form of a brochure that listed the adverse reactions of the medication they were taking. A control group was not provided the brochure. At the next visit, patients who received the brochure were able to name correctly more of the adverse reactions than control patients.

At the revisit, patients were also asked to report any new problems they experienced and whether they believed that the problems were caused by the medication. Seventeen health problems were specifically probed, some of which had been listed in the brochure as possible adverse reactions. There was no statistical difference between the groups in the number of problems reported. A power analysis confirmed that there was small likelihood that the provision of the adverse reaction information increased the number of problems experienced. However, there was a significant difference in the attribution of symptoms. Patients receiving the brochure were more likely to attribute experienced problems to the medication. Problems that were listed in the brochure were more likely to be attributed to the medication than problems that were not listed. However, even the unlisted problems were likely to be attributed to the medication by patients who received the brochure, especially problems that were similar to the ones listed in the brochure.

Thus, providing adverse reaction information promotes attribution effects rather than suggestion effects. If patients view their therapy as a source of health problems, they are more likely to discriminate adverse reactions from other naturally occurring states. Patients who are informed about drug adverse reactions may be better able to identify those effects and deal with them more appropriately if they occur. For example, if a patient perceives increased urination frequency as an adverse reaction of a medicine, that patient can rearrange the dosage schedule to ensure that the timing of the urination does not disrupt sleeping patterns or important occasions. Dodd (33) has shown that it is important to include self-care instructional techniques along with information about the occurrence of adverse reactions to assure that patients understand how to treat adverse reactions if they do occur.

However, the data also suggest that patients do not necessarily remember the precise names of adverse reactions and label bodily state changes with those names. Rather, patients appear to remember some vague sense of the adverse reactions that may occur and tend to attribute similar effects as adverse reactions of the medicine.

Thus, nondrug reactions could be attributed to the medicine. As the science of pharmacoepidemiology is imprecise, it is unlikely that scientists can necessarily correctly discriminate drug and nondrug reactions. Perhaps, more importantly, it is necessary to ask how the increased attribution of adverse reactions to the medicine influences drug taking and health care.

Attribution and Follow-up Compliance

A recent study by Myers et al. (34) suggested that informing patients about adverse reactions may increase the number of patients who drop out of treatment. In a multicenter study of medicines used to prevent angina, patients in two of the centers were informed that the medication could increase the occurrence of gastrointestinal adverse reactions, although at the third center, patients were told that the medicines were well-tolerated by most patients. There was no difference between the centers in the number of serious gastrointestinal adverse reactions experienced. However, the number of minor gastrointestinal adverse reactions experienced at the two centers where patients were preinformed was increased relative to the third center. Also, more patients in the two centers dropped out of treatment because of these minor gastrointestinal symptoms.

If patients informed about the risks of treatment attribute observed symptoms to the medicine, the possibility that these attributions lead to discontinuation of treatment must be considered. Studies of patients' compliance with therapeutic regimens indicate that many patients who stop their medication cite adverse reactions as the cause. In the study by Cartwright and Smith (31), 40% of the patients who stopped taking their medication cited the experience of adverse reactions as the major reason for discontinuation. Dodd's (33) research in which self-care information was provided along with the adverse reaction profile suggested that it is important to provide patients with viable options for dealing with adverse reactions.

RISK COMMUNICATION AND COMPLIANCE

Risk disclosures appear to have two distinct influences on patient compliance in medical care and in clinical trials. First, the inability to predict patient reactions to treatment and, in particular, the informed consent process forces the affirmative disclosure of uncertainty. In medical care, each course of illness may be viewed as a personal experiment, in which treatments are tried and their effects assessed. The purpose of a clinical trial is to test validly a "less than perfectly known" treatment. If one knew what to expect, there would be no reason for the trial. Physicians believe that the forced disclosure of risks reduces the perceived ability of the physician to select the best available treatment. Physician projections as well as patient reactions surely perpetuate this belief. Further, inherent in the design of most trials is a procedure that randomizes patients to treatments. Some of these treatments may be inert or ineffective.

Second, risk disclosure influences compliance through its motivational properties and because of the affirmative disclosure of specific adverse reactions. Risk disclosure energizes and directs patients toward important therapeutic goals. It also provides patients with a salient explanation for any bodily state changes that may occur.

Tailoring Coping Strategies

From the patient's perspective, risk disclosure highlights what is known and what is unknown when taking medication. The patient must actively cope with both the uncertainty and anxiety resulting from the illness and its therapy. Molleman et al. (35) suggested that two types of interventions can be used to allay problems associated with these dual concerns. To cope with uncertainty, greater information must be disclosed and more effectively shared in interactions between health care providers and patients. To cope with anxiety, social support systems must be provided, either directly by health care providers or indirectly by assuring that there are sufficient friends and family available to support the patient's needs.

Although information and social support are two primary ways of helping patients cope with their treatment, not all patients respond to treatment in the same fashion. For example, Morris et al. (36) catalogued patients' information-seeking proclivities regarding prescription drug therapy into four patterns. Some patients passively rely on their physician for drug information (40%), some passively rely on their pharmacist (17%), some aggressively seek information from multiple professional and lay information sources (7%), and some receive little information and see no compelling reason to seek it out (33%).

Different patients may cope with their illness and the threats resulting from its treatment in different fashions. Taylor (37) suggested that three themes underlie patients' cognitive and emotional adaptation to their illness and its treatment. First, patients seek to derive meaning from experience. Second, patients seek to restore self-esteem. Third, patients seek to regain some mastery and control over their environment. Different patients may seek to achieve these goals through totally different strategies. For example, the one-third of patients who remained uninformed about their treatments in the study by Morris et al. (36) may have sought to regain control over their treatment by transferring control to a more knowledgeable and powerful other, their physician. This group of patients was more likely than the other groups to endorse the statement that it is not necessary to learn about their therapy if they trust the physician. However, the active seekers of drug information may have coped with their treatment by taking an assertive, future-oriented perspective, actively evaluating and planning for contingencies as a primary method of coping with the risks of treatment.

Compliance itself may be perceived as a coping reaction. Many patients abhor taking medication, perhaps because it is a sign of weakness, depersonalization, or perhaps because of underlying values stressing drug avoidance (23). Lack of compliance may be a behavioral manifestation of these values.

There are a number of strategies to convince patients about the need to take medication. Further, compliance-inducing strategies may also seek to highlight or amplify alternate values that emphasize the patient's responsibility to maintain or regain their health. The "do it for them" campaign initiated by the National High Blood Pressure Educational Program sought to reinforce values of family responsibility as a means of increasing compliance with hypertension drug regimens.

An important area for future research is to investigate how the information provided to patients about their treatment is used as part of an efficacious coping strategy. Numerous coping mechanisms are possible that range from active planning to passive denial (38). Learning how to help patients understand the basics of their treatment and cope with the uncertainty and the risks undertaken could help assure their confidence and compliance.

ACKNOWLEDGMENTS

The authors would like to thank Dr. Janet Arrowsmith and members of the Division of Scientific Investigation and Division of Drug Advertising and Labeling, Food and Drug Administration for their thoughtful comments on earlier versions of this chapter. The views expressed are solely those of the authors and do not reflect the policy of the Food and Drug Administration or the Johns Hopkins School of Medicine.

REFERENCES

1. Starfield B, Wray C, Hess K, et al. The influence of patient–practitioner agreement on outcome of care. *Am J Public Health* 1981;71:127–131.
2. Ley P, Morris L. The psychology of written information for patients. In: Rachman S, ed. *Contributions to medical psychology.* New York: Pergamon Press, 1984.
3. Kraus N, Slovic P. Taxonomic analysis of perceived risk: modeling individual and group perceptions within homogeneous hazardous domains. *Risk Analysis* 1988;8:435–455.
4. Cassileth BR, Lusk EJ, Miller DS, et al. Attitudes toward clinical trials among patients and the public. *JAMA* 1982;248:968–970.
5. Mattson ME, Curb JD, McArdle R, et al. Participation in a clinical trial: the patients' point of view. *Controlled Clin Trials* 1985;6:157–167.
6. Barofsky I, Sugarbaker PH. Determinants of patient nonparticipation in randomized clinical trials for the treatment of sarcomas. *Cancer Clin Trials* 1979;2:237–246.
7. Williams GW, Snedecor SM, DeMets DL. Recruitment experience in the nocturnal oxygen therapy trial. *Controlled Clin Trials* 1987;8:121S–130S.
8. Hassar M, Pocelinko R, Wientraub M, et al. Free-living volunteer's motivations and attitudes toward pharmacologic studies in man. *Clin Pharmacol Ther* 1977;21:515–559.
9. DeVries BM, Hughes GS, Francom SF. Recruitment of volunteers for phase I and phase II drug development studies. *Drug Info J* 1989;23:699–703.
10. Taylor KM, Margolese RG, Soskoline CL. Physicians' reasons for not entering eligible patients in a randomized clinical trial for surgery for breast cancer. *N Engl J Med* 1984;310:1363–1367.
11. Taylor KM, Kelner M. Informed consent: the physicians' perspective. *Soc Sci Med* 1987;24:135–143.
12. Abram M. *Making health care decisions: the ethical and legal implications of informed consent in the patient–practitioner relationship.* Washington, DC: President's Commission for the Study of Ethical Problems in Medicine and Biomedical and Behavioral Research, 1982.
13. Morris LA. *Communicating therapeutic risks.* New York: Springer-Verlag, 1990.
14. Morris LA. A marketing perspective on quality of life measurement. In: Spilker B, ed. *Quality of life assessments in clinical trials.* New York: Raven Press, 1990.
15. Jeffery R. Risk behaviors and health. *Am Psychol* 1989;44:1194–1202.
16. Wertz D, Sorenson J, Heeren T. Interpretation of risks provided in genetic counseling. *Am J Hum Genet* 1985;39:253–264.
17. Moore MJ, O'Sullivan B, Tannock IF. How expert physicians would wish to be treated if they had genitourinary cancer. *J Clin Oncol* 1988;6:1736–1745.
18. Applebaum PS, Roth LH, Lidz CW, et al. False hopes and best data: consent to research and the therapeutic misconception. *Hastings Cent Rep* 1987;14:20–24.
19. Bujorian GA. Clinical trials: patient issues in the decision-making process. *Oncol Nurs For* 1988;15:779–783.
20. Nealon E, Blumberg BD, Brown B. What do patients know about clinical trials? *Am J Nurs* 1985;22:807–810.
21. Conrad P. The meaning of medications: another look at compliance. *Soc Sci Med* 1985;20:29–37.
22. Leventhal H, Cameron L. Behavioral theories and the problem of compliance. *Pat Ed Counsel* 1987;10:117–138.
23. Becker M, Maiman L. Sociobehavioral determinants of compliance with health and medical care recommendations. *Med Care* 1975;13:10–24.
24. Janz N, Becker M. The health belief model: a decade later. *Health Educ Q* 1984;11:1–47.

25. Job S. Effective and ineffective use of fear in health promotion campaigns. *Am J Public Health* 1988;78:163–167.
26. Loftus E, Fries J. Informed consent may be hazardous to your health. *Science* 1979;204:11.
27. Boyle J. *Patient information and prescription drugs: parallel surveys of physicians and pharmacists.* New York: Louis Harris and Associates, 1983.
28. Pogge R. The toxic placebo: I. Side and toxic effects reported during the administration of placebo medicine. *Med Times* 1963;91:773–778.
29. Reidenberg M, Lowenthal D. Adverse nondrug reactions. *N Engl J Med* 1968;279:678–679.
30. Shapiro A, Chassen J, Morris L, et al. Placebo induced side effects. *J Operat Psychiat* 1974;6:43–46.
31. Cartwright A, Smith C. *Elderly people, their medicines, and their doctors.* London: Routledge, 1988.
32. Morris L, Kanouse D. Informing patients about drug side effects. *J Behav Med* 1982;5:363–373.
33. Dodd M. Measuring informational intervention for chemotherapy knowledge and self-care behavior. *Res Nurs Health* 1984;7:43–50.
34. Myers M, Cairns J, Singer J. The consent form as a possible cause of side effects. *Clin Pharmacol Ther* 1987;42:250–253.
35. Molleman E, Krabbendam PJ, Annyas AA, et al. The significance of the doctor–patient relationship in coping with cancer. *Soc Sci Med* 1984;18:475–480.
36. Morris L, Grossman R, Barkdoll G, et al. A segmentational analysis of prescription drug information seeking. *Med Care* 1987;25:953–964.
37. Taylor S. Adjustment to threatening events: a theory of cognitive adaptation. *Am Psychol* 1983;38:1161–1173.
38. Carver C, Scheier M, Weintraub J. Assessing coping strategies: a theoretically based approach. *J Pers Soc Psychol* 1989;56:267–283.

PART II

Special Patient Populations

Patient Compliance in Medical
Practice and Clinical Trials
edited by J.A. Cramer and B. Spilker
Raven Press, Ltd., New York © 1991

7

Compliance with Pediatric Medical Regimens

Michael A. Rapoff and Martha U. Barnard

Department of Pediatrics, University of Kansas Medical Center,
Kansas City, Kansas 66103

Parenting often involves convincing children to behave in ways that do not seem natural (e.g., cleaning up their rooms, hanging up coats, and bathing regularly). The fact that children and adolescents have difficulty complying with medical regimens does not require empirical verification for most parents. The image of a child balking, with teeth and lips clenched tightly, as a parent attempts to administer a dose of medication is easily evoked for most parents.

This chapter will review the literature on pediatric medical compliance, including regimens for both acute and chronic conditions. Types of compliance problems, the prevalence and consequences of these problems, and patient/family, disease, and regimen factors related to compliance will be discussed and evaluated. Assessment and intervention strategies will also be examined with a concluding section on recommendations for clinical research.

DEFINITION AND PREVALENCE

The most widely quoted definition of compliance has been offered by Haynes (1): "the extent to which a person's behavior (in terms of medications, following diets, or executing lifestyle changes) coincides with medical or health advice." This definition has heuristic value in that it specifies the range of compliance behaviors required for different regimens (e.g., taking medications, following diets), an evaluation of the "extent" to which a patient complies with a regimen, and whether a given level of compliance coincides or agrees with accepted medical and health recommendations. Implied in this definition is that medical or health advice that has been offered will, when adequately complied with, lead to reductions in mortality, morbidity, and/or increased health promotion. This assumption may not be well-founded, as noted by Cousins (2):

> The history of medicine is replete with accounts of drugs and modes of treatment that were in use for many years before it was recognized that they did more harm than good.

It is incumbent on health professionals that they are requesting compliance with regimens with demonstrated efficacy that at least do more good than harm. As shall be discussed, it has not been shown for most pediatric regimens what degree of compliance is required to effect an adequate therapeutic outcome (3).

The prevalence of compliance problems varies depending on the method of assessment, the criteria used for defining acceptable compliance, the regimen prescribed, and the setting in which compliance has been assessed. An additional complication in pediatrics is that parental as well as child compliance is involved as parents are often responsible for administering or supervising regimens.

There is general agreement that overall compliance with acute regimens (e.g., 10-day courses of antibiotics) is higher when compared with chronic disease regimens (3). However, a wide range of compliance levels have been reported with regimens for acute conditions, with complete compliance during a 10-day regimen ranging from 5% at a university outpatient clinic primarily serving low-income families (4) to 63% in a private practice setting primarily serving middle-class families (5). In addition, compliance decreases over time with only about 20 to 30% of patients maintaining compliance after the fifth or sixth day of a 10-day antibiotic course (6,7).

Compliance with medication regimens for chronic diseases averages 50% (3,8,9). However, compliance rates vary across different diseases, regimens, and methods of assessing compliance. In two separate studies, 55% of patients were found to be compliant with salicylates in the treatment of juvenile rheumatoid arthritis as assessed by serum assays (10,11). Two studies have assessed (by urine assays) compliance with prednisone in the treatment of pediatric cancers and found that 58% (12) and 67% (13) of patients adequately complied. One study (14) reported on compliance levels (measured by patient/parent report corroborated by assays) to medications for cancer during approximately 1 year, with 81.2% of patients compliant at 2 weeks, 60.5% at 20 weeks, and 65% at 50 weeks after the initiation of treatment. About 32% of patients with a history of rheumatic fever on a long-term prophylactic antibiotic were found to be fully compliant as measured by urine assay and interviews (15). Compliance with phenobarbital in a sample of 25 patients with epilepsy was reported to be about 79% as measured by saliva assays (16). Compliance with antibiotic and vitamin regimens for cystic fibrosis was reported to be 90% in one study, but the sole measure of compliance was patient report (17).

Compliance with other types of regimens in the treatment of chronic diseases has also been reported in the literature, most notably compliance with diabetes regimens. Accuracy of urine glucose testing has been assessed in three separate studies. In one study (18), diabetic children correctly performed urine glucose testing only 45.7% of the time, whereas nurses and research technicians working with diabetic children were accurate only 61% of the time. In another study, diabetic children accurately tested an average of 5.17 standard urine samples of ten (19). Johnson et al. (20) found that 80% of 146 diabetic children made one or more serious errors in urine testing (i.e., errors that would result in incorrect readings). Problems have also been found with blood glucose monitoring. One study (21) found that spurious readings averaged 40%, underreporting of testing results averaged 18%, and accurate recording of test data averaged 73.8% in a sample of 18 children with diabetes. Compliance with a blood glucose monitoring schedule was assessed in one study (22) with compliance declining in a group of 12 patients with diabetes from a baseline value of 77.6%, to 67.2%, 59.7%, 51.2%, and 58.1% during four subsequent measurement occasions separated by 4 weeks.

Dietary compliance has also been assessed for children with diabetes. Lorenz et al. (23) examined dietary compliance in a sample of 90 children attending a camp for diabetic children. They found errors in the children's ability to recall appropriate diet plans (mean error rate, 0.21), to load their plates correctly to match a written meal plan (mean error rate, 0.28), to choose an appropriate meal from a restaurant menu (mean error rate, 0.51), and to choose actual intake at a meal as recorded by observers who compared their intake with a written diet plan (mean error rate, 0.35).

Compliance with factor replacement therapy by children with hemophilia has also been assessed by observation using a standard behavioral checklist (24,25). Gilbert and Varni (24) found a mean compliance rate of 80% across the four major steps in factor replacement therapy (reconstitution, syringe preparation, self-infusion, and equipment disposal) among seven children, with lower compliance rates (mean, 45%) for equipment disposal. This level of compliance was considered unacceptable because of the potential for inadvertent needle punctures and the spread of blood-related diseases to family members.

Compliance with therapeutic exercises has also been studied. The best compliance rates for exercise in the treatment of childhood obesity was found to be less than 75% in one study (26). Two survey studies have shown that patients with juvenile rheumatoid arthritis and/or their parents report greater compliance problems with prescribed therapeutic exercises as compared with medications (27,28).

CONSEQUENCES OF NONCOMPLIANCE

Potentially serious health and economic consequences can result from compliance failures (3,29). Compliance failures can compromise the efficacy of regimens and the health of patients. Cluss et al. (30) found that children with asthma who were noncompliant with their asthma medications were more likely than compliant patients to experience more days of wheezing and more variable peak expiratory flow rates. Incomplete compliance with antibiotic therapy may result in the emergence of resistant strains of organisms and a greater probability of recurrent infection (31,32). Compliance problems can also contribute to other types of morbidity and mortality such as failure of renal transplants from incomplete compliance with immunosuppressive medicines (33) and the possibility of death resulting from abrupt discontinuation of corticosteroids (32).

The cost-effectiveness of medical care can also be adversely affected by compliance failures (3). Money may be wasted on unused medications, physician visits and hospitalizations may be increased, and families may incur the expense of additional diagnostic and treatment procedures that may not have been necessary (34). These unnecessary expenses may add to the existing economic burden on families of chronically ill children and society in general, in the form of increased insurance premiums and taxes to cover these additional health care costs.

Variations in compliance can also adversely affect medical decisions and outcomes of clinical drug trials. Physicians, unaware of compliance problems, may incorrectly assume that poor therapeutic outcomes are due to inadequacies in the regimen and may prescribe more potent medicines with potentially more serious adverse reactions. Haynes and Dantes (35) suggested that intra- and interindividual variability in drug absorption, commonly reported in ambulatory drug trials, may be due to variability in compliance.

These potentially serious consequences of noncompliance illustrate the importance of discovering factors related to compliance and methods to assess and improve compliance. The potential benefits of these efforts are increased treatment efficacy; reductions in morbidity, mortality, and health care costs; and less-biased drug trials.

NONCOMPLIANCE FACTORS

Much of the compliance literature is concerned with identifying factors that either promote or impede compliance (3,36,37). This is done in several ways. Typically, correlation coefficients are computed between measures of compliance and factors presumed to be related to compliance, such as duration of treatment. Other studies attempt to test for significant between-group differences on various factors for patients classified as compliant and noncompliant. Stepwise or simple multivariate regression analyses can also be done with factors entered in separately as predictor variables to determine the relative proportion of variance in compliance accounted for by each factor and the total factors entered in the analysis.

Patient/family, disease, and regimen characteristics have been most frequently studied as factors related to compliance (see Table 7–1). Studies investigating compliance factors can be helpful in determining risk factors for compliance problems, even if these factors cannot be altered, and in suggesting variables that might be modified to improve compliance.

Patient/Family Factors

As noted by Meichenbaum and Turk (37), the search for stable factors that define the "typical" noncompliant patient has met with little success. No consistent relation with compliance has been found for such variables as age, sex, social class, or personality traits. However, a number of patient or family "states" may relate to compliance and are potentially modifiable (Table 7-1).

Low self-esteem has been found to correlate with poor compliance with medications for epilepsy (16) and juvenile rheumatoid arthritis (11), although in one study it was unrelated to compliance with vitamins for iron deficiency (38). Dysfunctional family characteristics (e.g., disharmony, conflicts, and poor parental coping and problem solving) have been correlated with poor compliance for both acute (39) and chronic (16,40) disease medication regimens. Increased family size has also been found to correlate with poor compliance (14,15), which may relate to the finding that decreased parental reminders to comply and limited parental supervision and vigilance correlates with lower compliance (38,39). A patient's or parent's initial reported intent to comply may also be a strong predictor of later compliance (38,39,41). Until recently, the relation of developmental factors to medical compliance in the pediatric population has not been studied. Wysocki et al. (42) surveyed diabetes professionals to obtain their estimates of appropriate ages for children with diabetes to master 38 self-management diabetes skills. Expectations between individual health professionals varied and estimated mastery ages were incongruent with American Diabetes Association recommendations for age-appropriate skills. Noncompliance might be directly related to the inability of children to carry out regimen requirements. Although causal directions cannot be demonstrated, these data suggest that dysfunctional family situations, limited parental supervision, the lack of com-

TABLE 7–1. *Nonadherence factors in the treatment of acute and chronic pediatric disease[a]*

Patient/family factors
    Low patient self-esteem
    Family dysfunction—disharmony, conflicts, and poor parental coping
    Increased family size
    Limited parental supervision of regimen
    Intent to adhere—patient or parent
    Oppositional child behavior in general
    Developmental stage and abilities
Disease factors
    Decrements in compliance over time
    Patient asymptomatic or in remission
    Younger age at disease onset
    Type of disease being treated
    Disease severity—as perceived by family
Regimen factors
    Longer duration of treatment
    Complex regimens
    Costly treatments
    Types of regimens—high demand (e.g., life-style changes)
    Lack of continuity of care
    Limited provider supervision of regimen
    Pharmacy errors—incorrect filling of prescriptions
    Regimen adverse reactions (e.g., pain when exercising)
    Shorter duration of subspecialty care for chronic diseases

[a]Adapted from ref. 9, with permission. See text for additional references.

mitment to comply, and developmentally inappropriate regimen requirements may be risk factors for poor compliance.

Disease Factors

There is consistent evidence for both acute and chronic conditions that compliance deteriorates over time, especially when the patient is asymptomatic or in remission (3,9). Compliance may be particularly difficult to sustain when patients feel well and when regimen adverse reactions are more troublesome than the asymptomatic condition being treated (e.g., when a patient whose arthritis is in remission is experiencing gastrointestinal irritation from anti-inflammatory medications) (9).

Duration of disease is also an important factor, as consistent compliance during a longer period is required, with more opportunities for lapses in compliance (9,10). The type of disease being treated may also relate to compliance. In one study, compliance with antibiotics was greater among patients treated for pharyngitis versus otitis media (7). The authors speculated that this difference may have been due to the family's perception that pharyngitis was a more serious disease than otitis media.

It is interesting to note that in some studies, disease severity as assessed by physicians has not been found to correlate with compliance (7), but degree of severity as perceived by parents has been related to compliance for both acute (39) and chronic (43) conditions. A possible explanation for this is that parents who perceive their children's disease status as severe or threatening will be more vigilant in administering and monitoring their children's regimens.

Longer disease duration, asymptomatic patient states, disease type, and parent perception of less severe disease status would appear to be risk factors for noncompliance.

Regimen Factors

The duration, complexity, costs, and types of regimens prescribed and the extent of parental or professional supervision of regimens may be important factors related to compliance (Table 1). As has been discussed, longer duration has been associated with poorer compliance. There is also consistent evidence that more complex and demanding regimens are associated with lower compliance (9). Therapeutic exercise and dietary regimens for chronic health conditions such as obesity (26), juvenile rheumatoid arthritis (27,28), and cystic fibrosis (17) may be especially problematic because of the degree of response costs associated with these regimens. For example, children with juvenile rheumatoid arthritis may be given range-of-motion exercises to maintain joint function that have to be integrated into their daily routine and may be painful yet without any apparent immediate beneficial effects (9).

The costs of treatments may also be prohibitive for some families, especially those with chronically ill children. A telephone survey of 138 parents of children with pediatric rheumatic diseases revealed that of those children who had a physician visit and purchase of medication in the month before the survey, 40.7% of the parents found it difficult to pay expenses related to physician visits and 25.3% had difficulty paying for medications (44).

The way health care is delivered and supervised and adverse reactions of treatments may also be important to compliance (3,9). Continuity of care has been associated with compliance to regimens for acute (39) and chronic diseases (10). Patients who see the same physician over time are more likely to be compliant. This may be due to the development of a personal and supportive relationship with a provider over time, which also allows for more consistent monitoring and supervision of the patient. Conversely, limited supervision of therapeutic regimens by providers and/or parents has been associated with lower compliance (9,10,15,27,37). With acute regimens (e.g., antibiotic therapy for otitis media), compliance may be adversely affected by underfilling or incorrect labeling of prescriptions (45). Adverse reactions of medications (e.g., bad taste, difficulty in swallowing pills for younger patients, and gastrointestinal disturbance) may also be associated with poor compliance (28,38).

There are numerous regimen characteristics that need to be considered as risk factors for noncompliance, particularly the demands placed on patients by the type of regimens prescribed and the way treatments are monitored and supervised. These factors may be particularly useful in that they suggest compliance can be improved by reducing the response costs of regimens and increasing monitoring and supervision of regimens in the context of a consistent and supportive relationship with a provider and/or parent. Research on factors related to compliance, particularly regimen factors, may suggest ways this can be done.

COMPLIANCE ASSESSMENT

Compliance assessment in pediatrics may be more complicated than in adult medicine as it involves not only assessment of the patient but also the parent or caretaker. A variety of methods has been reported in the literature, including assays, pill counts, observational methods, parent/patient reports, and automated devices (3,9). A total of 47 pediatric compliance studies were reviewed for this chapter, including studies reporting incidence figures, factors related to compliance, and compliance improvement studies (4–7,10–28,30,33,38–41,43,45–61). Of these 47 studies, 14 (30%) used assays to assess compliance (5–7,10–13,16,30,39,40,47–49), 10 (21%) used patient or parental reports (17,26–28,33,41,46,53,54,58), 10 (21%) used a multi-method approach such as assays and patient/parental reports (4,14,15,21,22, 38,43,56,57,59), 9 (19%) used an observational measure (18–20,23–25,50,52,55), and 4 (9%) relied solely on pill counts to assess compliance (45,51,60,61). Because there are disadvantages to each compliance assessment method (3,9), it is encouraging that ten of the 47 studies used more than one method to assess compliance. A discouraging note is that an equal number relied solely on patient or parental reports, which may be suspect because of poor recall or overestimating compliance levels to protect the relation with the practitioner (62).

Unfortunately, what may be a reliable and valid assessment method for research purposes may not be practical for clinical settings because of the need to be feasible, accessible, and sufficiently sensitive for early detection of compliance problems (63).

Drug Assays

Drug assays, the detection of drug levels, its metabolites, or pharmacologically inert substances can be detected in blood, urine, and in rare cases, saliva (3,64). Although this measure is quantifiable, relatively objective, and can be used to make adjustments in drug dosage levels, there are disadvantages and inaccuracies with this, as with all measures of compliance. Problems include expense, invasiveness, lack of availability, variability in absorption and excretion rates, type of drug preparation, and errors in collection procedures that can result in inaccurate assay results and thus inaccurate judgments regarding compliance. In addition, a medicine ingested or omitted immediately before assays may alter the result, thus resulting in inaccurate judgments being made regarding the patients' compliance status (3).

If assays are to be widely used in research and clinical practice, they need to be less invasive and expensive, readily available, and obtainable at more frequent intervals than periodic clinic visits. For example, urine or blood glucose assays have been developed for home use and can indirectly reflect the degree of compliance to diabetes regimens (19,22).

Pill Counts

Pill counts or volume measurements have been reported in compliance research, usually in conjunction with other measures such as patient/parent reports or assays (56,59). They are uncomplicated and can be done at repeated intervals to measure compliance during longer periods than other measures such as assays. However, the major disadvantage of pill counts is that pills removed are not necessarily pills ingested (3). They are also rarely used in clinical situations because patients may forget to bring medications to clinics, and it is impractical to make home visits to obtain pill counts. Volume measurements have been used to assess proper insulin administration, but these measurements may not reflect typical compliance behavior, as patients are aware of the purpose of such assessments and may alter their behavior accordingly. Pill counts have been obtained by phone (61), which may be more feasible for practitioners.

Observational Methods

Observational methods are infrequently used in compliance research because most studies investigate compliance with medications. They are the measure of choice for nonmedication regimens (e.g., therapeutic exercises) (3,9). Observational methods have been used with diabetic patients to detect significant errors in performing blood or urine glucose monitoring and in making appropriate dietary choices, all of which are necessary in successful self-management of a diabetes regimen (23,65). Parents have also been trained as observers and have obtained reliable and valid data on compliance with regimens for juvenile rheumatoid arthritis (55).

One major drawback of observational methods is that they can be reactive (3). That is, the patient may change their behavior when observed (usually in a socially desirable direction), and observations may not reflect typical compliance levels. To minimize reactivity, observations should be as unobtrusive as possible (3). When parents serve as observers, it is important to emphasize to them that they avoid verbally punishing their children for compliance lapses but remain neutral as they conduct their observations. If properly trained and provided with a relatively specific and simple observational strategy, parents can be an important source of valuable compliance information for practitioners.

Patient/Parental Reports

Patient and/or parental reports are the most practical and therefore most widely used compliance measure in clinical practice. However, there is general agreement that this is not an adequate measure of compliance, particularly when used alone (3,9,62). Patient and/or parental histories, however, represent an important source of diagnostic information in medicine (66), and this can be equally true for diagnosing compliance problems. When obtaining initial or follow-up patient histories, the practitioner can discern whether there are "red flags" indicating potential or actual compliance problems. The way patients and parents are asked about compliance problems may affect accurate and useful reporting. Questions about compliance should be nonjudgmental, specific, and time-limited. For example, one might say: "Mrs. Johnson, everyone has problems at times getting their children to take their medicine. Have you had any problems getting Mary to take her medicine in the past week? Do you ever forget to give a dose or does Mary ever have problems taking the medicine?" This type of approach is preferrable to a judgmental and global approach with no time referrent that may at best yield little useful information and at its worse may punish patients and parents for accurately reporting compliance problems.

Histories should also focus on the patients' health problem, the treatment, and their responses to treatment. Additionally, the practitioner should obtain information on other medical conditions and any concurrent treatment that has been prescribed. Barnard et al. (65) reported at a conference that one factor that interfered with compliance with juvenile diabetes regimens was another disease condition. These conditions, along with certain medications being used for that condition, might interfere with the ultimate outcome of attempts to follow a treatment program. For example, a diabetic reports that despite continued attempts to follow medical advice, he continues to have hypoglycemic episodes that "take him by surprise." A thorough history identified that the patient was placed on an antihypertensive medicine by another physician, which interfered with blood glucose levels. Because more abbreviated histories had been taken by the physician, this was not noted. Once adjustment was made for the types of medication, the masked hypoglycemic episodes resolved. Also, what became apparent with this case and others is the number of health professionals involved with one patient for one or more medical conditions. Because chronic illnesses are often treated by a variety of health professionals, a variety of explanations and treatments can be given to patients that may or may not be congruent. A thorough history should identify and resolve any inconsistencies in the medical advice given to patients and their families.

In addition to a medical history, a thorough psychosocial history should be obtained, including information about family stability, financial and other stressors, developmental factors, and other information that relates to potential risk factors for compliance problems (see Table 7–1). Medical and psychosocial history data can be collated and evaluated to identify risk factors for compliance problems.

Patient self-monitoring of specific compliance behaviors as opposed to global ratings of compliance may be a more useful and accurate way of obtaining self-report compliance data (3). To improve the accuracy and honesty of self-monitoring, Mahoney and Arnkoff (67) recommended that (a) target behaviors to be monitored are clearly specified; (b) the self-monitoring strategy is simple to use; (c) the practitioner emphasizes the importance of accuracy and honesty in self-reports; (d) the self-monitoring strategy be demonstrated by the practitioner; (e) the patient is given supervised practice in self-monitoring; (f) the practitioner and patient agree to allow occasional and unannounced checks on self-monitoring accuracy (e.g., by parents or the practitioner); and (g) other measures be used to evaluate the accuracy of self-reports (e.g., pill counts or assays).

Another method for obtaining patient reports is through telephone interviews. Reports have appeared in the literature indicating the practical use of telephone interviews for both research and practice (22,68). In an unpublished telephone interview study, Freund et al. reported correlations averaging at least 0.80 between parent–child pairs on five compliance factors in diabetes management. Although the possibility exists that both parents and children will be equally inaccurate in their reports, telephone interviews may allow practitioners to assess compliance at more frequent intervals than is possible with clinic interviews and can allow the practitioner to identify and resolve any problems with the regimen that are impeding compliance.

In addition to patient or parent reports of compliance, assessment of knowledge-based information may be useful. Information about patient/parent understanding of the illness and treatment can be obtained through structured interviews. However, reliable and valid knowledge measures that are behaviorally based should be used to supplement interview information. Notable examples reported in the literature include urine or blood glucose testing procedures in diabetes (19,22) and a behavioral checklist to assess factor replacement skills in hemophilia (24,25). Although increasing knowledge *per se* may not be sufficient as a means of improving compliance, a basic understanding of the illness and the treatment is necessary to initiate compliance with a treatment protocol.

Automated Devices

Computerized pill counts have been recently reported in the literature (69), with microcircuitry built into pill bottle caps that automatically and unobtrusively record the time containers are opened. This is a definite improvement on traditional pill counts, but its feasibility for use in clinical settings is yet to be determined. In addition, it suffers from the same problem as traditional pill counts (i.e., removing the cap off a pill container, like removing pills from a container, does not guarantee ingestion of the prescribed number of pills).

Home blood glucose monitoring is another example of a potentially useful automated system for assessment. Using reflectance meters with memories, diabetic patients can perform and store up to 382 blood glucose determinations with the date and time of individual determinations stored in the memory (22). The results are printed out during clinic visits. Although there is some promise in the use of computer technology in the assessment of compliance, patients have found ways to falsify results. For example, adolescent patients with diabetes have reported using the blood of nondiabetic peers for glucose determinations to appear more compliant with their regimens. Others have intentionally or unintentionally placed too small a drop of blood on a blood strip, thus obtaining lower blood glucose values than what actually was the case.

Treatment Outcome

Practitioners may be tempted to view outcomes as indirect indicators of patient compliance. Treatment outcomes (e.g., pulmonary function tests with asthmatic children) are different phenomena than compliance behaviors and need to be assessed separately. Treatment outcomes do not necessarily correlate with compliance behaviors (3,37). Should treatment outcome be less than adequate in the presence of adequate compliance, then other disease- and treatment-related variables need to be assessed to determine the reasons for poor outcomes. Also, medical and behavioral researchers need to determine what level of compliance is necessary for particular regimens to effect an adequate therapeutic outcome (3). This has not been done for most acute and chronic pediatric illnesses.

COMPLIANCE IMPROVEMENT STRATEGIES

Compliance improvement strategies can be broadly classified as educational, organizational, and behavioral (70). Educational strategies primarily rely on verbal and written instructions designed to inform patients and their parents about the illness, regimen requirements, the importance of consistent compliance, and strategies for improving compliance. Organizational strategies involve changes in the health care delivery system (e.g., greater accessibility of health care services, simplified regimens, and increased supervision of patients by health care providers). Behavioral strategies refer to procedures designed to alter specific compliance behaviors that make up the components of regimens (e.g., patient or parental monitoring of compliance, behavioral rehearsal of regimen components, contracting, and reinforcement). Studies have used these types of strategies alone but usually in combinations to improve compliance.

Review of Compliance Improvement Studies

Table 7–2 provides details on compliance improvement studies conducted with pediatric patients who were acutely or chronically ill. The list includes controlled studies using single-subject or between-group designs with the exception of two studies (24,58), which were included because they employed a baseline, treatment, and follow-up condition and were unique in the literature in that they were the only studies reporting on compliance improvement with regimens for hemophilia.

A review of Table 7–2 clearly shows that educational strategies have generally been effective in improving compliance with regimens for acute diseases (45,46,48,56), with the exception of one study in which the control condition incorporated elements of previous intervention studies such as an instructional booklet and monitoring form thus yielding compliance rates the same as the intervention conditions. Educational strategies have not been helpful components of compliance interventions for chronic disease regimens because they are part of routine long-term care and have obviously been ineffective with chronically ill patients recruited for compliance intervention studies.

Only two studies employed organizational strategies to improve compliance. In one study, increased supervision by a health care provider in the form of a home visit and special instructions was not effective in improving compliance with physical therapy regimens for developmentally delayed children (53). In the other study, a sustained release form of theophylline resulted in significantly higher compliance when compared with short-acting theophylline, suggesting that simplification of a regimen may be beneficial for some patients.

The majority of studies on improving compliance with chronic disease regimens have successfully employed behavioral procedures, which is in agreement with reviews of the adult literature (71). These studies have used specific instructions for improving compliance, monitoring, prompting, contingent performance feedback, and reinforcement strategies (Table 7–2). The most common behavioral strategy has been the use of token reinforcement programs implemented by allied health care providers or parents (19,49,50,55,58,60). This strategy involves monitoring and reinforcing compliance behaviors with tokens (e.g., plastic chips), which are traded for special privileges and activities. Although behavioral strategies seem to be effective in improving compliance with chronic disease regimens, most of the studies have employed small patient samples. In addition, the more complicated behavioral strategies (e.g., token systems) require specially trained personnel (e.g., psychologists) to implement and are not feasible for routine use in most pediatric settings (59). Therefore, the generalizability and feasibility of behavioral procedures need to be established with larger samples in randomized control group designs. Using this review and clinical and research experience as a foundation, practical suggestions for clinicians can be developed to refine and incorporate compliance improvement strat-

TABLE 7-2. *Compliance improvement studies in pediatrics*

Ref. no.	Population Setting Diagnosis	Design	Medical regimen	Compliance strategies	Compliance measures	Outcome
46	N = 274 Pediatric outpatient Various acute illnesses	Random assignment to experimental and control groups	Varied according to diagnosis Acute	Experimental group—met with family health management specialist who provided special counseling, coordinated services and clinic Control group received usual nursing services	Interviews and case records	69% experimental group consumed adequate meds compared with 18% of the controls Significant difference (in favor of experimental group) in appointment keeping and knowledge regarding children's illness and treatment
48	N = 300 Pediatric outpatient Streptococcal pharyngitis	Random assignment to 3 treatment groups	Acute Pencillin	Group I = IM penicillin Group II = PO penicillin and routine instructions Group III = PO penicillin and extended counseling regarding use and written instructions	Repeat throat cultures; urine assay (9th day of treatment)	87% compliance = Group I 58% compliance = Group II 80% compliance = Group III No significant difference in treatment failures. Significantly higher relapse rate in Group II vs Groups I and III
45	N = 233, (1–12 yr) Pediatric outpatients Otitis media	Experimental/group (N = 33) 200 concurrent controls No random assignment	Acute oral antibiotic	Education by hospital pharmacy personnel gave parent verbal and written instructions regarding medications, calibrating/measuring device, and a calendar monitoring form	Level of remaining liquid medicine measured at end of therapy	Compliance = 51% in experimental as compared with 8.5% in 200 concurrent controls (significant difference)
56	N = 73 (6 mo–6 yr) Pediatric outpatient Otitis media	Random assignment to experimental control groups	Oral antibiotics	Educational handout about ear infections, self-monitoring calendar, and midregimen telephone reminder	Unannounced pill count and urine assay on home visit	Compliance = 82% experimental group vs 49% control group (significant difference) No difference in resolution of otitis media
57	N = 90 (2–24 mo) Hospital-based pediatric outpatient clinics Otitis media	Randomized 3-group design Group I, baseline intervention group (control) Group II, slidetape group Group III, phone follow-up group	PO liquid amoxicillin	Information pamphlet, self-monitoring reminder sticker; slide-tape or phone follow-up	Parental reports of missed doses, number of boxes checked on reminder record Volume measurement Urine assay in the home on 8th day of regimen	Home visits completed on 85 (94%) of 90 patient–parent pairs No significant differences between groups on all compliance measures

	Sample/Setting	Design	Target Regimen	Intervention	Measures	Results
47	$N = 77$ Pediatric outpatient Rheumatic fever	Random assignment to 2 groups Continuous care or traditional care	Oral prophylaxis penicillin daily	Continuous care (saw same physician who provided all medical care and available by phone) Traditional care (specialty clinic, did not see same physician, general medical care not provided)	Urine assay	After 15 mo—no significant difference in compliance between 2 groups
49	$N = 4$ Pediatric inpatient Renal failure Subj I = 13 yr; Subj II = 11 yr; Subj III = 13 yr; Subj IV = 18 yr.	Reversal design (single subject)	Dietary regimen	Token point system	Weight, blood urea nitrogen (BUN), potassium level (indirect measure)	Adequate weight gain compared with baseline conditions BUN improved
50	$N = 1$ (9-yr-old) Home setting Insulin-dependent diabetes mellitus	Multiple baseline across behaviors (foot care, urine testing, and diet) (single subject)	Urine testing Meal plan Foot care	Instructions given Token point system	Urine testing for glucose and acetone Diet adherence Foot care Observed by parent and sibling	Instructions were effective with diet compliance Token system increased compliance in the following: urine testing from $\bar{x}$ 16% to 97%; foot care from $\bar{x}$ 72% to 100%
51	$N = 20$ (11–18 yr) Pediatric outpatient Asthma	Random assignment to 1 of 2 medication groups Short-acting theophylline (SAT) q 6 hr or sustained-release theophylline (SRT) q 12 hr for 6 weeks then switched to 2nd study drug	Daily theophylline either q 6 or q 12 hr	Sustained-release tablet to be given q 12 hr Instructions given to both groups re: frequency of medication and exact number of tablets to be given during 2 weeks	Serum theophylline levels Pill counts	Significantly higher compliance with sustained-release vs short-acting by pill counts No significant difference between theophylline levels of 2 drugs
19	$N = 19$ (12–18 yr) Outpatient setting Insulin-dependent diabetes mellitus	Multiple baseline (single subject)	Diet Exercise Injections Insulin	Point token system and praise for improvement of diabetic management skills	Urine assay for glucose	Negative urines 27% baseline to 39% posttreatment with 45% at follow-up

TABLE 7-2. Continued

Ref. no.	Population Setting Diagnosis	Design	Medical regimen	Compliance strategies	Compliance measures	Outcome
52	$N = 17$ (6–18 yr) Outpatient setting Insulin-dependent diabetes mellitus	Random assignment to 2 treatment groups after screening procedure to determine which patients met 50% accuracy criterion when determining glucose concentration	Urine testing for glycosuria	Assignment to feedback group or a practice group Feedback group, tested 20 test tubes of various glucose concentrations; each was informed of concentration after each of the 20 testing trials Practice group, tested various glucose concentrations in 20 testing trials but no feedback re: actual concentration	Urine assay for glucose concentration	A significant decrease in error rate in the patients who were trained with feedback when compared with subjects who were trained in practice group Increase in accuracy from 36–72%
22	$N = 42$ (13–16 yr) Pediatric endocrine clinic Insulin-dependent diabetes mellitus	Random assignment to 2 groups for 30 patients: (1) meter alone group (MA); (2) meter and contract group (MC) Control group, $N = 12$ using conventional therapy (CT)	Standard diabetic regimen Multiple daily insulin injections, meal plan, and daily blood glucose monitoring	MA group earned $20 at each 4 subsequent data collection sessions MC group signed contract to earn up to $20 at each 4 subsequent sessions, with amount earned in proportion to compliance with prescribed self-monitoring of blood glucose	Pre/Post-blood glucose by memory reflectance meter Glycosylated hemoglobin Insulin adjustments 24-hr recall by telephone	Mean blood glucose 237.3 mg/dl = baseline to 193.1 mg/dl for MA and MC groups Neither MA or MC groups achieved blood glucose in normal range Mean increase of GHb: MC, 0.3%; MA, 0.7%; CT, 1.3% 24-hr recall interviews showed trend toward noncompliance
53	$N = 18$ mother/ infant (<36 mo) Home Developmental delay	Random assignment Experimental or control group	Physical therapy	Both groups were given demonstration of exercises Experimental group: (1) home visit; (2) list of exercises; (3) journal for recording exercises; (4) supplies	Structured interview Parental reports Count of treatment supplies remaining	No significant differences in compliance between groups Home visit patients had significantly greater improvements in motor development vs controls
54	$N = 4$ Pediatric outpatient Insulin-dependent diabetes mellitus	Multiple baseline	Urine glucose testing	Behavioral contracting	Percentage of daily urine tests done 4 times a day	Compliance averages increased from 9% in baseline to 74% in treatment

No.	Sample/Setting	Design	Medical regimen	Intervention	Measures	Results
55	N = 1 (7-year-old) Home Juvenile rheumatoid arthritis	Multiple baseline across behaviors with follow-up when token procedures withdrawn	(1) Aspirin (10 gr qid), prednisone (15 mg qod), penicillamine capsule (120 mg qd) (2) Wrist or knee splints to be worn at night (3) lying prone on firm surface (qd for 5 min)	Token system Tokens exchanged for routine and special privileges	Daily observations by parents and recording: (1) meds taken, (2) % of nights splints worn; (3) % of days prone lying	Introduction of token reinforcements increased compliance with treatment components B, baseline; T, tokens; M, meds; S, splints; PL, prone lying Follow-up—after withdrawing token procedures, compliance was maintained at: M = 90%; S = 91%, PL = 80%
58	N = 10 (8–15 yr) Physical therapy, outpatient and patient's home Hemophilia	Baseline, treatment, and 6–9 mo follow-up	Home therapeutic exercise program	Instructions for home exercises, behavioral contracting, token point system, positive reinforcement by therapist and parents	The percentage of: (1) therapeutic exercises performed—recorded by child and checked by parent; (2) exercise records returned; (3) sessions attended	Baseline compliance averaged 55% and increased to 96% during treatment; 94% average compliance during treatment phase for all 3 parameters; 84% and 66% averages on all 3 parameters during 6–9 mo follow-up
24	N = 1 (10-yr-old) Home Hemophilia	Baseline, treatment and 4½-mo follow-up	IV—factor replacement therapy	Modeling, behavioral rehearsal, praise and corrective feedback	Performance of factor replacement therapy as observed and rated by nurse on behavioral checklist	At 4½-mo follow-up, child demonstrated 100% compliance

Detail table (row 55 results):

	B	T
M	59%	95%
S	0%	77%
PL	0%	71%

TABLE 7-2. *Continued*

Ref. no.	Population Setting Diagnosis	Design	Medical regimen	Compliance strategies	Compliance measures	Outcome
61	N = 3 (11–18 yr) Pediatric rheumatology clinic Systemic lupus erythematous or dermatomyositis	Multiple baseline Across subjects (single subject)	Prednisone on alternate days	Feedback and education monitoring strategies Instruction—included review of patient's disease, medication, and reasons to comply with their regimen	Weekly pill counts by phone— parents of patients provided number of pills remaining in bottle	Compliance improved for taking prednisone over baseline levels in all patients

P	B	T	FU
1	38%	89%	A
2	7%	67%	Na
3	33%	88%	A

P, patient; B, baseline; T, treatment; FU, follow-up; NA, not available; A, accepted ranges (80–100%) |
| 59 | N = 3 (3–13 yr) Outpatient rheumatology clinic Juvenile rheumatoid arthritis | Multiple baseline across patients (single subject) Baseline, treatment, and 4-mo follow-up | Daily medications Subject 1 and 2 took Naproxen (250 mg bid) Subject 3 took 14 baby aspirins tid until week 5—switched to Tolmetin sodium qid | Home visit, using written handouts about medication and on how to improve compliance (close monitoring and positive reinforcement for compliance) Standard monitoring form mailed in on weekly basis | Pill counts also done in clinic by investigator Pill counts by weekly phone calls via parents and 1 pill count done in clinic where parent and investigator counted to determine agreement | Pill count

P	B	T	FU
1	44	49	24
2	38	97	56
3	54	92	89

Compliance ratings

P	B	T	FU
1	2.4	2.2	3.0
2	3.4	5.0	3.5
3	3.3	4.1	4.8

60	N = 1 (14-yr-old) Pediatric rheumatology clinic Juvenile rheumatoid arthritis	Withdrawal design (single subject) 9-mo follow-up	Tolmedin sodium (400 mg qid)	Weeks 5–12, change in medication dosage from qid to tid, the token system introduced—for appropriate behaviors but not medication compliance Weeks 13–22, token system applied to medical compliance Weeks 23–29, token system withdrawn for medication compliance Weeks 30–36, token for medical compliance reinstated Weeks 37–45, maintenance (token system withdrawn)	Parental global compliance ratings obtained by weekly phone contact before pill count on 5-point scale with 1 = noncompliant and 5 = very compliant Pill counts by weekly phone calls via patient's mother	Baseline $\bar{x}$ = 44%; simplified regimen $\bar{x}$ = 59%; token system $\bar{x}$ = 100%; token withdrawal $\bar{x}$ = 77%; Second token system $\bar{x}$ = 99% Maintenance $\bar{x}$ = 92% 9-mo follow-up $\bar{x}$ = 97%

egies for pediatric practice. These recommendations are appropriate for different types of regimens but are particularly relevant to the management of chronic diseases.

Recommendations for Improving Compliance

Treatment Goals

Setting medical treatment goals in collaboration with patients and their families is a common sense but neglected aspect of clinical practice. As shown with parents of juvenile diabetic patients (72), health care providers and parents may have different medical treatment goals, which could affect patient compliance. A more effective clinical alliance can be formed if goals of clinicians, patients, and their families are at least made explicit, even if they are not always shared (72). With adolescent juvenile rheumatoid arthritis patients, their goals may be related to functional outcomes (e.g., returning to active involvement in sport activities), whereas the health care provider's goals may be related to controlling disease activity and minimizing joint damage. These different goals may conflict, as resuming some activities (e.g., sports) may lead to further joint damage. Patients may be less inclined to comply consistently with regimens that do not address their goals of returning to functional activities. Health care providers should address patient and family goals and attempt to incorporate these with their goals of medical treatment. For example, patients with juvenile rheumatoid arthritis may need to shift to a different type of sport (e.g., swimming) to fulfill their goals and also address the health care provider's goal of minimizing trauma to affected joints.

Organizational Strategies

Although it seems obvious that compliance can be affected by organizational factors (e.g., the waiting time for clinic appointments, the talents and personalities of health professionals, and the complexity of medical regimens), these factors are seldom addressed when patients are considered to be noncompliant. The tendency is to find something in the patient (usually patient or family psychopathology) to explain noncompliance. Health professionals might first look outside the patient to determine what part the organization of the clinical setting plays in stimulating noncompliant behavior. Patients may need to wait several hours before being seen in the clinic and may anticipate seeing one health professional and end up seeing students or other staff before or instead of being seen by their regular provider. These factors may lead to patient dissatisfaction and confusion as incongruent advice is given and result in noncompliance. This is not an uncommon scenario, at least in teaching hospitals, and patients are rarely prepared for this at the beginning of their care. Patients and their parents need to be taught from the beginning the policies and procedures of the clinical setting and what course of action they can take if they are not satisfied with the care they are receiving. Helping patients and their families to anticipate what they can expect and to have some control over the process is an important step in obtaining their cooperation.

Differences in personality characteristics and expertise among health professionals may also influence patient compliance. There may not always be a good match, in terms of communication and interaction styles, between providers and patients/ families. In addition, complex chronic disease conditions requires the expertise and unique contribution of different health professionals to address medical and psycho-social concerns that can impact patient compliance and treatment outcome. Collab-oration among psychologists, physicians, therapists, and nurses has been beneficial for patient care as well as clinical research. This type of team approach can be of value in addressing the multitude of factors that can affect patient compliance.

The complexity of regimens can also be important in patient compliance. Health professionals should assess typical daily schedules of patients to determine how the prescribed regimen can be tailored to the patients' daily routines. It is usually easier to alter regimens than to alter established patient routines. For example, younger children with juvenile rheumatoid arthritis can perform their therapeutic exercises (e.g., lying prone) while watching their favorite television shows in the late afternoon.

Educational Strategies

The content of educational materials needs to be expanded to include not only information about diseases and their treatments but specific information about prac-tical strategies for improving and maintaining optimal patient compliance (59,61). A pamphlet is available from the first author of this chapter for parents of children with juvenile rheumatoid arthritis, which specifically addresses strategies for improving compliance (e.g., cueing, reinforcement, and discipline procedures). This type of information can be developed and tailored to specific types of diseases and treat-ments and integrated with disease and medical treatment information.

Educational practices also need to be expanded to include modeling, behavioral rehearsal, and performance feedback. To insure that patients can demonstrate the necessary skills for carrying out prescribed regimens, they need opportunities to observe correct performance of skills, practice these skills, and receive contingent feedback and correction from a skilled health professional. This has been done in an exemplary way with diabetes (19,22,52) and hemophilia (24,58) regimens.

Finally, the medical concept of education needs to be expanded. Education is not a one-time experience when patients are first diagnosed. It is an ongoing and adap-tive process, which may require intensive "booster" sessions periodically. This is particularly important in chronic disease management. When patients are first di-agnosed, they and their parents may be too anxious to attend to and retain complex information. Also, most chronic disease regimens are periodically altered, thus re-quiring changes in the education of the patient and family.

Monitoring/Supervision

The critical dimension of most compliance interventions may be that parents and/ or health professionals are more closely monitoring what patients are doing. Also, teaching patients to self-monitor is an important self-management strategy. This can take many forms, including keeping written records, the use of automated devices (e.g., reflectance meters for blood glucose monitoring), and regular updates deliv-ered to the health professional in the form of mailed-in records or phone calls. As noted by Wright (73), compliance procedures need to be standardized. Barnard et al. (65) standardized monitoring of diabetic patients by having them or their parents call a patient report line, which they have been instructed to use at regular intervals to report on treatment progress and any compliance problems. Telephone answering machines are ideal for this purpose, and patients and their families can be instructed on standard reporting procedures. If the patient or family does not call at regular intervals or has any problems, the provider can phone the patient to troubleshoot any problems or address specific questions.

Incentives to Comply

In an ideal situation, a patient is prescribed an effective treatment, which rapidly and pervasively resolves or controls their health problem. Thus, the incentive to comply is that the patient gets and feels better. However, this is not congruent with the experience of most patients, families, and providers. For example, nonsteroidal anti-inflammatory medications in the treatment of juvenile rheumatoid arthritis may not effectively control symptoms for at least 8 weeks from the initiation of therapy (9). To provide more immediate incentives for compliance, behavioral procedures such as token systems can bridge the gap between initial compliance and the long-range benefits of compliance (9). If compliance can thus be sustained, maximal therapeutic effects may be obtained and provide the necessary incentives (in the form of improved health and function) to further maintain compliance.

General Compliance Problems

Medical compliance problems may be symptomatic of compliance problems in general. A child may be oppositional and noncompliant with any or all parental requests, not just regimen compliance requests. This argues for clinical interventions for general compliance problems before tackling the problem of medical compliance (cf. 55). Effective behavioral procedures for child oppositional behavior have been developed, including shaping and reinforcing cooperative behavior and disciplinary procedures such as time-out for noncompliance (74). Targeting and improving general oppositional behavior first may make it easier (or unnecessary) to manage medical noncompliance.

Patient/Family Psychopathology

In a small percentage of cases, medical compliance problems may be symptomatic or exist concurrently with patient and/or family dysfunction. For example, a chronically depressed patient may feel helpless to alter their negative attitudes and behavior patterns, which is likely to impact medical compliance adversely. These psychological problems need to be addressed by competent mental health personnel who have extensive experience with children in medical settings. Effective management of psychological problems may result in improved compliance or may allow the health professional to address medical compliance problems effectively. However, underlying patient or family dysfunction is rarely the primary cause of medical noncompliance. Health professionals would do well to look elsewhere unless their assessments reveal the presence of significant patient or family dysfunction.

RECOMMENDATIONS FOR CLINICAL RESEARCH

This review illustrates the need for further research on compliance prediction and improvement. Methodological refinements and replications are necessary to establish the reliability and validity of assessment and intervention strategies in compliance research. The following recommendations are suggested to improve future research.

Patient Samples

Pediatric diseases, especially chronic ones, are diverse in their onset, duration, severity, and treatment. Patient samples should be selected to control for these factors and their possible influence on compliance. Relatively homogeneous samples can help determine the generality of research findings (e.g., on compliance improvement strategies).

Sackett (75) recommended the use of "inception cohorts" in compliance research (i.e., recruiting samples that include all newly diagnosed patients initially prescribed a particular regimen for a particular disease, including those who quit or drop out of treatment). This type of sample would provide more accurate information about compliance rates with various treatments and would allow for introduction of compliance enhancement strategies at the point when compliance rates begin to decline. When relatively homogeneous samples are not feasible, factors thought to influence compliance can be controlled methodologically (e.g., stratifying samples) or statistically (e.g., covariate analyses).

Compliance Assessment

All measures of compliance, even more "objective" methods, have disadvantages as well as advantages (3). Reviews, including this one, continue to show that too many compliance studies rely on less objective methods to assess compliance (e.g., patient report) (3,9,62). Caron (62) suggested that it may be fallacious to believe that good staff–patient relations will lead to truthful compliance reports, as patients may be less than truthful to protect a relationship they value. Valid interview methods that minimize biases in patient reports have not yet been developed (62).

The use of multiple measures may yield a more complete assessment of compliance (3,29,37). Patient reports should never be the sole measure of compliance and should be supplemented by other measures (e.g., direct observations or assays) (3). With proper training and occasional monitoring by a professional, parents can also provide independent and reliable observations of their childrens' compliance (55).

All measures of compliance share one major disadvantage: If patients are aware of when and how assessments are being obtained, their rate of compliance can be altered at least temporarily (3). This may be circumvented by obtaining measurements at random and/or unannounced times (with informed consent by patients and parents) in a clinic setting or at patients' homes or schools (3,62).

Clinical Outcome Assessment

Clinical outcomes need to be assessed, particularly with chronic diseases, to determine which patients are achieving treatment goals and the effect of compliance on outcome. Standard clinical outcomes include clinical findings based on physical examinations, laboratory tests, and roentgenographic results. However, these "hard" measures of clinical outcome have their own reliability and validity problems. As noted by Feinstein (76): "Just as all that glistens is not gold, all data that are "hard" are not necessarily reliable." Traditional outcome measures fail to assess the functional impact of diseases or therapies (77).

Functional impact measures have been developed in the adult literature, most notably for rheumatoid arthritis (78). Two attempts have been made to validate downward-scaled versions of adult functional status measures for children with juvenile rheumatoid arthritis (79,80), but some of the scales from the adult version may not be appropriate for children (e.g., the Mobility Scale). Development of a generic functional impact measure, applicable for a variety of chronic diseases, would be useful for research on compliance and chronic disease impact.

Another difficulty with traditional measures of outcome is the limited frequency at which they can be obtained. Patients with chronic diseases may be treated at tertiary care settings that serve patients from an extensive geographical area, which may limit visits to these settings for repeated outcome assessments. If reliable and valid measures of disease activity and functional impact could be obtained from patients or parents, it would be possible to monitor outcome at regular and repeated intervals. For example, in an unpublished study, Rapoff et al. found that parental ratings of juvenile rheumatoid arthritis symptoms were significant predictors of active joint counts determined by a rheumatologist. Moderate test–retest reliability coefficients were also obtained during a 3-week period.

Compliance Improvement Research

Much of the literature on compliance has been correlational (3,9). There is a clear need for prospective and controlled experimental manipulations of variables to improve compliance. The research on compliance improvement might best be described as being in the technique-building phase (3). That is, investigators are attempting to determine which strategy components and combinations can reliably improve compliance with different types of regimens. Single-subject (within-subject) designs may be most appropriate during this phase of research (3). These types of designs are more flexible than traditional between-subject designs, in that they allow investigators to adjust compliance improvement strategies according to the individual responses of patients. They also accommodate smaller numbers of patients and allow for repeated assessment of compliance and clinical outcome over time, which are ideal design features for studying chronic diseases that affect relatively few patients and have variable disease courses (81). Single-subject investigations can isolate effective compliance enhancement strategies, which can then be compared with each other or with control conditions in conventional randomized, prospective between-group trials.

This and other reviews (3,9,29) would suggest that educational strategies may be sufficient for improving compliance with acute regimens. However, they may be necessary but not sufficient to improve compliance with chronic disease regimens. More complex interventions, which contain elements of regular monitoring by parents and/or health professionals and prompts and reinforcement for compliance, may be needed for improving compliance to more demanding chronic disease regimens.

Before intervening to improve compliance, health professionals should be certain that they are dealing with true noncompliance. What appears to be noncompliance may in reality be pseudo-noncompliance (65). This may occur when poor patient outcomes are due to prescribing an inadequate treatment regimen or the lack of optimal professional care, guidance, and education rather than patient noncompliance.

Collaborative, Multicenter Trials

There is clearly a need for multicenter collaborative compliance research, particularly with regimens for chronic pediatric diseases. Treatment centers often do not have enough patients to accommodate large-scale clinical trials required to validate compliance assessment and improvement strategies. Multicenter collaboration will present some interesting but potentially frustrating challenges (e.g., obtaining agreement on the types of measures used to assess compliance and clinical outcome). However, our compliance knowledge base will not expand efficiently and effectively without this type of collaboration just as the current knowledge base about treatments for chronic diseases could not have been established without collaborative, multicenter trials.

One potential benefit of this type of effort would be the development of a "compliance data base." Standard measures of compliance and clinical outcome could be obtained at regular intervals across several centers to assess these variables (and their interactions) over time and to serve as baseline measures in compliance improvement studies. Patients and their parents have the most to gain from collaborative efforts, as they are not engaged in an academic exercise but in a daily struggle to cope with the demands of chronic diseases and their treatments.

REFERENCES

1. Haynes RB. Introduction. In: Haynes RB, Taylor DW, Sackett DL, eds. *Compliance in health care*. Baltimore: Johns Hopkins University Press, 1979;1–7.
2. Cousins N. *Anatomy of an illness as perceived by the patient*. New York: Bantam Books, 1979.
3. Rapoff MA, Christophersen ER. Compliance of pediatric patients with medical regimens: a review and evaluation. In: Stuart RB, ed. *Adherence, compliance and generalization in behavioral medicine*. New York: Brunner/Mazel, 1982;79–124.
4. Dickey FF, Mattar ME, Chudzik GM. Pharmacist counseling increases drug regimen compliance. *Hospitals* 1975;49:85–88.
5. Schwartz RH, Rodriquez WJ, Grundfast KM. Pharmacologic compliance with antibiotic therapy for acute otitis media: influence on subsequent middle ear effusion. *Pediatrics* 1981;68:619–622.
6. Bergman AB, Werner RJ. Failure of children to receive penicillin by mouth. *N Engl J Med* 1963;268:1334–1338.
7. Charney E, Bynum R, Eldredge D, et al. How well do patients take oral penicillin? A collaborative study in private practice. *Pediatrics* 1967;40:188–195.
8. Jay S, Litt IF, Durant RH. Compliance with therapeutic regimens. *J Adolesc Health Care* 1984;5:124–136.
9. Rapoff MA. Compliance with treatment regimens for pediatric rheumatic diseases. *Arthritis Care Res* 1989;2:S40–S47.
10. Litt IF, Cuskey WR. Compliance with salicylate therapy in adolescents with juvenile rheumatoid arthritis. *Am J Dis Child* 1981;135:434–436.

11. Litt IF, Cuskey WR, Rosenberg BA. Role of self-esteem and autonomy in determining medication compliance among adolescents with juvenile rheumatoid arthritis. *Pediatrics* 1982;69:15–17.
12. Lansky SB, Smith SD, Cairns NU, Cairns GF. Psychological correlates of compliance. *Am J Pediatr Hematol Oncol* 1983;5:87–92.
13. Smith SD, Rosen D, Trueworthy RC, Lowman JT. A reliable method for evaluating drug compliance in children with cancer. *Cancer* 1979;43:169–173.
14. Tebbi CK, Cummings KM, Zevon MA, Smith L, Richards M, Mallon J. Compliance of pediatric and adolescent cancer patients. *Cancer* 1986;58:1179–1184.
15. Gordis L, Markowitz M, Lilienfeld AM. Why patients don't follow medical advice: a study of children on long-term antistreptococcal prophylaxis. *J Pediatr* 1969;75:957–968.
16. Friedman IM, Litt IF, King DR, et al. Compliance with anticonvulsant therapy by epileptic youth: relationships to psychosocial aspects of adolescent development. *J Adolesc Health Care* 1986;7:12–17.
17. Passero MA, Remor B, Salomon J. Patient-reported compliance with cystic fibrosis therapy. *Clin Pediatr* 1981;20:264–268.
18. Epstein LH, Coburn PC, Becker D, Drash A, Siminero L. Measurement and modification of the accuracy of determination of urine glucose concentration. *Diabetes Care* 1980;3:535–536.
19. Epstein LH, Beck S, Figueroa J, et al. The effect of targeting improvements in urine glucose on metabolic control in children with insulin dependent diabetes. *J Appl Behav Anal* 1981;14:365–375.
20. Johnson SB, Pollak RT, Silverstein JH, et al. Cognitive and behavioral knowledge about insulin-dependent diabetes among children and parents. *Pediatrics* 1982;69:708–713.
21. Wilson DP, Endres RK. Compliance with blood glucose monitoring in children with type 1 diabetes mellitus. *J Pediatr* 1986;108:1022–1024.
22. Wysocki T, Green L, Huxtable K. Blood glucose monitoring by diabetic adolescents: compliance and metabolic control. *Health Psychol* 1989;8:267–284.
23. Lorenz RA, Christensen NK, Pichert JW. Diet-related knowledge, skill and adherence among children with insulin-dependent diabetes mellitus. *Pediatrics* 1985;75:872–876.
24. Gilbert A, Varni JW. Behavioral treatment for improving adherence to factor replacement therapy for children with hemophilia. *J Compliance Health Care* 1988;3:67–76.
25. Sergis-Deavenport E, Varni JW. Behavioral assessment and management of adherence to factor replacement therapy in hemophilia. *J Pediatr Psychol* 1983;8:367–377.
26. Epstein LH, Koeske R, Wing RR. Adherence to exercise in obese children. *J Cardiac Rehabil* 1984;4:185–195.
27. Hayford JR, Ross CK. Medical compliance in juvenile rheumatoid arthritis: problems and perspectives. *Arthritis Care Res* 1988;1:190–197.
28. Rapoff MA, Lindsley CB, Christophersen ER. Parent perceptions of problems experienced by their children in complying with treatments for juvenile rheumatoid arthritis. *Arch Phys Med Rehabil* 1988;66:427–429.
29. Varni JW, Wallander JL. Adherence to health-related regimens in pediatric chronic disorders. *Clin Psychol Rev* 1984;4:585–596.
30. Cluss PA, Epstein LH, Galvis SA, Fireman P, Friday G. Effect of compliance for chronic asthmatic children. *J Consult Clin Psychol* 1984;52:909–910.
31. Mattar ME, Yaffe SJ. Compliance of pediatric patients with therapeutic regimens. *Postgrad Med* 1974;56:181–188.
32. Ruley EJ. Compliance in young hypertensive patients. *Pediatr Clin North Am* 1978;25:175–182.
33. Korsch BM, Fine RN, Negrete VF. Noncompliance in children with renal transplants. *Pediatrics* 1978;61:872–876.
34. Smith M. The cost of noncompliance and the capacity of improved compliance to reduce health care expenditures. In: *Improving medication compliance: proceedings of a symposium*. Washington, DC: National Pharmaceutical Council, 1985;35–44.
35. Haynes RB, Dantes R. Patient compliance and the conduct and interpretation of therapeutic trials. *Controlled Clin Trials* 1987;8:12–19.
36. Haynes RB. Determinants of compliance: the disease and the mechanics of treatment. In: Haynes RB, Taylor DW, Sackett DL, eds. *Compliance in health care*. Baltimore: Johns Hopkins University Press, 1979:49–62.
37. Meichenbaum D, Turk DC. *Facilitating treatment adherence: a practitioner's guidebook*. New York: Plenum Press, 1987.
38. Cromer BA, Steinberg K, Gardner L, Thornton D, Shannon B. Psychosocial determinants of compliance in adolescents with iron deficiency. *Am J Dis Child* 1989;143:55–58.
39. Becker MH, Drachman RH, Kirscht JP. Predicting mothers' compliance with pediatric medical regimens. *J Pediatr* 1972;81:843–854.
40. Fehrenbach AMB, Peterson L. Parental problem-solving skills, stress, and dietary compliance in phenylketonuria. *J Consult Clin Psychol* 1989;57:237–241.

41. Litt IF. Know thyself—adolescents' self-assessment of compliance behavior. *Pediatrics* 1985;75: 693–696.
42. Wysocki T, Meinhold P, Cox DJ, Clark WL. Survey of diabetes professionals regarding developmental changes in diabetes health care. *Diabetes Care* 1990;13:65–68.
43. Radius SM, Becker MH, Rosenstock IM, Drachman RH, Schuberth C, Teets KC. Factors influencing mothers' compliance with a medication regimen for asthmatic children. *J Asthma Res* 1978;15:133–149.
44. McCormick MC, Stemmler MM, Athreya BH. The impact of childhood rheumatic diseases on the family. *Arthritis Rheum* 1986;29:872–879.
45. Mattar MF, Markelio J, Yaite SJ. Pharmaceutic factors affecting pediatric compliance. *Pediatrics* 1975;55:101–108.
46. Fink D, Malloy MJ, Cohen M, Greycloud MA, Martin F. Effective patient care in the pediatric ambulatory setting: a study of the acute care clinic. *Pediatrics* 1969;43:927–935.
47. Gordis L, Markowitz M. Evaluation of the effectiveness of comprehensive and continuous pediatric care. *Pediatrics* 1971;48:766–776.
48. Cochler IS, Bass JW. Penicillin treatment of streptococcal pharyngitis: a comparison of schedules and the role of specific counseling. *JAMA* 1972;222:657–659.
49. Magrab PR, Papadapoulou ZL. The effect of a token economy on dietary compliance for children on hemodialysis. *J Appl Behav Anal* 1977;10:573–578.
50. Lowe K, Lutzker JR. Increasing compliance to a medical regimen with a juvenile diabetic. *Behav Ther* 1979;10:57–64.
51. Tinkelman DG, Vanderpool GE, Carrol MS, Page EG, Spangler DL. Compliance differences following administration of theophylline at six- and twelve-hour intervals. *Ann Allergy* 1980;44:283–286.
52. Epstein LH, Figueroa J, Farka GM, Beck S. The short-term effects of feedback on accuracy of urine glucose determinations in insulin dependent diabetic children. *Behav Ther* 1981;12:560–564.
53. Mayo NE. The effect of a home visit on parental compliance with a home program. *Phys Ther* 1981;61:27–32.
54. Gross AB. Self-management training and medication compliance in children with diabetes. *Child Family Behav Ther* 1982;4:17–25.
55. Rapoff MA, Lindsley CB, Christophersen ER. Improving compliance with medical regimens: case study with juvenile rheumatoid arthritis. *Arch Phys Med Rehabil* 1984;85:267–269.
56. Finney JW, Friman PC, Rapoff MA, Christophersen ER. Improving compliance with antibiotic regimens for otitis media. *Am J Dis Child* 1985;139:89–95.
57. Williams RL, Maiman LA, Broadbent DN, et al. Educational strategies to improve compliance with an antibiotic regimen. *Am J Dis Child* 1986;140:216–220.
58. Greenan-Fowler E, Powell C, Varni JW. Behavioral treatment of adherence to therapeutic exercise by children with hemophilia. *Arch Phys Med Rehabil* 1987;68:846–849.
59. Rapoff MA, Purviance MR, Lindsley CB. Educational and behavioral strategies for improving medication compliance in juvenile rheumatoid arthritis. *Arch Phys Med Rehabil* 1988;69:439–441.
60. Rapoff MA, Purviance MR, Lindsley CB. Improving medication compliance for juvenile rheumatoid arthritis and its effect on clinical outcome: a single subject analysis. *Arthritis Care Res* 1988;1:1–5.
61. Pieper KB, Rapoff MA, Purviance MR, Lindsley CB. Improving compliance with prednisone therapy in pediatric patients with rheumatic disease. *Arthritis Care Res* 1989;2:132–135.
62. Caron HS. Compliance: the case for objective measurement. *J Hypertension* 1985;3:11–17.
63. McKenney JM. The clinical pharmacy and compliance. In: Haynes RB, Taylor DW, Sackett DL, eds. *Compliance in health care.* Baltimore: Johns Hopkins University Press, 1979;260–277.
64. Dubbert PM, King A, Rapop SR, Brief D, Martin JE, Lake M. Riboflavin as a tracer of medication compliance. *J Behav Med* 1985;8:287–299.
65. Barnard M, Jackson RL, Guthrie D. Psychosocial adjustment and compliance of child with diabetes. In: Jackson RL, Guthrie D, eds. *The physiological management of diabetes in children.* New York: Medical Examination Publishing Co., 1986;194–210.
66. Feinstein AR. *Clinical judgment.* New York: Robert E. Krieger Publishing Co., 1967.
67. Mahoney MF, Arnkoff DB. Self-management. In: Pomerleau OF, Brady JP, eds. *Behavioral medicine: theory and practice.* Baltimore: Williams & Wilkins, 1986;75–96.
68. Johnson SB, Silverstein J, Rosenbloom A, Carter R, Cunningham W. Assessing daily management in childhood diabetes. *Health Psychol* 1986;5:545–564.
69. Cramer JA, Mattson RH, Prevey ML, Scheyer RD, Ouellette VL. How often is medication taken as prescribed: a novel assessment technique. *JAMA* 1989;261:3273–3277.
70. Dunbar JM, Marshall GD, Hovell MF. Behavioral strategies for improving compliance. In: Haynes RB, Taylor DW, Sackett DL, eds. *Compliance in health care.* Baltimore: Johns Hopkins University Press, 1979;174–190.
71. Haynes RB. Strategies to improve compliance with referrals, appointments, and prescribed med-

ical regimens. In: Haynes RB, Taylor DW, Sackett DL, eds. *Compliance in health care*. Baltimore: Johns Hopkins University Press, 1979;121–143.

72. Marteau TM, Johnston M, Baum JD, Bloch S. Goals of treatment in diabetes: a comparison of doctors and parents of children with diabetes. *J Behav Med* 1987;10:33–48.

73. Wright L. The standardization of compliance procedures, or the mass production of ugly ducklings. *Am Psychol* 1980;35:119–122.

74. Forehand R, McMahon RJ. *Helping the noncompliant child: a clinician's guide to parent training*. New York: Guilford Press, 1981.

75. Sackett DL. Methods for compliance research. In: Haynes RB, Taylor DW, Sackett DL, eds. *Compliance in health care*. Baltimore: Johns Hopkins University Press, 1979;323–333.

76. Feinstein AR. Clinical biostatistics. XLI. Hard science, soft data, and the challenges of choosing clinical variables in research. *Clin Pharmacol Ther* 1977;22:485–498.

77. Meenan RF, Anderson JJ, Kazis LE, et al. Outcome assessment in clinical trials: evidence for the sensitivity of a health status measure. *Arthritis Rheum* 1984;27:1344–1352.

78. Meenan RF, Gertman DM, Mason JH, Dunaif R. The arthritis impact measurement scales: further investigations of a health status measure. *Arthritis Rheum* 1982;25:1048–1053.

79. Coulton CJ, Zborowsky E, Lipton J, Newman AJ. Assessment of the reliability and validity of the arthritis impact measurement scales for children with juvenile arthritis. *Arthritis Rheum* 1987;30:819–824.

80. Varni JW, Wilcox KT, Hanson V. Mediating effects of family social support on child psychological adjustment in juvenile rheumatoid arthritis. *Health Psychol* 1988;7:421–431.

81. Barlow DH, Hersen M. *Single case experimental designs: strategies for studying behavioral change*, 2nd ed. New York: Pergamon Press, 1984.

Patient Compliance in Medical
Practice and Clinical Trials
edited by J.A. Cramer and B. Spilker
Raven Press, Ltd., New York © 1991

8

Behavioral Strategies to Increase Compliance in Adolescents

Barbara A. Cromer

The Ohio State University College of Medicine, Department of Adolescent Medicine,
Children's Hospital, Columbus, Ohio 43205-2696

As awareness of noncompliance as a common problem in clinical practice has increased during the past 30 years, research in this area has blossomed. Many of these investigative efforts have focused on attempting to establish personality characteristics that describe the noncompliant patient. This is obviously an important goal, as such indicators would aid the clinician in identifying the patient at risk for noncompliant behavior. To date, however, no such consistent personality profile has been found. In fact, what is remarkable is the wide variety in demographic background and psychosocial characteristics of noncompliers reported in the literature (1). The inconsistent findings from study to study may in part be accounted for by variations in study design that include differences in the definition of compliance, a wide range of techniques to measure compliance, and a large variety of medical conditions and age groups under study.

An additional problem in the clinical application of research findings to date has been that many of the psychosocial constructs evaluated are relatively stable personality traits and, thus, would likely be difficult to change. Examples of such psychosocial variables include self-esteem, affective states, body image, and locus of control (a measure of self-determination). Although there certainly is a place for research to define further these underlying issues, more recent focus is now turning to the identification of other personal and environmental variables that are potentially more responsive to behavioral manipulation. Thus, the present discussion represents a selected review of research that identifies some of these variables that have direct clinical application. These include effective family involvement, patient's initial stated intent to comply, quality of the physician–patient relation, and characteristics of the treatment regimen. The major focus of the chapter will be in research performed with adolescents, but additional comments will be directed toward information obtained from adults and younger children.

EFFECTIVE FAMILY INVOLVEMENT

Family involvement has been shown to have a significant impact on an adolescent's adjustment to chronic illness and compliance with daily treatment regimens (1–3). For example, Myers et al. (4) reported, in a group of adolescent girls instructed to perform exercises and wear a brace for treatment of scoliosis, that the family's ongoing support was crucial for the girls' successful use of the brace. The potentially positive aspects of effective parental reinforcement are echoed in a study of adolescent diabetics and their mothers by Babrow et al. (5). They found that the compliant patients who managed the self-care program in conjunction with their mothers did so more effectively and in a less confrontative manner than the noncompliant families (5). In another study (6), simple reminders from parents to adolescents to take prescribed medication for iron deficiency was shown to be associated with enhanced compliance. Other evidence for the usefulness of parental involvement comes from two studies (7,8) that found adolescents more compliant if their parents were involved in appointment-making and attendance at the clinic visit.

Effective support systems may extend beyond parents and may include friends or, more common in adults, spouses. A much needed area of investigation is the potential support derived from peers close to the adolescent and the effect of that support on the adolescent's compliant behavior. In the adult population, the role of significant others may be an important contributor to enhancing patient compliance. For example, Schlenk and Hart (9) found a positive correlation between social support, from either family members or friends, and compliance scores among adult diabetics. The strength of this relation was underscored on regression analysis by the large amount of variance (50%) in compliance scores explained by social support and another variable, health locus of control.

Despite the large body of data that implicate the positive aspects of effective family involvement on patient compliance, the findings are not universal. In their study of hyperactive children on stimulant medication, Brown et al. (10) reported that intact families had a higher dropout rate than the single-parent families; additionally, the compliant, as well as partially compliant, children had families who reported a significantly higher degree of family conflict than those who dropped out from the study. It was postulated that high levels of family stress may have stimulated action by the parent to decrease one potential contributor to that stress (i.e., controlling irritating behavior of the child) (11). The unusual finding may also relate to a need for the family to admit the presence of conflict as a prerequisite for compliance in this clinical situation (10). An additional caveat to social support was provided by Shenkel et al. (12). Specifically, they assessed compliance with a diabetic dietary regimen in a mixed adolescent and adult population according to the patient's perceived expectations from significant others and his or her consequent motivation to comply. Interestingly, these behavioral attitudes were strongly correlated with the intention to comply with diet; however, they failed to predict actual behavior successfully.

The lack of parental involvement has been demonstrated as exacerbating noncompliant behavior in adolescents. In a study of mostly adolescent renal transplant patients, Beck et al. (13) reported that every child who was found to be noncompliant had assumed sole responsibility for managing his or her medications properly. Moreover, these noncompliant children were most likely to come to clinic without a parent (13). The importance of family support is underscored in an investigation of another group of young renal transplant patients, which found noncompliance related to the adolescent feeling "closest to someone outside the family" or "helped most in adaptation to illness experiences by a non-family member" (14).

An interesting observation was made by Deaton (15), who studied the families of preadolescent asthmatics and found that therapeutic outcome was more related to perceived expertise by the parent in accurately adjusting dosage than to the actual level of compliance. In other words, the most effective parental involvement is one that can transcend the literal recommendations and modify them to improve the outcomes of the child.

In summary, most of but not all the available data suggests that parental involvement is potentially an effective and inexpensive strategy to increase compliance in a young patient. This source of support may not be limited to parents; any significant person who provides support to patients who are chronically ill may improve compliance and that particular person may be identified by the patient and, if possible, included at a clinic visit to learn the treatment schedule as well as at follow-up to review interim problems with compliance.

PHYSICIAN–PATIENT RELATION

A good physician–patient relation has traditionally been recognized as integral in establishing appropriate behavioral response to therapeutic recommendations. The few studies that have been conducted in this area in general support this contention. In a seminal study by Francis et al. (16), noncompliance was highest among mothers who were "grossly dissatisfied" with their interaction with their child's physician. Dissatisfaction occurred when the physician was viewed as unfriendly and when perceived expectations were not met. Similarly, in a group of adolescents with rheumatoid arthritis, Geersten (17) reported compliance with medication and appointments significantly higher in those patients who felt that the physician employed a "personal," rather than "business-like," approach and who felt that the physician spent enough time with them.

The provision of a consistent caregiver is a relatively easy intervention to institute and has been demonstrated as enhancing compliance. Charney et al. (18) in their study of young children treated with penicillin found that compliance of the mothers administering the medication was associated with "years cared for by that doctor" and "whether seen by own doctor or by partner." Becker et al. (19) presented data to suggest that this arrangement is also more satisfying to physicians and staff. Increased supervision in the form of longer and more frequent appointments appears to enhance patient compliance. In these instances, improved cooperation may be a function of the additional caring and attention from the health care team, rather than from the actual instructions provided during these visits. Additional evidence for improving physician–patient rapport is found in a study by Radius et al. (20), in which mothers prescribed medication for their asthmatic children were more compliant if they felt better when heeding the physician's advice.

A significant impediment to compliance in many cases is discrepancy between the outlooks on the disease and its optimal treatment between the patient and care provider. As pointed out by Amarasingham (21), "We should distinguish between disease as a biological entity and illness as a social experience." Physicians tend to underestimate the potential social limitations incurred by certain behavioral and pharmacologic regimens. "The patient experiences his illness not only as a biological fact but also as it impinges on his experiences and interactions as a social being" (21). The recognition of the patient as the primary decision maker in his or her self-health care, rather than as a passive vessel for prescriptive advice, is crucial for the establishment of effective negotiation involving both the physician and patient (22).

The exchange during such a discussion should include query into the patient's understanding of the disorder; if the patient interpretation involves an alternative explanatory model, it may be helpful to frame future explanations using the same model (23). In addition, the physician is only one potential source for information; the patient may consult several other sources of health information before deciding on a particular health-related behavior. Therefore, initial discussion of a patient's understanding of his or her disease may clear up misinformation, facilitate the physician–patient relation, and improve compliance (24).

INTENT TO COMPLY

There is no more straightforward approach toward assessing the risk of noncompliance than by simply asking the patient if he or she anticipates any difficulty in following the prescribed regimen. For those patients who predict a potential problem with compliance, immediate negotiation may be performed, which, hopefully, leads to a more workable treatment plan.

Surprisingly, little research attention has been directed toward examination of how frequently patients will admit to future noncompliance. Twenty years ago, Davis (25) conducted a study in which a group of adult patients attending a general medical clinic were interviewed during 8 months as to their various behavioral responses to prescribed medical advice. Of those who were eventually identified as noncompliers (37% of the total group), almost half admittedly had had no intention of complying from the outset. In a recent report of adolescents prescribed medication for iron deficiency, patients, on the average, predicted 2 of the following 7 days as probably noncompliant (6). Additionally, there was a significant positive correlation between the number of days predicted for noncompliance and actual level of compliance as measured by home pill counts.

A related issue to the intent to comply is the generalizability of compliant behavior over time as well as across other clinical situations. There are some data to support that a patient's past behavioral response is predictive of future such behavior. For example, Chacko et al. (26) reported a higher return rate in follow-up appointments among those adolescents who had kept the previous appointments compared with those who had not. Among overweight children, Israel et al. (27) found that "anything but high adherence" to a weight loss program during a preliminary period was associated with dropout from the later full treatment program. There are also data to support the patient tendency to have a consistent approach in terms of compliant behavior irrespective of the clinical problem. Davis (28) evaluated the level of self-reported compliance among adult cardiac patients who were prescribed modifications in their work regimens, personal habits, and exercise programs. He found compliance with the recommended work program correlated with either both the other regimens or the one that posed the least inconvenience for the patient. Litt et al. (29), in their study of adolescent girls taking oral contraceptives, reported that those who were compliant not only had exhibited similar behavior in the past but also described themselves as generally more well-organized than the noncompliant group. This suggests that compliance may emanate from certain stable personality traits from which develop a generally consistent approach from medical condition to condition.

In summary, initial inquiry into a patient's intent to comply is warranted in every case so that a forum for future effective communication can be established. This technique is most helpful for those patients who are willing to admit their lack of positive intent (25). The problem is among those patients who profess positive intentions but who fail to follow through successfully. As mentioned earlier, there may be positive intent without effect on actual compliant behavior (12). In cases of discrepancy between self-report and subsequent clinical appearance, more objective measurements of compliance (e.g., blood or urine assays) may be performed as well as counseling of the patient then based on the test results. In all cases, physician–patient negotiation should take the form of collegial problem-solving rather than directives delivered by the doctor.

TREATMENT REGIMEN

Several behavioral strategies involving the treatment regimen itself have been developed to improve compliance. Although the ultimate solution is to obviate the issue of compliance altogether, by providing one-dose treatment at the clinic or office site, few drug regimens have the potential to be reduced to a single dose. It seems empirically obvious that minimizing the frequency of dosing schedule would improve drug compliance. Evidence in support of this contention comes from a study by Jordan (30), who reported that adult men with genital gonorrhea given tetracycline (four doses per day) had five times the risk of positive posttreatment culture as those men treated with doxycycline (two doses per day). In a group of adolescents with chronic arthritis, Wasner et al. (31) found a linear, negative relation between the number of pills prescribed per day and the degree of compliance. Compliance also appears to decrease when the number of prescribed medications exceeds three (32). Although complex regimens are not always associated with poor compliance, certainly choosing simpler rather than more complex drug regimens, as well as a review of the total patient pharmacologic schedule, is in order.

Adverse reactions as a possible deterrent to successful compliance must also be considered. For example, Emans et al. (33) evaluated the level of compliance with oral contraceptives in a large group of adolescents; drug compliance at approximately 1 year after initial prescription was associated with the absence of adverse reactions. In another study, the occurrence of adverse reactions among adolescents treated for an asymptomatic condition had a significantly negative impact of the likelihood of compliance (6). Using physician estimates to measure compliance, Dolgin et al. (34) reported nausea and vomiting as two of the symptoms that interfered with patient continuance of oral chemotherapy for cancer. It is an empirical observation that adolescents who experience adverse reactions, rather than mention this to the care provider, will simply stop treatment. Thus, it is incumbent on the physician to explore the possibility of adverse reactions in the ostensibly noncompliant patient, especially in this age group.

The cost of a specific regimen may also be a significant deterrent to successful compliance. Although the use of doxycycline has been associated with better compliance versus the use of tetracycline because of decreased frequency of dosing (30), the former can cost four times more than the latter, thus representing a potential barrier to filling the prescription for some patients. The cost of complying with a therapeutic regimen may also be viewed in personal lifestyle and social terms. The traditional thought is that the less interference with normal daily habits, the higher the likelihood of compliance.

The standard rule concerning the positive effects of minimizing the complexity of the treatment regimen is not without exception. In a study of children treated for streptococcal pharyngitis, Colcher and Bass (35) found the same low recidivism rate for the group treated with a single dose of intramuscular penicillin and the group treated with a 10-day course of oral penicillin whose parents were given explicit instructions regarding the treatment schedule. A higher rate of treatment failures was noted in the group prescribed oral penicillin without family instruction.

In summary, several aspects of the treatment regimen can potentially be modified to suit the needs of the individual patient. These include decreasing the number and frequency of the dosing schedule, choosing drugs that minimize adverse reactions (and explanation of anticipated reactions), and considering the cost to the patient, from both a financial and social perspective.

ACKNOWLEDGMENT

The author would like to thank William Hritsko, B.S.I.M., for his diligence and continued assistance in the completion of this chapter.

REFERENCES

1. Haynes RB, Taylor DW, Sackett DL, eds. *Compliance in health care*. Baltimore, London: Johns Hopkins University Press, 1979.
2. Cromer BA, Tarnowski KJ. Noncompliance in adolescents: a review. *J Dev Behav Pediatr* 1989;10:207–215.
3. Friedman IM, Litt IF. Promoting adolescents' compliance with therapeutic regimens. *Pediatr Clin N Am* 1986;33:955–973.
4. Myers BA, Friedman SB, Weiner IB. Coping with a chronic disability. *Am J Dis Child* 1970;120:175–181.
5. Babrow ES, Avruskin TW, Siller J. Mother–daughter interaction and adherence to diabetes regimens. *Diabetes Care* 1985;8:146–151.
6. Cromer BA, Steinberg K, Gardner L, et al. Compliance in adolescents with iron deficiency. *Am J Dis Child* 1989;143:55–58.
7. Scher PW, Emans SJ, Grace EM. Factors associated with compliance to oral contraceptive use in an adolescent population. *J Adolesc Health Care* 1982;3:120–123.
8. Irwin CE, Millstein SG, Shafer MAB. Appointment-keeping behavior in adolescents. *J Pediatr* 1981;99:799–802.
9. Schlenk EA, Hart LK. Relationship between health locus of control, health value, and social support and compliance of persons with diabetes mellitus. *Diabetes Care* 1984;7:566–574.
10. Brown RT, Borden KA, Clingerman SR. Adherence to methylphenidate therapy in a pediatric population: a preliminary investigation. *Psychopharmacol Bull* 1985;21:28–36.
11. Dunbar J, Waszak L. Patient compliance: pediatric and adolescent populations. In: Gross AM, Drabman RS, eds. *Handbook of clinical behavioral pediatrics*. New York: Plenum, 1990;365–382.
12. Shenkel RJ, Rogers JP, Perfetto G, Levin RA. Importance of "significant others" in predicting cooperation with diabetic regimen. *Int J Psychiatry Med* 1985–86;15:149–155.
13. Beck DE, Fennell RS, Yost RL, et al. Evaluation of an educational program on compliance with medication regimens in pediatric patients with renal transplants. *J Pediatr* 1980;96:1094–1097.
14. Korsch BM, Fine RN, Negrete VF. Noncompliance in children with renal transplants. *Pediatrics* 1978;61:872–876.
15. Deaton A. Adaptive noncompliance in pediatric asthma: the parent as expert. *J Pediatr Psychol* 1985;10:1–14.
16. Francis V, Korsch BM, Morris MJ. Gaps in doctor–patient communication. Patients' response to medical advice. *N Engl J Med* 1969;280:535–540.

17. Geersten HR. Patient non-compliance within the context of seeking medical care for arthritis. *J Chron Dis* 1973;26:689–698.
18. Charney E, Bynum R, Eldredge D, et al. How well do patients take oral penicillin? A collaborative study in private practice. *Pediatrics* 1967;40:188–195.
19. Becker MH, Drachman RH, Kirscht JP. Continuity of pediatrician: new support for an old shibboleth. *J Pediatr* 1974;84:599–605.
20. Radius SM, Becker MH, Rosenstock IM, et al. Factors influencing mothers' compliance with a medication regimen for asthmatic children. *J Asthma Res* 1978;15:133–149.
21. Amarasingham LR. Social and cultural perspectives on medication refusal. *Am J Psychiatry* 1980;137:353–357.
22. Kleinman A. Clinical relevance of anthropological and cross-cultural research: concepts and strategies. *Am J Psychiatry* 1978;135:427–431.
23. Stimson GV. Obeying doctor's orders: a view from the other side. *Soc Sci Med* 1974;8:97–104.
24. Conrad P. The meaning of medications: another look at compliance. *Soc Sci Med* 1985;20:29–37.
25. Davis MS. Physiologic, psychological and demographic factors in patient compliance with doctors' orders. *Med Care* 1968;6:115–122.
26. Chacko MR, Wells RD, Phillips SA. Test of cure for gonorrhea in teenagers. Who complies and does continuity of care help? *J Adolesc Health Care* 1987;18:261–265.
27. Israel AC, Silverman WK, Solotar LC. Baseline adherence as a predictor of dropout in a children's weight-reduction program. *J Consult Clin Psychol* 1987;55:791–793.
28. Davis MS. Predicting non-compliant behavior. *J Health Soc Behav* 1965;6:265–272.
29. Litt IF, Cuskey WR, Rudd S. Identifying adolescents at risk for noncompliance with contraceptive therapy. *J Pediatr* 1980;96:742–745.
30. Jordan WC. Doxycycline versus tetracycline in the treatment of men with gonorrhea: the compliance factor. *Sex Transm Dis* 1981;8:105–109.
31. Wasner C, Britton MC, Kraines G, Kaye RL, Bobrove AM, Fries JF. Nonsteroidal anti-inflammatory agents in rheumatoid arthritis and ankylosing spondylitis. *JAMA* 1981;246:2168–2172.
32. Blackwell B. Drug therapy. Patient compliance. *N Engl J Med* 1973;289:249–252.
33. Emans SJ, Grace EA, Woods ER, et al. Adolescents' compliance with the use of oral contraceptives. *JAMA* 1987;257:3377–3381.
34. Dolgin MJ, Katzer S, Doctors SR, et al. Caregivers' perceptions of medical compliance in adolescents with cancer. *J Adolesc Health Care* 1986;7:22–27.
35. Colcher IS, Bass JW. Penicillin treatment of streptococcal pharyngitis. *JAMA* 1972;222:657–659.

*Patient Compliance in Medical
Practice and Clinical Trials*
edited by J.A. Cramer and B. Spilker
Raven Press, Ltd., New York © 1991

9

Improving Compliance in the Older Patient

The Role of Comprehensive Functional Assessment

*Norma J. Owens, *E. Paul Larrat, and **Marsha D. Fretwell

*College of Pharmacy, University of Rhode Island, and **Brown University Program
in Medicine and Department of Medicine, Roger Williams General Hospital,
Providence, Rhode Island 02910

Many clinicians believe that a high rate of noncompliance exists in the older population of patients, resulting in problems with medication use. In this chapter, it is proposed that the research methodology used most often in the past measured the quantitative issues of noncompliance without constructing a satisfactory model for the process of prescribing by physicians or medication-taking habits of the patient. Thus, it may be known with greater certainty *who* will not adhere to a medication regimen, but there is little understanding *why* this behavior occurs. After briefly reviewing medication issues that are important to the older group of patients and the research that has been performed on noncompliance in the older patient, a framework will be provided for the study of the process of prescription and acceptance to medication regimens. This chapter concludes with a description of the application of comprehensive functional assessment for the specific purposes of improving the differences between physician prescription and patient acceptance of medication regimens.

BACKGROUND

Our society is aging. Today, about 12% of the United States population is 65 years of age or older, and in the next 10 years this age group will increase by 20% while the number of school age children will drop by 10% (1). Although this shift seems dramatic, it is even more startling when compared with the statistics of different groups of older people. For instance, in the three decades between 1930 and 1960 the mortality rate of the very aged, those individuals older than 85 years, decreased by 10%. In the next single decade, their mortality decreased again by another 26%. By the year 2000, the 65 to 74 age group will increase by 20% to 17.4 million people. However, the 75- to 84-year-old population will increase by almost 50% to 10.6 million, and the very old age group of people (older than 85 years) will increase by 80% to 3.8 million people (2,3).

MEDICATION USE IN THE OLDER PERSON

Many of the medical issues that arise in the course of caring for elderly patients are no different from those that potentially exist for patients of any age. However, practitioners will be faced with dilemmas more often because older patients have greater needs for medical care at all levels.

Older patients are prescribed more medications than other groups of patients. They consume about 25% of all prescription medications and take, on average, 11 medicines annually (4,5). This is due in part to their greater burden of illness, especially chronic illnesses such as hypertension, atherosclerosis, and arthritis. The approach to medical care has been studied for frail older patients who are admitted to a general community hospital for treatment of an acute illness. Data published about this older population show that persons 75 years of age or older report taking an average of 4.5 ± 3.0 medications before hospitalization. These same patients have on average 7 ± 2.7 diseases listed by their primary physician and are prescribed an average of seven to eight medications on a given day during hospitalization. Six weeks later, these same frail older patients who reside either at home or in a nursing home are consuming an average of six to seven medications per day (6). This is striking when one considers the functional abilities of these frail patients 6 weeks after hospitalization: almost 50% have more than three dependencies in activities of daily living, only 20% score as intact on measures of cognitive ability, and almost 20% of the patients who are cognitively intact are depressed (7). Approximately one-third of these patients reside in nursing homes. However, this means the majority of these frail older patients who have had a recent hospitalization for treatment of an acute illness must manage their own medications at home.

The number of medications an older patient takes has been correlated with adverse patient outcomes. In the hospital setting, an increased incidence of iatrogenic problems is seen with increasing numbers of medications prescribed. Types of complications encountered include aspiration pneumonia and infection (8). In the outpatient setting, Shimp et al. (9) reported an average of 11 medication-related problems in a selected group of patients referred by their physician or social service agency. The medication-related problems were directly correlated to the number of medications the older patient took, and many of these problems were issues of inappropriate medication administration (9).

The number of medications an older patient takes is also correlated to adverse functional effect. For instance, the chance of an older patient falling is correlated to the number of medications taken (10), and drug-associated cognitive impairment is nine times more likely to occur in outpatients who take more than four prescription medications (11).

Older patients also have enhanced susceptibility to adverse drug reactions from both altered pharmacokinetic and pharmacodynamic changes that occur with age. Research shows that the overall incidence of adverse drug reactions in the elderly is about two to three times higher than that found in younger patients (12). The medications most often implicated in these adverse drug reactions are those most commonly used in the older patient: digoxin, thiazide diuretics, antihypertensive medications, nonsteroidal anti-inflammatory agents, theophylline, and benzodiazepines (13,14).

It is not surprising then that the number of medications a patient takes is also associated with issues of noncompliance. As will be discussed later in this chapter, noncompliance is not necessarily linked to older patient age. Intuitively, one might expect to see increased noncompliance with increased use of medications as a rational response to the prescription of too many medications. Noncompliance should really be viewed as an adverse event for the physician and should not be added to the list of risk factors of medication concerns in the older patient.

In summary, issues of noncompliance may be especially critical in older patients because they have a complex medical history, receive multiple medications to treat their illnesses, are often functionally impaired, and are at higher risk for adverse drug reactions. Their increased risk for adverse drug reactions stems from both an increased use of medications and also age-associated changes in pharmacokinetics and pharmacodynamics.

GENERAL ISSUES OF MEDICATION COMPLIANCE IN THE OLDER PATIENT

Medication compliance is traditionally defined in a patient as someone who takes his or her medicines as prescribed: in the correct dose and at the correct time. Whether this occurs depends on a complex interaction between the patient, his or her illness, the physician, and the medication prescribed.

The literature is inconsistent in showing whether age is correlated to noncompliance. For instance, age appeared to be a factor in noncompliance by patients at both ends of the lifespan. Noncompliance was higher in children not supervised by their parents and adolescents and in those older than 60 (especially if they live alone) (15). However, the majority of published literature does not support the association between age and noncompliance (16). Clinicians may expect to see a high incidence of noncompliance issues in older patients because of the associations between age and the number of medications taken.

As will be discussed in the following sections, patient characteristics that predict noncompliance with medication regimens have been well-studied. However, the prescriber may have little control over many of these variables in the older patient. For instance, one cannot change a patient's age, economic status, or his or her overall burden of illness. Interventions to understand a person's behavior with respect to noncompliance may result in improvements in medication regimens by the patient's physician. Research into a patient's behavior with respect to medication-taking is less well-studied but potentially more valuable in developing mechanisms for altering behavior that places an older patient at high risk for an adverse outcome.

Intelligent Noncompliance

Because noncompliance is traditionally defined as a lack of compliance to recommendations, little consideration is given to the rational act of noncompliance. Some patients lower a dosage of a medication or discontinue a medication because of adverse reactions or a large amount of inconvenience caused by the medical regimen. Intelligent noncompliance can be defined as a rational act of altering prescribed therapy by patients who do not suffer adverse consequences as a result (17). Most research in the field of compliance does not take into account the deliberate discontinuation or alteration of a medication by a patient, although some information is available. For example, Spriet et al. (18) reported on compliance to pentoxyphylline in 1,662 geriatric patients being cared for by general practitioners in clinical practices. They found no correlation between any predictor variable and compliance (including age, sex, packaging type, or memory aid stickers on medication vials) and reported that patients who achieved a good therapeutic outcome continued their medication regimen and those who experienced adverse reactions discontinued therapy or reduced the prescribed dose (18). Cooper et al. (19) also measured "intentional noncompliance" in 111 older patients and found that 52% lowered their dose of medication because they felt they did not need that much medication and that 15% lowered their doses because they experienced adverse reactions. Clinicians must acknowledge that patients will and probably should apply basic pharmacological principles to their own therapeutic regimens (i.e., lower a medication dose when experiencing an adverse reaction).

The Patient

Issues of concern in the patient include functional, physical, and social abilities necessary to ensure compliance. Examples of functional abilities include one's cognitive and sensory state. Physical abilities describe whether a patient can manage a medication regimen (e.g., opening the prescription vial or taking out the tablets). Social factors that are of importance to ensuring patient compliance include those that affect a patient's values and beliefs regarding treatment of a disease in addition to economic or other barriers that may inhibit a patient from taking his or her medication as prescribed.

Understanding a medication regimen is necessary to ensure compliance. Recent evidence may suggest that certain groups of older persons are functionally impaired, particularly with respect to cognitive ability. Evans et al. (20) studied the prevalence of Alzheimer's disease in a community population of older persons. Using a defined community of 32,000 persons residing in East Boston, they showed that the prevalence rate for probable Alzheimer's disease in persons 65 to 74 years of age was 3.0% (95% confidence limits 0.8 and 5.2), 75 to 84 years of age was 18.7% (95% confidence limits 13.2 and 24.2), and in those older than 85 years was 47.2% (95% confidence limits 37.0 and 63.2). Thus, many older individuals residing in the community may not have the cognitive ability to manage their medication regimens properly. This may mean the cognitively impaired older patients are not as able to learn about a medication change (registration of new information) or to remember whether they have taken the day's dose (short-term memory impairment). They also may not recognize or recall their own compliance problems when visiting their physician or pharmacist. Noncompliance resulting from mistakes caused by cognitive or emotional impairment is particularly serious in the older patient residing at home alone.

To achieve compliance with medication regimens, a patient must have a sufficient degree of functional ability. That is, they must be able to purchase their medication, which involves both getting to a pharmacy and paying for the medication. They must be able to open the prescription vial, take out the prescribed dose, and swallow the medication. Many patients may be partly impaired in their activities of daily living and rely on family members or other caregivers for help. Meyer et al. (21) studied the functional abilities of 93 older patients to perform medication-taking tasks. The skills assessed included the ability to read and interpret labels of prescription vials, to open and close prescription vials, to remove tablets, and to identify tablet colors. Patients who were responsible for their own medications were more likely to be able to read and understand medication directions, remove tablets, and to identify colors.

Patients who had cognitive impairments were less likely to be able to perform these activities. One interesting result discovered in this study was that motor skills were not correlated to cognitive skills (i.e., patients who were cognitively impaired could open and close and remove tablets from prescription vials). The loss of color discrimination for medications was also confirmed recently by Cady et al. (22), who showed an association between age and an inability to discern medication colors in older patients with diabetes. They advised pharmacists and physicians to avoid referring to medications by their color when counseling older patients.

Additional functional risk factors for noncompliance in older patients is the ability to read computer-printed directions for medication use on prescription vials and to remove vial tops of medication containers. Misinterpreting prescription directions may arise not so much from an inability to read or understand directions, but from smudged or lightly printed labels (23). Many people have some degree of difficulty opening child-resistant containers, but in addition to this common problem, older patients also have difficulty opening vials with flip-off-type container tops. In this same study by Murray et al., 16% of patients who did not comply with prescription directions could not open flip-off tops and 36% could not open the child-resistant vial lids.

Becker and Maiman (24) reviewed some of the social and behavioral determinants of compliance to medical recommendations. They suggested that understanding a patient's risk or propensity for noncompliance to a medical regimen will do little to help alter the situation and does not explain what factors help to motivate the larger group of patients who do comply with recommendations, even in the face of inconvenience and other adverse reactions. It is necessary to understand why noncompliance occurs rather than merely to predict who will exhibit the behavior. These researchers have used value-expectancy models to explain behavior under conditions of uncertainty. Thus, they feel the behavior can be predicted by understanding the value of an outcome to an individual and from the individual's belief that a given action will result in that outcome.

A "health belief model" can be developed (see Fig. 9–1), which suggests that the motivation to achieve an action depends on how much one desires the action plus

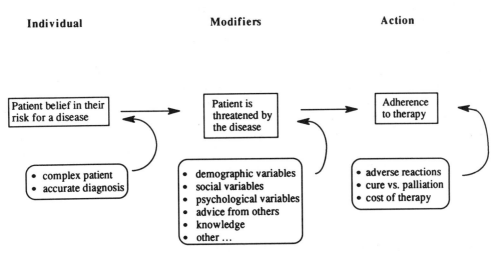

FIG. 9–1. Health belief model as a predictor of behavior for older patients.

the person's belief regarding the likelihood of achieving that outcome. Put simply, an older patient will comply with their antihypertensive medication regimen if they believe they are at risk for a complication from their hypertension, if they desire to prevent that complication, and if they believe the medication will correct or reduce the hypertension without adverse reactions. The patient's perceived susceptibility for a disease or outcome of the disease has been studied in areas of preventive medicine (e.g., cancer screening or immunizations). Persons who believe they are vulnerable are more likely to comply. After a diagnosis is made, perceived susceptibility must be modified somewhat to include the patient's belief in the accuracy of the diagnosis, belief about recurrence of the disease, and one's overall perception of their health vulnerability. In older patients who are medically complex, an accurate diagnosis becomes more difficult to make, so that uncertainty modifies this variable.

This model asserts that even when a patient believes in their diagnosis, an action will not occur unless they also believe becoming ill will have serious repercussions that they wish to avoid. Research on perceived severity shows that low levels are not sufficiently motivating, whereas high levels produce fear and are inhibiting. An older patient may define "serious repercussions" in a different manner than younger patients. For instance, maintenance of mobility, mental state, and continence, or what is loosely termed as *function*, become major positive outcomes for older patients, whereas successful treatment may mean a cure for patients of other ages. Older patients may desire symptomatic relief rather than a cure or may not desire a treatment at all. It is therefore of greater importance in older patients to discuss what their expectations are from "treatment" of a disease. This leads to the final modifier of the health belief model, which is a patient's readiness to accept therapy.

Perceived benefits of the therapy must be present in a patient, whereas the barriers of treatment should be minimal for compliance to take place. Barriers of the treatment would include potential adverse reactions of medications; financial cost of the therapy; the extent the therapy will change work, family, or other social environments; and the complexity and duration of the proposed regimen. Older patients may experience more barriers to therapy because of their increased risk for adverse drug reactions, increased complexity of medication regimens when treating multiple illnesses, and economic situation. Becker and Maiman (24) suggested that individuals holding a combination of these beliefs would be more likely to adhere to treatment recommendations.

Another area of a patient's psychological make-up that needs to be addressed is motivation. One can consider a patient's desire to reduce severity of illness as the "pull" toward compliance and motivation as the "push." Motivation has been studied by focusing on a patient's desire or intent to comply with a therapeutic regimen. The belief that patients "should do what the doctor tells them" is significantly associated with compliance. There are also some other positive behaviors in patients who are seen as motivated to comply with therapy. For instance, patients already committed to weight reduction and a low-salt diet to control hypertension may be more likely to take antihypertensive medication.

The Patient–Physician Relation

Variations in patients' compliance with physicians' advice has been investigated to determine the major social and psychological factors of importance during the physician–patient visit (25). Assumptions that guide this type of research are (a) that patients seek medical advice for a problem but differ in their personal characteristics, (b) that these personal characteristics are used by the physician in developing a therapeutic regimen for the patient, (c) that patients discuss these therapeutic regimens with other influential persons in their lives whose opinions they value, and (d) that these outside influences are interactive with the patient's personal characteristics and the nature of the physician–patient relation, which produce differing patterns of compliance with physician's orders. Thus, the complexity of the patient, the patient's illness, and the physician–patient relation are great and may lead to barriers and breakdowns in communication and compliance to treatment regimens.

Types of patterns of patient–physician breakdown have been studied in 154 patients who attended a total of 223 primary physician visits and revisits by audiotaping the interactions (25). Thirty-seven percent of the patients disregarded their physician's recommendations. Dimensions of the patient–physician visit that were associated with noncompliance were malintegrative behavior, authoritative patient–permissive doctor, nondirective antagonism by the physician, and nonreciprocal information-seeking by the physician. Malintegrative behavior exists when both the patient and physician exhibit negative social and emotional interactions. Both persons appear formal, show passive rejection, and withhold help from the other. Also negatively associated with compliance was the pattern of communication between an authoritative patient and a physician who passively acccepts this position. The authors feel these patients provide their own analysis of the problem and solution and do not accept what the physician contributes. Nondirective antagonism is suggestive of a physician who neglects to give the patient information, explanation, or orientation. The physician confines his or her activity to expressing opinions and feelings about the situation. And finally, nonreciprocal information-gathering reflects the way in which physicians collect information from a patient to make a diagnosis without providing feedback to the patient.

Compliance was positively associated when tension-release mechanisms were used during the patient–physician visit. In this case, malintegrative behaviors that have built up during the visit are released through joking, laughing, and showing some satisfaction with the relationship. It is interesting to note that the authors measured congruence during the visit [evidence that the patient and physician were on "the same wavelength" (i.e., agreed on what was desirable, right, and proper)], but this activity was unrelated to the patient's later compliance. Thus, although some behaviors that led to barriers between the patient and physician are associated with noncompliance to physician's recommendations, evidence of positive social interactions that occur during a visit do not guarantee later compliance to recommendations.

Physicians who interact and care for older patients learn that "care" sometimes means supporting patients in their efforts to comply with their own choices rather than the choices provided by the traditional medical approach to treatment of an illness (26). This arises because the traditional medical approach to treatment of an illness occurs when decisions are made rapidly without much discussion with the patient. This works well in younger patients because there is less disagreement about the desired outcome. Older patients, however, have often thought about their mortality and express some degree of fear about the prospect of a medical intervention "imposed" on them when they cannot speak for themselves. Thus, if the prescriber is not aware of a patient's preferences for treatment, dissatisfaction with an outcome may occur by both physician and patient alike.

The Patient, The Illness, and the Medication Regimen

The Brown Bag Prescription Evaluation Program was developed in 1982 by the University of Rhode Island College of Pharmacy as a community outreach project (27–29). The program provides counseling and education by a pharmacist to consumers about their medication regimens in a community setting. After systematic collection of patient demographic and prescription information, intervention by the pharmacist takes place when medication-related problems are discovered. Risk factors for prescription-related compliance problems were thus examined in 1,017 ambulatory patients. Associations between medication-related problems and patient characteristics were also studied.

The average age of the sample population was 71 years, 74% were female, and most individuals were interviewed in senior citizens centers. Patients reported the following common medical diagnoses: cardiovascular diseases 72.6%, musculoskeletal diseases 34.5%, endocrine/metabolic diseases 23.4%, and neurologic diseases 13.6%. Table 9–1 lists the medication problems observed in this study and the intervention that the pharmacist provided to the patient.

During the course of the interview, the pharmacist attempted to correct any medication-taking problems discovered and summarized his or her level of intervention. As listed in Table 9–1, this activity ranged in depth from no intervention to an intervention that required communication with another health care provider and follow-up contact with the patient. Most patients, however, required an intermediate level of intervention, such as reinforcement of the patient's proper medication-taking activities, clarification that provided information to enhance an existing level of knowledge, or education that meant the patient required information that was essential for correcting medication problems. The education intervention exceeded the provision of directions for use or purpose of the pharmacotherapy.

Bivariate and multivariate relations were assessed between the independent variables and the measures of noncompliance to determine which patient characteristics might predict compliance problems. A multivariate model was also developed to

TABLE 9–1. *Types of medication problems and interventions in the Brown Bag Prescription Project*

Type of medication problems encountered/intervention required	Percentage of participants
Medication	
Problems with medicines that sound alike	0.6
Improper drug administration	5.5
Contraindications or drug interactions	5.6
Duplication of drug product	5.9
Change in directions	6.8
Adverse reactions	8.0
Other problems	8.1
Under- or overuse	12.5
No understanding of drug therapy	19.1
Intervention	
None	14.9
Reinforcement	38.6
Clarification	34.7
Education	39.4
Follow-up	6.3

determine the relative risk for each risk factor after controlling for the other risk factors. Neither age, sex, or type of health insurance was associated with noncompliance. Thus, our research supports the studies published that do not show a correlation between compliance problems and age.

A patient's understanding of the medication regimen was the single most critical variable associated with compliance problems. The relative odds ratio calculated for this variable (while controlling for other variables in the multivariate model) was 9.87. Thus, patients who do not understand the purpose of their drug therapy are almost ten times more likely to have compliance problems than patients who do understand their medication regimen. Many studies in the literature also document a lack of knowledge regarding drug therapy as a risk factor, although relative risk of this variable had not previously been determined (30).

Patients who consume a large number of medications and who do not understand their medication directions are also at significantly greater risk for medication compliance problems. Reducing polypharmacy in the elderly should therefore be a desirable outcome to both the patient and prescriber. The literature shows, however, that it is often difficult to achieve physician compliance to recommendations for improvements in pharmacotherapy. For instance, Kroenke and Pinholt (31) surveyed 272 older persons and discovered 89 (33%) who were taking five or more prescription medications. Recommendations were formulated to simplify these patients' medication regimens, and 59% were implemented by the prescriber. A small, but significant reduction in total number of medications was achieved (5.9 ± 0.2 versus 5.4 ± 0.2). Types of recommendations most often followed included those to simplify the medication regimen (100%), to substitute a medication for a different choice (62%), and to discontinue a medication (40%). In this study, physicians stated that they were reluctant to discontinue a medication that another physician had originally prescribed (31).

Two other important predictors for patient noncompliance discovered in the Brown Bag Prescription Project was the length of time since the last physician visit and the length of time taking the medication. The longer the time interval since the patient's last physician visit the greater the risk of noncompliance. The specific type of noncompliance affected was under- or overuse of a prescribed medicine. The relative odds ratio for this variable in the multivariate model indicated that those patients who visited their physician at longer intervals than 6 months were at 1.5 times greater risk of compliance problems. An inverse relation was seen for duration of medication use: Patients were more likely to be noncompliant with medications that had been prescribed for less than 1 year. Better compliance was achieved with medications prescribed for longer than 1 year.

The analysis of data from this ongoing project includes the identification of patients with differing types of diseases and their association to compliance problems and an assessment of noncompliance and therapeutic class of medication. For instance, patients reporting the presence of respiratory disease were at least two times more likely to be under- or overusing their medications, misadministering their medications, or taking the same medication under more than one name. Patients who were suffering with neurologic conditions were at 2.45 times greater risk for developing adverse drug reactions to their prescription medications (e.g., drowsiness and confusion). The therapeutic class of the medication was also associated with compliance problems. Patients taking respiratory medications, anti-infectives, or blood modifiers showed the greatest number of compliance problems.

Conclusions reached from the Brown Bag Prescription Project include recommendations for continued education for the patient during regularly scheduled physician visits with reinforcement provided by nurses and pharmacists. The pharmacist should especially focus on patients who present with respiratory or neurologic diseases and medications because these groups of patients appear to have a greater degree of difficulty with compliance and experience more adverse drug reactions.

METHODS TO ENHANCE COMPLIANCE IN OLDER PATIENTS

Some research has been conducted to try to improve compliance. Patients with memory impairment may benefit from devices like written material or medication organizational boxes. Studies give conflicting results as to whether these aids actually improve compliance (16). One particular difficulty with studies designed to improve compliance is that they generally target only one type of intervention. Thus the method used for improvement is not tailored to the patient nor does it allow for the benefit that one would experience from using multiple methods (e.g., personal communication with written material in addition to a medication organizational box).

Other research in this area shows that many patients adapt their own methodologies to improve compliance. When asked how one ensures compliance, many patients reported that they store their medication on the kitchen counter or a night stand (rather than in a bathroom medicine cabinet). This is not because they are trying to avoid the humidity and subsequent medication deterioration problems but rather that they find being able to see their prescription vials serves as a reminder for compliance. When further questioned as to how they specifically remember to take more than one medication or a medication with multiple dosing, patients report adopting specific methods. Some patients, for instance, reported that they remove the day's dosages of all medications prescribed and place them into glasses on the kitchen table. These patients prevent themselves from overusing a medication but perhaps increase their difficulty with medications requiring multiple daily dosing.

It has been studied whether counseling a patient to reinforce medication knowledge and prescription-taking skills at the end of a hospital stay will prevent the loss of medication knowledge. Thirty-two patients with an average age of 82 years, who were admitted from home and who were cognitively intact were randomized to receive a pharmacist counseling session or the customary education received by patients in an inpatient setting. The medication counseling session provided the patient was individualized to meet the needs of the patient and used multiple methods of instruction. For instance, the pharmacist explained the medication regimen to the patient, counseled regarding adverse reactions of therapy and when to call their physician with problems, and provided printed medication education. Six weeks later, patients who received the intervention gained more knowledge (50% versus 15%) and fewer lost knowledge (17% versus 55%) than did control patients ($p<0.01$) (32). Thus, it has been shown that the variable most highly associated with noncompliance (knowledge of a medication and regimen) can be both preserved and improved in the frail older patient if a health professional (in this instance, a pharmacist) intervenes to instruct the patient.

RECOMMENDATIONS FOR IMPROVING COMPLIANCE IN OLDER PATIENTS

Recommendations can be developed to aid compliance by using those factors that health care professionals and patients can and want to change. Prescribers must recognize that much of the research into patient nonacceptance to physicians' recommendations has dealt with identifying variables in the patient that predict this noncompliance, but are not easily changed. By using a comprehensive functional assessment in evaluating a patient, the prescriber can form a treatment plan that patients can agree to because it incorporates their desires and wishes. Physicians will also be comfortable with the treatment plan as it is formulated with a complete patient database. Comprehensive functional assessment is now considered to be the preferred method of evaluating older patients who have complex medical, social, and psychological issues that are interdependent (33,34).

1. Assess patients with both medical and psychosocial goals in mind. Understanding the patients' values and beliefs regarding health and treatment is the first step to developing a treatment regimen that will be successful. Reevaluate patients to learn of changes in attitudes or values regarding treatment at periodic intervals. Ask patients about their outside sources of health information that they value and life experiences that have altered their health knowledge. Elicit patients' support in a partnership for successful treatment of their health problems.

2. Educate patients about their disease. Be sure patients understand the repercussions of treatment or no treatment. Tell them the expectations of their disease course given differing treatment options. Provide time for patients to express opinions and attitudes about these options.

3. Keep medication regimens as simple as possible. This means limiting the number of medications to as few as possible to reduce the likelihood of drug interactions, adverse drug reactions, and errors in compliance to a medicine regimen. Also, medications that can be prescribed once or twice daily rather than multiple times per day will be easier for patients to comply with.

4. Set priorities for which medications are critical to patients' health. Improve the patients' belief in the treatment of their illness by explaining to patients one's own belief in the treatment. Describe how long it will take to experience a benefit, anticipated adverse reactions, and the potential value to the patient of treatment.

5. Assure patients that there will be diligent monitoring for unexpected and expected adverse reactions. If an unexplained decline in patient status occurs or an unexplained symptom is present, assume it is an adverse drug reaction. The problem could arise from a medication mistake (either an omission or excessive use), some other issue of noncompliance, or an idiosyncratic adverse drug reaction.

6. Educate patients (and caregivers if appropriate) as to the name, dose, and indication for every medication. Reinforce this knowledge at each contact with the patient: by nurses and physicians during office visits, by pharmacists when prescriptions are being filled, and by health personnel who come into contact with hospitalized patients.

7. Ask patients what techniques they have developed to remind themselves to take their medications. Offer medication organizational boxes if appropriate for the patient.

8. Provide printed educational materials for reinforcement of patient knowledge.

9. Give patients an opportunity to ask questions. This serves as a time to reassess the patients' understanding of the medication regimen and as reinforcement of the knowledge they have learned.

10. Ask patients to repeat medication names and instructions for use to allow for reiteration of newly acquired medication knowledge.

By understanding a patient's value system, his or her expectations from a medical encounter, and his or her medical and functional history and present illnesses, a therapeutic plan can be developed and presented to the patient. After discussion and modification with the patient as to what is right for him or her, education regarding the illness and its treatment will reinforce and encourage the patient to adhere to the therapeutic plan. Reevaluation and refinement must occur over time to monitor for effectiveness and adverse reactions and to reinforce desirable behavior.

REFERENCES

1. Lamy PP. Drugs and the elderly: a new look. *Fam Community Health* 1982;5:34–44.
2. Brotman HB. The aging society: a demographic view. *Aging* 1981;315:2–5.
3. Soldo BJ. America's elderly in the 1980's. *Popul Bull* 1980;3:3–47.
4. McCormick WC. Perceptions of the elderly regarding pharmacies, drugs, and pharmacists. *Pharmacy Management* 1979;151:90–95.
5. Baum C, Kennedy DL, Forbes MB, et al. Drug use in the United States in 1981. *JAMA* 1984;251:1293–1297.
6. Owens NJ, Sherburne NJ, Silliman RA, Fretwell MD. The Senior Care Study: the optimal use of medications in acutely ill older patients. *J Am Geriatr Soc* (*in press*).
7. Fretwell MD, Raymound PM, McGarvey ST, et al. The Senior Care Study: a controlled trial of a consultative/unit based geriatric assessment program in acute care. *J Am Geriatr Soc* (*in press*).
8. Steel K, Gertman PM, Crescenzi C, Anderson J. Iatrogenic illness on a general medical service at a university hospital. *N Engl J Med* 1981;304:638–642.
9. Shimp LA, Ascione FJ, Glazer HM, Atwood BF. Potential medication-related problems in non-institutionalized elderly. *Drug Intell Clin Pharm* 1985;19:766–772.
10. Hindmarsh JJ, Estes EH. Falls in older persons. Causes and interventions. *Arch Intern Med* 1989;149:2217–2222.
11. Larson EB, Kukull WA, Buchner D, Reigler BV. Adverse drug reactions associated with global cognitive impairment in elderly patients. *Ann Intern Med* 1987;107:169–173.
12. Nolan L, O'Malley KO. Prescribing for the elderly. Part 1: Sensitivity of the elderly to adverse drug reactions. *J Am Geriatr Soc* 1988;36:142–149.
13. Williamson J, Chopin JM. Adverse drug reactions to prescribed drugs in the elderly: a multicentre investigation. *Age Ageing* 1980;9:73–80.
14. Grymponpre RE, Mitenko PA, Sitar DS, Aoki FY, Montgomery PR. Drug associated hospital admissions in older medical patients. *J Am Geriatr Soc* 1988;13:1092–1098.
15. Blackwell B. The drug defaulter. *Clin Pharmacol Ther* 1972;13:841–848.
16. Fincham JE. Patient compliance in the ambulatory elderly: a review of the literature. *J Geriatr Drug Ther* 1988;2:31–52.15.
17. Weintraub M. A different view of patient compliance in the elderly. In: Vestal RE, ed. *Drug treatment in the elderly*. Balgowlah, Australia: ADIS Health Science Press, 1984;43–50.
18. Spriet A, Beiler D, Dechorgnat J, Simon P. Adherence of elderly patients to treatment with pentoxyphilline. *Clin Pharmacol Ther* 1980;231:1–8.
19. Cooper JK, Love DW, Raffoul PR. Intentional nonadherence (non-compliance) in the elderly. *J Am Geriatr Soc* 1982;30:329–333.
20. Evans DA, Funkenstein H, Albert MS, et al. Prevalence of Alzheimer's disease in a community population of older persons. *JAMA* 1989;262:2551–2556.
21. Meyer ME, Schuna AA, William S. Assessment of geriatric patients' functional ability to take medication. *Drug Intell Clin Pharm* 1989;23:513–514.
22. Cady PS, Hurd PD, Bootman JL. The effects of aging and diabetes on the perception of medication color. *J Geriatr Drug Ther* 1989;4:113–121.
23. Murray MD, Darnell J, Weinberger M, Martz BL. Factors contributing to medication noncompliance in elderly public housing tenants. *Drug Intell Clin Pharm* 1986;20:146–152.

24. Becker MH, Maiman LA. Sociobehavioral determinants of compliance with health and medical care recommendations. *Med Care* 1975;13:10–24.
25. Davis MS. Variations in patient's compliance with doctor's advice: an empirical analysis of patterns of communication. *Am J Public Health* 1968;58:274–288.
26. Jahnigen DW, Schrier RW. The doctor/patient relationship in geriatric care. *Clin Geriatr Med* 1986;2:257–264.
27. Taubman AH, Truncellito M, Mattea EJ, Larrat EP. *The Brown Bag Prescription Evaluation Clinic Practice manual.* Boston: New England Institute for Healthcare Services Research, 1986.
28. Larrat EP, Taubman AH, Willey C. Compliance related problems in the ambulatory population. *Am Pharm* 1990;NS30:18–23.
29. Larrat EP, Taubman AH, Willey C. Identification and prevention of medication compliance related problems utilizing a risk assessment model. (*submitted*).
30. Klein LE, German PS, McPhee SJ, et al. Aging and its relationship to health knowledge and medication compliance. *Gerontologist* 1982;22:384–387.
31. Kroenke LK, Pinholt EM. Reducing polypharmacy in the elderly. A controlled trial of physician feedback. *J Am Geriatr Soc* 1990;38:31–36.
32. Sherburne NJ, Owens NJ, Silliman RA, Fretwell MD. A controlled trial of the effect of pharmacist medication counseling on medication knowledge. *Pharmacotherapy* 1988;8:127.
33. Fretwell MD. Comprehensive functional assessment (CFA) in everyday practice. In: Hazzard WR, Andres R, Bierman EL, Blass JP, eds. *Principles of geriatric medicine, and gerontology.* New York: McGraw-Hill, 1990;218–224.
34. National Institutes of Health Consensus Development Conference Statement. Geriatric assessment methods for clinical decision-making. *J Am Geriatr Soc* 1988;36:342–347.

PART III

Monitoring Techniques for Specific Therapies

*Patient Compliance in Medical
Practice and Clinical Trials*
edited by J.A. Cramer and B. Spilker
Raven Press, Ltd., New York © 1991

10

Monitoring Compliance with Antiepileptic Drug Therapy

Joyce A. Cramer and Richard H. Mattson

*Epilepsy Center, Department of Veterans Affairs Medical Center, West Haven,
Connecticut 06516; and Department of Neurology, Yale University School of Medicine,
New Haven, Connecticut 06510*

Treatment of epilepsy depends on a compliance with a drug regimen and periodic assessment of progress (1). Taking extra doses, omitting doses, or using erratic dosing patterns can diminish drug action or cause adverse reactions. Despite the potential for physical harm and serious adverse ramifications caused by unexpected seizures, epilepsy patients frequently omit medication. Irregular adherence to a treatment regimen not only has an adverse effect on medical care but also greatly confounds evaluation of drug effects during clinical trials.

BACKGROUND

Epilepsy

Epilepsy is an appropriate model for studies of compliance with medications because it is not a silent disease. All patients diagnosed as having epilepsy have experienced two or more seizures. They know that seizures are usually frightening to observers and dangerous for themselves, lead to loss of work and driving privileges, and require long-term follow-up coupled with medication, often for a lifetime. The need for drug therapy is discussed with patients at the time of their diagnosis and reiterated at each follow-up visit with reinforcement by attention to drug serum concentration and dose adjustment. If the patient has no more seizures, action need not be taken if the drug serum concentration is below the desired "therapeutic range." When seizures occur in no discernible relation to precipitating factors, an investigation of the dosage requirements for that patient is initiated. The next step is usually to assess the regularity of medication dosing.

Eisler and Mattson (2), recognizing that partial compliance is a major factor contributing to lack of seizure control, interviewed epilepsy patients about their pill-taking habits. Seventy-two percent of their patients reported having missed doses. This was ascribed largely to forgetfulness; inadequate understanding of the need for regular dosing; or confusing medical advice, adverse reactions, fear of addiction, or ineffectiveness. In more recent analyses of the medical and psychosocial backgrounds of newly treated adults with epilepsy, the probable medication defaulter can be described as one who (a) doubts his or her diagnosis, (b) questions the need for medication, (c) suggests that his or her schedule is too complex for follow-up visits, (d) has no social support system at home or work to help him or her identify epilepsy and drug-related problems, or (e) is overly concerned about the complexity of the medication regimen (3). Many such patients can be converted into excellent adherers by medical staff who target their attention on those issues known to be important for specific epilepsy patients (4). These topics are discussed in Chapter 1, *this volume*.

Good seizure control often leads to complacency by patients about the need to take medicine daily. Realization that a seizure did not occur after a missed dose or even several missed doses may suggest a "cure" to some patients and lead to irregular drug use or even discontinuation. Unfortunately, such remissions in the incidence of seizures are usually brief. The risk of seizure recurrence depends on many factors, which is why most neurologists prefer to maintain drug therapy until the patient has been seizure-free for at least 2 years. Some 30–70% of patients can remain seizure-free long-term using antiepileptic drugs (5), but it is unknown how many had breakthrough seizures during periods of careless or planned dose omission. The clinical impact of missed medication was estimated using data from the Department of Veterans Affairs Epilepsy Cooperative Study (5). Documentation of 1,050 seizures showed that 28% occurred at or before reports of inadequate drug levels (i.e., sub- or low therapeutic range) (1). This undoubtedly was a conservative estimate because many patients took extra doses or resumed their assigned dosage schedule after the seizure and before the blood test. Similar figures of 31% and 38% of seizures related to missed medication or subtherapeutic levels were found in patients with uncontrolled seizures (6,7).

Compliance Estimates in Epilepsy

Patient interviews have been the traditional method to ask about dosing. With the development of pharmacies and dispensing records, review of prescription refills or actual counting of leftover pills became feasible methods for checking drug consumption. By 1970, the ability to measure drug concentration in blood and urine developed into a therapeutic drug monitoring system for many medications in epilepsy. Recent advances in computer technology have allowed miniature recording devices to be adapted to medication dispensers to record dosing.

METHODS

Medication Event Monitoring System

Medication Event Monitoring Systems (Aprex Corporation, Fremont, California) were used to observe doses taken by epilepsy patients. Medication Event Monitoring System bottles are standard 15- or 30-dram pill bottles fitted with caps that contain a microprocessor that can record as many as 1,000 openings. Opening and closing of the bottle is recorded electronically as a presumptive dose. Data are collected from the units by connection to a microcomputer and are sent to Aprex for analyses. Epilepsy patients were invited to use a Medication Event Monitoring System bottle after a full explanation in the informed consent that the bottle would record dosing events. They were asked to fill the bottles once a week, to remove only one dose at a time, and to use only the Medication Event Monitoring System bottle for all medication dosing. The plan was to observe how often patients took the prescribed number of doses each day (from 3:01 AM to 3:00 AM to cover early morning and late night dosing). Noncompliance was defined as omission of a scheduled dose, including taking double pills at a later time to make up for a missed dose, or taking an extra dose the following day, or omitting the dose altogether.

Compliance Rate

A compliance rate was calculated for each patient as follows:

$$\frac{\text{Number of days during which doses were taken as prescribed}}{\text{Number of days observed}} \times 100\%$$

Analysis of variance and Student's *t* tests with Bonferroni multiple comparison corrections were used for group comparisons.

Population

Fifty-five patients (55% male) were recruited from the Veterans Affairs Seizure Clinic (42%) and Yale Medical Center Seizure Clinics and local referrals. Patients aged 18 to 68 years were grouped by prescribed dosage regimen of one, two, three, or four daily doses. One-third of the patients received extensive counseling during participation in a research protocol, including the importance of taking medication regularly. Patients from the general epilepsy clinic, although not having formal compliance counseling, had medication instructions reinforced during years of treatment. All patients knew that a blood sample would be drawn at every visit to check drug serum concentration.

DATA

Overall Compliance By Dose Schedule

Table 10–1 lists the rates of compliance with prescribed one, two, three, or four daily dosage regimens, including 7,266 days of observation of 15,679 doses for 55 patients taking 72 medications. Eleven patients used individual Medication Event

TABLE 10–1. *Compliance rates for prescribed dosing regimens*

Number doses daily	Total number of days observed	Number of patients	Compliance		
			Rate (%)	SD (%)	Range (%)
1	987	6	86	10	73–99
2	4,618	41	80	15	44–100
3	1,188	14	76	14	46–94
4	473	11	53	23	3–85
All	7,266	72	75	19	3–100

Monitoring System units for each of two drugs, and six patients were observed using two different dosing regimens. The average length of monitoring was 14 weeks (range 2–45 weeks). The overall rate of compliance with dosing regimens was 75%. Mean compliance rates were similar for one, two, and three daily doses at 86%, 80%, and 76% declining to 53% for four doses. The distribution of compliance rates for individual patients is shown in Fig. 10–1. Drug serum concentrations checked on clinic day were in the therapeutic range or were reasonable based on low dose, providing no clue to intervisit dose omissions. Coefficients of variation in drug concentration averaged $19 \pm 8\%$, poorly correlating with compliance rates ($r = 0.07$, $p = 0.6$) (8).

Variable Compliance Between Visits

Data from a subset of 20 patients for whom data were available for clinic visits at least 2 months apart were reviewed for differences in compliance during three periods:

1. The 5 days before a clinic visit
2. The 5 days after a clinic visit
3. The 5 days that were 1 month after or before the visit

Figure 10–2 depicts an example of variability of dosing between visits. Overall, the group averaged 88% and 86% compliance rates before and after seeing the physician. However, mean compliance declined significantly to 73% ($p = 0.01$) as the visit became remote. Dosage regimens of twice and three times daily both show the same pattern of significant decline a month after a visit ($p < 0.05$ and $p < 0.025$, re-

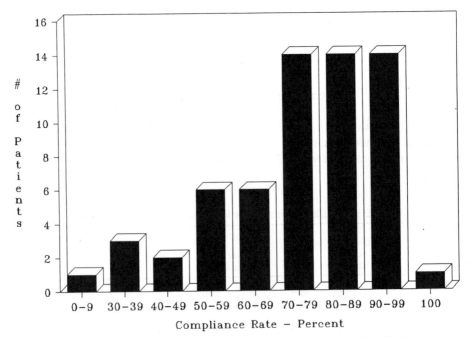

FIG. 10–1. Distribution of individual compliance rates for 55 patients.

```
M    T    W    T    F    S    S

               2    2    2    2
2    2    2    2    2    2    2
2    2    3    2    0    3    2
1    2    2    2    1    3    2
2    2    2    1    2    2    2
2    1    2    2    2    0    2
2    2    1    0    0    3    3
2    2    1    1    1    2    2
1    2    2    2    2    1    2
2    2    2    1    2    1    1
2    3    2    2    1    1    3
2    2    2    2    1    3    2
2


# DOSES    0    1    2    3
_____

# DAYS     4    16   54   8

        BID = 65%
```

FIG. 10–2. Calendar plot listing number of doses taken each day demonstrates variable compliance during 3-months observation. Compliance rate is 65% for the prescribed twice-daily schedule; doses were taken incorrectly on 35% of days.

spectively) (9). Observation of individual dosing records shows examples of erratic compliance between visits with resumption of regular dosing of short half-life medicine soon enough to achieve drug levels in the midtherapeutic range when tested. Eight of nine patients whose interim compliance was less than 70% showed marked improvement before the visit.

Undercompliance Versus Overcompliance

Seventy percent of dosing errors were found to be neglect of the dose rather than overcompliance with extra doses. Fifteen patients taking two daily doses of antiepileptic medication were observed for an average of 134 days to determine whether the morning (5–11 AM) or evening (4 PM–3 AM) dose was omitted most frequently. The evening dose was taken more regularly by 80% of patients, with a significantly higher compliance rate of 98% compared with 69% ($p<0.005$) for the morning dose (10). Patients taking three daily doses had a similar preponderance of missed morning doses.

Interdose Intervals

To compare the ability of patients to take doses according to time intervals based on pharmacokinetic principles (i.e., half-life), analyses were made of the number of doses taken at appropriate time intervals. Standard interdose intervals were established as 10 to 14 hr for two daily doses and 6 to 10 hr for three daily doses, and expanded intervals were established as 6 to 18 hr for two daily doses and 4 to 14 hr for three daily doses. For two or three daily doses, only 40% and 38% of doses were taken within the standard time range. This compares with 87% and 81% of doses taken within the wider time frame (both $p<0.001$). Thus, taking the appropriate number of pills might not fulfill the intent of the physician's prescription if periods between doses are longer than the duration of drug effect. Similarly, doses taken too close together could cause transient adverse reactions.

Seizures Related to Missed Medication

During the course of continuous microelectronic monitoring, seven patients reported occasional seizures (range 1–7 seizures for each patient). Data revealed missed medication before seizures in five of these seven patients and provided information about lack of sleep that could have precipitated events in two patients. Overall, the data helped explain 15 of 19 (79%) seizures: 11 were linked to noncompliance and four to sleep deprivation. The data clearly showed that the lengthy period of time from last dose to the seizure allowed drug levels to decline to the subtherapeutic range based on drug half-life.

An example is shown in Fig. 10–3. Patient AP-09 usually took carbamazepine doses twice daily at approximately 7 AM and 10 PM. He forgot to take the Wednesday bedtime and Thursday morning doses, leaving a 38-hr period without medication. A seizure occurred Thursday evening at 10 PM, after which he took medication. Assuming a 16-hr half-life for carbamazepine, his drug serum concentration likely declined to 18% (over 2 half-lives) of usual steady state. Dosing data documented that the seizure occurred at a time when drug concentration was negligible.

Availability of continuous monitoring may provide the opportunity to link events such as seizures with specific medication dosage patterns. A desktop unit has been developed that "reads" the data collected in a Medication Event Monitoring System unit and prints a report of dosage pattern (dose calendar) with the number of doses taken each day and a listing of the time of each dose. This reader-display-printer (Aprex Corporation, Fremont, California) is a rental unit that can be used in an office or clinic. The immediate review of the date of a seizure and medication dosing during the few days before allows the physician and patient to discuss whether missed pills could have contributed to the breakthrough seizure (see Chapter 1, *this volume*).

Data Summary

Despite the potential for socially unacceptable and medically dangerous consequences, the population of epilepsy patients studied took only an average of 76% of their medication as prescribed. Drug serum concentrations did not reflect the periods of noncompliance determined by the Medication Event Monitoring System between visits. Pill counts also suggested greater compliance than what was documented by Medication Event Monitoring System reports (92% versus 76%). The specific, timed microelectronic recording of medication intake not only provided evi-

MON	TUE	WED	THU
7:30AM	7:40AM	8:45AM	----
9:30PM	1:40AM	----	*10:15PM

*Seizure at ~10pm Thursday
dose interval = 38 hours

FIG. 10–3. Patient AP-09 omitted two doses of carbamazepine (half-life approximately 16 hr) before having a seizure on Thursday evening prior to the medication dose.

dence of noncompliance, but also allowed correlation with clinical events (i.e., seizures and adverse reations). These pilot data can help one to approach several major questions, as discussed below.

COMMENTARY

How Widespread is Noncompliance?

Finding that overall noncompliance approximated one-fourth of doses prescribed indicated that it was a pervasive pattern among men and women of a wide range of ages, socioeconomic backgrounds, intellectual capacities, and treatment plans. This population was extensively educated about the disorder and need for medication and was closely followed. Additionally, they knew their dose schedule was being observed, which should have improved compliance. The complexity of a regimen was associated with noncompliance in this small group, although the statistically nonsignificant differences in rates of compliance among one, two, or three daily doses indicated that none of these regimens was ideal and that even a single daily dose could be missed. Nevertheless, some patients did overcomply occasionally as shown in the dose calendar. A rare report in the literature of mean 109% compliance with short-term antibiotic use for otitis media was attributed to extensive counseling and home visits (11).

Wide ranges of partial compliance are commonly reported for patients with a variety of medical disorders including painful or life-threatening as well as benign or silent diseases. Self-reports of missed antiepileptic medicines have ranged from 40 to 49% (2,12). For example, with antacid use, a comparison of physician estimates of missed doses (71%) and patient reports (89%) both differed from the actual pill count of 47% (13). A prospective survey of medical residents and interns found that predictions of compliance were worse than by chance. Only 35% of noncompliers were predicted correctly based on pill counts (14). Kass et al. (15) found 76% compliance for use of pilocarpine and 83% for timolol eyedrops (documented by electronic monitoring) by glaucoma patients, although they reported skipping only 3% of doses. Thirty percent of depressed patients on a two-daily-dose regimen failed to take up to one-fourth of their medication (documented by pill count), with a higher frequency of missed pills as the number of daily doses increased (16). When Fletcher et al. (17) asked patients with heart failure about digoxin use, they found that 19% did not take their medicine correctly as measured by pill counts. Takaki et al. (18) reported that 19% of epilepsy patients had wide fluctuations (>35%) in phenobarbital levels, indicating erratic compliance, with the teenage group having the highest rate. Long periods of seizure control correlated with increasing noncompliance.

How Can Noncompliance Be Documented?

Patient interviews, drug serum concentrations, and pill counts have been used as traditional methods for compliance assessment. Each method measures a different aspect of compliance, and none is considered a "gold standard." Microelectronic monitoring reports add a fourth dimension by determining the presumptive total number of doses, the presumptive number of doses taken daily, and whether the prescribed schedule was used. Details of timing and frequency of dose-taking also can be used to understand drug serum concentrations and link seizures to missed doses.

Ask the Patient

The simplest estimate of compliance is to ask the patient and family directly. Although many patients want to please the physician by telling him or her what they think he or she wants to hear, self-reports of erratic or partial compliance can be helpful. Asking adolescent patients how much medication they planned to take correlated well with outcome, particularly if the teenager expected not to comply (19). Self-reports of failure to take medication are generally accurate, whereas denial of noncompliance is often erroneous.

Asking patients to record missed doses in a diary or on their seizure calendar would be helpful if patients remembered to do so. However, not only might the patient be embarrassed to report such neglect to the physician, but it is improbable that he or she would *remember* to make note of a dose that had been *forgotten*. Assuming that the patient has overcome the initial concerns about chronic need for medication and has accepted the diagnosis, forgetfulness is not willful noncompliance. These patients consciously try to adhere to the plan but are not always successful because of issues that compete for their attention or for reasons lying in their subconscious. Controlled epilepsy can lull some patients into a sense of well-being so that scrupulous attention to daily dosing becomes less important to those patients. Diaries are helpful both for the patient and interviewer for documentation of events and missed or extra doses. However, the concordance of written records with electronic data is not good. Gonder-Frederick et al. (20) found that only 43% of diaries maintained by adult diabetics matched electronic records from glucose reflectance meters. Both omissions and extra tests were listed in the diaries. The major problem was poor recordkeeping habits rather than an intention to deceive the physician.

Drug Serum Concentration

Use of biological markers such as drug serum concentration testing has been widely accepted for more than a decade as a method to evaluate patient compliance. Antiepileptic drug monitoring was one of the disease areas in which therapeutic monitoring was pioneered. Estimates of the therapeutic range for antiepileptic medicines helps physicians decide which dose provides adequate medication to minimize or prevent seizures and minimize the occurrence of troublesome adverse reactions. Therapeutic drug monitoring was developed to provide the physician with a measure of active medicine and metabolites to guide dosing. Biological samples showing low or absent drug concentrations have been a valuable aid in suggesting noncompliance (1). However, use of single drug levels to estimate compliance is subject to numerous flaws including assumed half-life and individual clearance rates; time of last dose and absorption characteristics; dose adjustments for adverse reactions; or tolerance and low efficacy. Knowledge that patients may take pills more carefully before an anticipated blood test (9) could explain why most drug levels are or tend to be in the therapeutic or expected range in this group. Enhanced compliance during the 5 days before a blood test yields "steady-state" levels that are not necessarily representative of the patient's usual pattern. Missed doses and longer dose intervals during normal usage could result in transient subtherapeutic drug serum concentrations. These data suggest that continuous electronic compliance monitoring is a valuable adjunct to therapeutic drug monitoring in the understanding of how patients actually take their medications every day.

The anticipation of a medical appointment and the knowledge that blood will be drawn to check levels are factors that could increase the likelihood of taking medications as prescribed in advance of the visit. Remembering the appointment and willingness to attend suggest an intention to follow the physician's instructions. Not only could the heightened awareness of medical instructions before the visit significantly improve compliance for attenders (9), but also the reinforcement of the visit could sustain compliance for several days thereafter.

When a seizure occurs, the patient frequently reports no knowledge of having missed doses. Unless a blood sample is obtained immediately after the seizure, most patients will take a dose of antiepileptic medicine as soon as possible thereafter, making later blood level checks unrepresentative of the status at the time of the seizure. By the time the patient is evaluated by his or her physician, his or her attention to careful dosing usually has brought the drug serum concentration into the appropriate range, suggesting that medication has been used regularly throughout the prior weeks but that the medicine failed.

Immediate determination of a drug level at the time of a seizure, albeit rare, is valuable to understand the reason for occurrence of a seizure or adverse reaction. The inability to extrapolate beyond several half-lives when interpreting drug levels diminishes its usefulness in assessing the amount of medication the patient actually takes during a long period (21). Electronic dose verification reports revealed numerous occasions when drug serum concentrations would have been subtherapeutic during intervals between visits, despite consistently good results when tested at regularly scheduled visits.

Leppik et al. (22) proposed a coefficient of variation based on three or more drug levels to provide a long-term view of drug levels, but this method is influenced by dose time and frequency. It has been found that coefficients of variation were similar among all medicines, ranging from 7 to 34%, and did not correlate with either compliance rates or pill counts. Variability of drug levels in patients taking medication once or twice daily who were good compliers can be explained by the long dose interval for short half-life medicines. A patient with 99% compliance with a once-a-day regimen had a 20% coefficient of variation for phenytoin, probably because the 18 to 24 hr drug half-life allowed marked changes in serum concentrations to be measured. Conversely, stability of drug levels in erratically compliant patients taking medication three or four times a day allowed less fluctuation because of frequent dosing and a relatively stable steady state before the test. A patient who had 46% compliance with his three-times-a-day regimen had a 12% coefficient of variation for carbamazepine. This was attributable to a consistently lower serum concentration. Although neither individual drug levels nor coefficients of variation estimated compliance or pill counts, Medication Event Monitoring System reports explained the levels, particularly when the coefficient of variation was high. Finding a drug serum concentration within the therapeutic range or small variation in scheduled blood test results cannot be assumed to reflect good patient compliance. Continuous dose observations bridged the gap between occasional therapeutic drug monitoring and potential novel drug delivery systems that could provide medication independent of patient action.

Pill Counts

The medical literature shows heavy reliance on pill counts for documentation of compliance. Although pill counts have been used traditionally in clinical trials and in compliance studies to measure the compliance of patients to a regimen, pill counts provide only approximate information that the patient had consumed more or less than a certain number of pills during the time interval between visits. The methodology of assessing compliance with pill counts is flawed because it cannot be determined (a) on which days patients took their pills, (b) whether they took the appropriate number, more, or fewer pills than were prescribed, or (c) whether pills were discarded before the visit to enhance the appearance of having complied with the regimen (23). Although our epilepsy patients used an average of 92% of pills by count, they did not take these pills according to instructions based on pharmacokinetic or pharmacodynamic rationales designed for their safety.

The unreliability of pill counts because of discarded pills has been anecdotal among researchers, although lack of methods to test this hypothesis has hindered analysis. Rudd et al. (24) noted large inter- and intrasubject variance in pill counts even in a selected group of patients participating in a research program. Pullar et al. (25) demonstrated the unreliability of pill counts in three studies of pill counts and level–dose ratios using tiny doses of phenobarbital as a marker. Tracer levels documented that pill counts failed to identify 87% of low compliers. Fletcher et al. (17) also demonstrated overestimation of compliance by pill count based on measuring serum digoxin levels. These reports show a trend similar to data from the population described above (8). Pill counts were increasingly erroneous as electronically documented noncompliance declined, demonstrating the sensitivity of continuous dose monitoring. For example, a patient taking daily morning doses but forgetting evening doses half the time would have a pill count of 75%, although the twice-a-day regimen was maintained on only 50% of days. Unfortunately, the same pill count can be derived by a patient who forgets all doses on 25% of days or skips many doses and takes extra pills occasionally (8). The frequency of over- and underdosing, as revealed by dose verification reports, would have suggested much higher compliance rates based on pill count than was actually seen with Medication Event Monitoring System reports. Pill counts remain a useful measure in research to account for the dispensing of pills, but they have never been widely used in clinical practice. Electronic dose counts may be convenient for use by clinicians particularly with a desktop reader, in addition to their use as a more accurate compliance measure in research.

Prescription refills can provide some information about overall drug usage in clinical practice. Epidemiological studies have used this method to estimate the pattern of medication compliance (26) (see Chapter 2, *this volume*). For example, if a prescription is written for 120 pills to be taken as four pills daily, with two refills, absence of a request to renew the prescription at this or another pharmacy after 3 months can be taken to indicate missed doses, but the pattern of noncompliance is not defined. The pills could be unused and stored, taken at a lower dose to last longer, or taken only for a given period and then stopped.

Automated Devices

Early attempts to use automated devices to record doses were hampered by insufficient technology. Azrin and Powell (27) used an alarm clock dispenser that provided a single tablet when the alarm was stopped but provided no report of how many and when doses were taken. Moulding (28) developed a cumbersome system of a radioactive exposure on photographic paper at each bottle opening that provided a record of the frequency and approximate time of each dose. An eyedropper medication bottle integrated into a device to document dosing of liquid medication was first developed by Norell (29) and later refined by Kass et al. (15). By 1987, technological advances had merged use of tiny microprocessors with standard pill bottles to provide an unobtrusive and accurate dose-counting device. A list of microelectronic monitoring systems are described in Chapter 1, *this volume*.

Apparatus is available for microelectronic recording of doses from nebulizers that dispense aerosolized medication (see Chapter 12, *this volume*), eyedroppers for liquid medication (see Chapter 13, *this volume*), and boxes or bottles for solid dosage formulations (see Chapter 11, *this volume*). These devices count each opening as a presumptive dose. A major drawback to interpretation of data is the inability to assume that the patient swallowed the correct number of tablets or capsules. However, review of daily dosage patterns for patients indicates high likelihood that medication was removed from the bottles regularly.

Calendar plots (Fig. 10–2) and detailed listing of actual dates and times of every bottle opening (Fig. 10–3) document missed and extra doses. Some safeguards are programmed into the software to filter excess, sequential openings (e.g., when the user checks that the caps is tightly closed). Extra openings at unusual times are easily noted in the reports. Unusual patterns would lead the interviewer to ask the patient directly about unscheduled events. Most importantly, errors of omission far outnumber errors of extra dosing. Bias toward overreporting of extra openings is trivial in comparison with the accuracy of observed underdosing.

Although other methods have specific use, only continuous microelectronic monitoring reports provide several levels of information about individual habits. The sensitivity and specificity of this technology over pill counts and drug level method was demonstrated by revealing the patterns of missed doses, quantification of medication taken as prescribed, as well as poor correlation with individual and serial blood levels. Use of a reflectance meter with a microprocessor did not influence glucose testing habits by adult diabetes patients (20). Patients who knew about the electronic recording of data made the same number of diary errors as the group unaware of the recording. However, the glucometer device not only relieved the patients of the burden of compulsively recording every test but also benefited the physician by providing an accurate and reliable record of the frequency and results of all glucose monitoring.

The clinical value of continuous microelectronic monitoring is the ability to link exacerbations of medical disorders to periods of missed medication. Providing clinicians with information about the patient's actual pill-taking habits would offer possible explanations for precipitating factors leading to seizures or other emergent medical events. Physicians could use these objective data in the same manner that drug serum concentration test results and other laboratory measures help guide the treatment plan.

What Dose Schedule Is Optimum for Good Compliance?

The commonly used antiepileptic medicines carbamazepine and valproate have relatively short half-lives of 6 to 12 hr when used in multiple drug treatment plans, thereby requiring multiple daily doses. Physicians occasionally prescribe three, four, or five daily doses to dampen drug concentration peaks and avoid adverse reactions. With recent emphasis toward using a single agent, the extended drug half-life allows more patients to use a twice-a-day schedule.

Similar compliance rates for regimens have been found in studies of other types of medication. Jacobs et al. (30) reported that nonsteroidal anti-inflammatory drugs were taken at rates of 78, 72, 64, 60, and 44% for regimens of one, two, three, four, and more than four daily doses, averaging 65% overall compliance. Although other data showed lower mean compliance rates as dose frequency increased, no significant differences were found among one-, two-, or three-daily-dose schedules. In agreement with Pullar et al. (31), daily dosing is *not* preferred for antiepileptic drug usage. Stretching dose interval to the half-life of the medicine (e.g., one dosing for a medicine with an 18–24-hr half-life) could result in low drug serum concentrations in patients with rapid clearance and in wide swings from peak to trough levels. More importantly, omission of a single daily dose likely causes decline in drug concentration below the desired minimum range. The small decrease in mean compliance rate from one dose (87%) to two doses (81%) in the current study suggested little loss in use of a twice-daily schedule. Minor decline to 77% for three doses does not preclude use of that schedule as needed for pharmacokinetic reasons. The small sample size does not provide sufficient power to recommend an optimum schedule other than to demonstrate the inferiority of four-times-a-day dosing. However, ruling out one dose because of the danger of missing a full day's dosing in one missed dose, and three doses as unnecessary for medicines with greater than or equal to 12-hr half life, two doses is the preferred schedule.

Does Counseling Make a Difference?

All epilepsy patients who routinely see physicians in developed countries are educated about their diagnosis and the need for medication. The emphasis on drug serum concentration testing in many patients throughout their long-term follow-up reaffirms physicians' belief that the correct dose minimizes seizures and adverse reactions. Frequent clinic visits during initiation of new antiepileptic medication appeared to provide the type of counseling and feedback that assisted newly diagnosed patients to achieve moderately good compliance. Wannamaker et al. (32) reported that the more frequently a patient visits a physician, the more likely that drug serum concentrations would be within the therapeutic range. Counseling patients on discharge from a medical ward significantly decreased noncompliance to 15% compared with noncounseled patients (24%, $p < 0.01$) (33). Similarly, Bond and Monson (34) were able to document sustained improvement in the use of antihypertensive medication after counseling by a nurse and pharmacist. The fraction of patients following the prescription and maintaining normal blood pressure rose from 29% in controls to 69% in counseled patients during 9 months.

Previous analyses found no difference in compliance among groups of patients who were recently diagnosed or who were long-term. Only a mixture of a complex dose changing plan coupled with three- and four-times-a-day dosing led to decreased compliance, despite extensive counseling (8). Finding almost as good compliance in the new onset group was with the patients who had uncontrolled seizures for many years suggests, albeit in an uncontrolled fashion, that counseling does help patients to develop reasonable habits for taking their medications regularly (4,8). Although these analyses did not include a population who had been treated with antiepileptic medicines long-term but had well-controlled epilepsy, it is reasonable to expect to find lower compliance in this group in which the negative feedback of breakthrough seizures was a less imminent threat. Recognition of patterns and extent of noncompliance allows a practitioner to help his or her patients plan effective strategies that fit their life-style (3,35).

How May Dose Monitoring Information Be Used?

Providing clinicians with information about a patient's actual pill-taking habits would offer possible explanations for precipitating factors leading to events such as seizures, asthma attacks, diabetic coma, or congestive heart failure. Physicians could use these objective data in the same manner that drug serum concentration test results and other laboratory measures help guide individual treatment plans.

It would be useful to have microelectronic monitors available as a laboratory test that could be prescribed by the physician. Patients could be requested to use a unit for a month or more and return it for analysis during the office visit so the physician would have a detailed report to better understand why treatment has not been fully successful. Patient safety would be enhanced by preventing unnecessary dose increases or drug changes. Electronic monitors would become an element of patient care for a physician to ascertain degree of compliance or actual dose usage before recommending or instituting changes in therapy.

CONCLUSION

In conclusion, multiple methods for compliance monitoring are useful to assess reasons for inadequate therapeutic outcomes. Each system is based on a different concept. Continuous microelectronic compliance monitoring is a sensitive tool that can complement therapeutic drug monitoring (36), particularly for epilepsy. Dose time listings and calendar plots of daily dosing can be used to interpret therapeutic failures (e.g., breakthrough seizures) between blood tests. Data can explain whether the medicine failed or whether the patient failed to take enough of the medicine to provide adequate and steady concentrations. The translation of a test's methodology into data that are useful in improving patient care is the ultimate triumph of such technology. Standard medical practice could someday include long-term compliance monitoring for follow-up assessment of patients who appear to be refractory to drug therapy.

ACKNOWLEDGMENT

This work is supported by the Department of Veterans Affairs Medical Research Service and the National Institute of Neurological Disorders and Stroke grant no. 5PONS06208-24.

REFERENCES

1. Mattson RH, Cramer JA, Collins JF, VA Epilepsy Cooperative Study Group. Aspects of compliance in epilepsy: taking drugs and keeping clinic appointments. In: Schmidt D, Leppik IE, eds. *Compliance in epilepsy,* Amsterdam: Elsevier, 1988;111–117.
2. Eisler J, Mattson RH. Compliance in anticonvulsant drug therapy. *Epilepsia* 1975;16:203.
3. Cramer JA, Collins JF, Mattson RH. Can categorization of patient background problems be used to determine early termination in a clinical trial? *Controlled Clin Trials* 1988;9:47–63.
4. Cramer JA, Russell ML. Strategies to enhance adherence to a medical regimen. In: Schmidt D, Leppik IE, eds. *Compliance in epilepsy,* Amsterdam: Elsevier, 1988;163–175.
5. Mattson RH, Cramer JA, Collins JF, et al. Comparison of carbamazepine, phenobarbital, phenytoin, and primidone in partial and secondary generalized tonic-clonic seizures. *N Engl J Med* 1985;313:145–151.
6. Stanaway L, Lambie DG, Johnson RH. Non-compliance with anticonvulsant therapy as a cause of seizures. *N Z Med J* 1985;98:150–152.
7. Sherwin AK, Robb JP, Lechter M. Improved control of epilepsy by monitoring plasma ethosuximide. *Arch Neurol* 1973;28:178–181.
8. Cramer JA, Mattson RH, Prevey ML, Scheyer R, Ouellette V. How often is medication taken as prescribed? A novel assessment technique. *JAMA* 1989;261:3273–3277.
9. Cramer JA, Scheyer R, Mattson R. Compliance declines between clinic visits. *Arch Intern Med* 1990;150:1509–1510.
10. Cramer JA, Ouellette VL, Mattson RH. Which medication dose is missed most frequently? *Epilepsia* 1989;30:640.
11. Williams RL, Maiman LA, Broadbent DN, et al. Educational strategies to improve compliance with an antibiotic regimen. *Am J Dis Child* 1986;140:216–220.
12. Peterson GM, McLean S, Millingen KS. A randomised trial of strategies to improve patient compliance with anticonvulsant therapy. *Epilepsia* 1984;25:412–417.
13. Roth HP, Caron HS. Accuracy of doctors' estimates and patients' statements on adherence to a drug regimen. *Clin Pharmacol Ther* 1978;23:361–370.
14. Mushlin AI, Appel FA. Diagnosing potential noncompliance. *Arch Intern Med* 1977;137:318–321.
15. Kass MA, Meltzer DW, Gordon M, Cooper D, Goldberg J. Compliance with topical pilocarpine treatment. *Am J Ophthalmol* 1986;101:515–523.
16. Ayd FJ. Single dose of antidepressants. *JAMA* 1974;230:263–264.
17. Fletcher SW, Pappius EM, Harper SJ. Measurement of medication compliance in a clinical setting. *Arch Intern Med* 1979;139:635–638.
18. Takaki S, Kurokawa T, Aoyama T. Monitoring drug noncompliance in epileptic patients: assessing phenobarbital plasma levels. *Ther Drug Monit* 1985;7:87–91.
19. Cromer BA, Steinberg K, Gardner L, Thornton D, Shannon B. Psychosocial aspects of compliance in adolescents with iron deficiency. *Am J Dis Child* 1989;143:55–58.
20. Gonder-Frederick LA, Julian DM, Cox DJ, Clarke WL, Carter WR. Self-measurement of blood glucose accuracy of self-reported data and adherence to recommended regimen. *Diabetes Care* 1988;2:579–585.
21. Spector R, McGrath P, Uretsky N, Newman R, Cohen P. Does intervention by a nurse improve medication compliance? *Arch Intern Med* 1978;138:36–40.
22. Leppik IE, Cloyd JC, Sawchuk RJ, Pepin SM. Compliance and variability of plasma phenytoin levels in epileptic patients. *Ther Drug Monit* 1979;1:475–483.
23. Norell SE. Methods in assessing drug compliance. *Acta Med Scand* 1983;683:35–40.
24. Rudd P, Byyny RL, Zachary V, LoVerde ME, Mitchell WD, Titus C. Pill count measures of compliance in a drug trial: variability and suitability. *Am J Hypertension* 1988;1:309–312.
25. Pullar T, Kumar S, Tindall H, Feely M. Time to stop counting the tablets? *Clin Pharmacol Ther* 1989;46:163–168.
26. Cooper JK, Love DW, Raffoul PR. Intentional prescription nonadherence (noncompliance) by the elderly. *J Am Geriatr Soc* 1982;30:329–333.
27. Azrin NH, Powell J. Behavioral engineering: the use of response priming to improve prescribed self-medication. *J Appl Behav Anal* 1969;1:39–42.
28. Moulding TS. Commentary: the unrealized potential of the medication monitor. *Clin Pharmacol Ther* 1979;25:131–136.
29. Norell SE. Improving medication compliance: a randomised clinical trial. *Br Med J* 1979;2:1031–1033.
30. Jacobs J, Goldstein AG, Kelly ME, Bloom BS. NSAID dosing schedule and compliance. *Drug Intell Clin Pharm* 1988;22:727–728.
31. Pullar T, Birtwell AJ, Wiles PG, Hay A, Feely MP. Use of a pharmacologic indicator to compare compliance with tablets prescribed to be taken once, twice, or three times daily. *Clin Pharmacol Ther* 1988;44:540–545.

32. Wannamaker BB, Morton WA, Gross AJ, Saunders S. Improvement in antiepileptic drug levels following reduction of intervals between clinic visits. *Epilepsia* 1980;21:155–162.
33. Kellaway GS, McCrae E. The effect of counseling on compliance-failure in patient drug therapy. *NZ Med J* 1979;89:161–165.
34. Bond CA, Monson R. Sustained improvement in drug documentation, compliance, and disease control. *Arch Intern Med* 1984;144:1159–1162.
35. Lima J, Nazarian L, Charney E, Lahti C. Compliance with short-term antimicrobial therapy: some techniques that help. *Pediatrics* 1976;57:383–386.
36. Peck CC. Qualitative aspects of therapeutic decision making. In: Melmon KL, Morelli HF, eds. *Clinical pharmacology: basic principles in therapeutics*. New York: Macmillan Publishing Company, 1978;1063–1083.

*Patient Compliance in Medical
Practice and Clinical Trials*
edited by J.A. Cramer and B. Spilker
Raven Press, Ltd., New York © 1991

11

Monitoring Compliance

The Sine Qua Non of Assessing Therapeutics in the Elderly

*R. John Dobbs, *Sylvia M. Dobbs, and **J. Dickins

*Therapeutics in the Elderly, Research Group and **the Division of Bioengineering,
Clinical Research Centre, Northwick Park Hospital, Harrow,
Middlesex, HA1 3UJ, United Kingdom*

From the foundation of the Therapeutics in the Elderly, Research Group, it was obvious that variable compliance with the prescribed drug regimen was to be a major problem in the management of the elderly. Macdonald and Macdonald (1) found that only 26% of elderly patients were "compliant" 6 weeks after discharge from the hospital. This was despite their generous criteria for compliance of between 50 and 200% of prescribed tablets being taken and their use of pill counting as the measure of compliance. If useful data are to be collected from patient groups that include such "miscreants", everything possible must be done to encourage and monitor compliance.

The number of tablets remaining in a patient's medicine container does not reveal when tablets were removed or if they were swallowed. Spot checks on drug concentrations in blood or urine can only reflect compliance over a short period, dependent on the half-time of the medicine, and the interpretation of these data is complicated by inter- and intraindividual variation in drug handling. Remote monitoring of tablet-taking habits, using an electronic monitor coupled to a tablet container, should resolve some of the difficulties in assessment of compliance.

The present chapter describes our initial studies of remote monitoring, placing particular emphasis on the clinical consequences of variation in compliance.

Both studies reported (2,3) relate to the thorny question of antibacterial dosage: how much for how long? Are current antibacterial regimens unnecessarily demanding on the patient? Many studies (4–7) have demonstrated that the compliance of the patient decreases with time. This seems to occur over both the short time course of antibiotic treatment of acute infection (8,9) and the long duration of treatment for tuberculosis (10–13). The issue in question is whether detailed compliance data should be a routine requirement in trials of the comparative efficacy of different regimens and of different antibacterials?

THE PILL BOX

It is likely that if a pill box is opened according to a recurrent pattern, its contents are being swallowed. An obvious advantage of the monitored pill box described below (14) is that it may be used with any size or shape of tablet or capsule. A limitation is that it only records box openings and does not give information as to the number of "pills" removed at any one opening: Interpretation of the "memory" of the box in the light of interviewing the patients and of pill counts is necessary.

A brightly colored plastic box [110 × 90 × 35 (height) mm] with a hinged lid (The Plastic Box Co. Ltd., Lincolnshire, United Kingdom) and an inner container is used (Fig. 11–1). A portion of the lid of the inner container is cut away, to allow easy removal of tablets, by placing the thumb and index finger inside or by tilting the box and decanting them; the rest of the lid serves to minimize spillage. The box is held closed by two bar magnets, one fixed to the lid, the other to the body of the box. Protruding ledges on the lid and body facilitate opening. The pill boxes are clearly labeled as to contents and the dosage regimen. There is a printed reminder to close the lid on the inner container. In coming to such a design, it was taken into account that the patient's ability to comprehend and recall instructions about medication may be reduced in the elderly (15) and that ability to open child-resistant containers certainly is reduced (16).

The monitor records the number of times that the pill box is opened in time periods of predetermined length. One-hour periods are used, which with a 1K memory, allow 42 complete days of recording. The trigger to the recording system is a reed switch, which is operated by the two bar magnets each time the box is opened. Each opening is recorded as data in an "event counter." At the end of each hour, an "hours counter" is incremented by one and the static memory is "enabled" to read the event

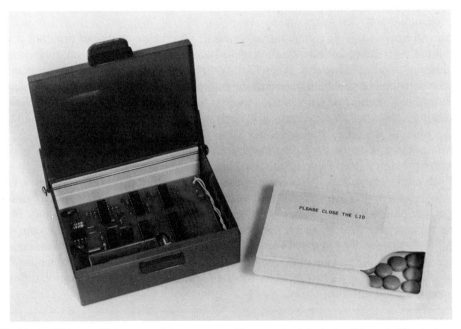

FIG. 11–1. Pill box with inner container removed to reveal printed circuit board. (Cost of components, approximately £30 per box.)

counter into the appropriate memory location. The event counter then resets to zero. Given the overall current consumption of the monitor, the battery would be capable of several months use. The batteries used are inexpensive and readily available. A microcomputer with a short program, written in Basic, and a simple interface are the only extras required to operate a complete system with many pill boxes. Interrogation of the memory and its resetting takes only a few minutes per box.

DISPLAY AND EDITING OF DATA

Figure 11–2 shows a comprehensive analysis of data. Two patients, A and B, were dispensed a 7-day course of cephalexin, to be taken four times daily.

The simplest method of displaying the data is illustrated at the bottom of the display for patients A and B. Each box opening is represented by a solid bar above the horizontal line. The position of the bar along the line corresponds to the day and hour when the opening occurred. Broader bars would represent single openings in 2 consecutive hours. More than one opening in any 1 hour would have resulted in a proportionally taller bar. Patient A complied well with the four times daily medication regimen. Patient B was not as good a complier, as can be seen from the gaps

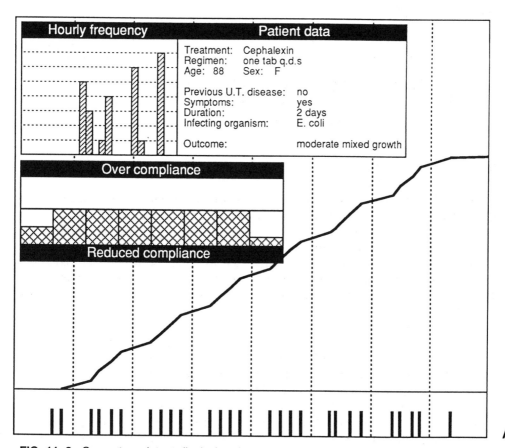

FIG. 11–2. Computer printout displaying data on compliance in two subjects, **A** and **B**, with widely different "pill"-taking habits. **FIG. 11-2.** *Continues.*

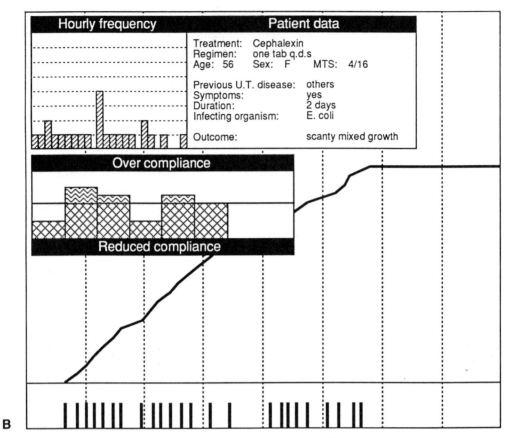

FIG. 11–2. *Continued.* Subject **B.**

between openings. However, when she missed a daily dose, she compensated by taking an extra tablet on the next day.

Above this simple display of the time course of box openings is a cumulative plot of the number of openings during the 7-day period. In the inset are some patient details and two histograms. The lower histogram shows the number of tablets taken each day. Patient A started her course halfway through a day and two openings occurred that day. Thereafter the required four openings occurred each day, until the last half day. The upper histogram shows the cumulative number of tablets taken plotted against the hour of the day. The model patient, A, was very regular in her tablet-taking habits. Other, more poorly compliant patients, such as B, did not show any pattern with respect to the time of day.

For the purpose of the work described below, only one opening per hour was regarded as representative of the removal of a dose of medication from the box. Two events in adjacent hourly memory locations were held to represent a single administration time, which straddled a time change, and the second event was ignored. Experience showed that there were often excessive openings when patients first received a pill box. This presumably resulted from curiosity provoked by the boxes in patients and/or their friends and relatives. This discrepancy becomes small when the full 6-week capacity of the memory is used to monitor maintenance therapy.

MEASURES OF COMPLIANCE FOR USE IN THE
ANALYSIS OF CLINICAL TRIALS

"Totality" of compliance may be assessed in terms of both the recorded number of tablets removed from the box and the number of times the box was opened, each being expressed as a proportion of the number expected had compliance been perfect. An index of the consistency of dosage intervals, namely the proportion of the total number of intervals between box openings, which were of a predetermined "ideal" length, can also be calculated. The latter provides a new dimension to compliance measurements, not available before the introduction of monitored pill containers. Hermann (17) had suspected, as a result of interviewing patients, that they often interpreted a dosage schedule differently from the physician. In particular, three- and four-times-daily regimens seemed to contain an interval of around 12 hr, corresponding to the "overnight gap." Alfredsson and Norell (18) and Kass et al. (19) were able to confirm this suspicion using medication monitors. The later study also revealed that the morning dose tended to be administered with great regularity, while the noon, evening, and nighttime doses were frequently omitted.

APPLICATION OF THE PILL BOX IN A CLINICAL
TRIAL AND IN ROUTINE THERAPY

Two studies in which the pill box was used to monitor compliance of the patient with antibacterial therapy are described. These studies had been approved by the local ethics committee. Informed consent for monitoring the outcome of treatment was obtained, but patients were not made aware of the presence of the recording device in the pill box. They were, however, asked to evaluate the suitability of the pill box for use by the elderly or disabled. Encouragingly, the great majority of our patients aged 50 years or older stated a preference for the pill box over a standard screw top (but not childproofed) plastic bottle.

Comparison in the Community of the Use of 7-day Courses of Two Antibacterial
Preparations in the Treatment of Urinary Tract Infection

A single large dose of an antibacterial can be as effective in treating urinary tract infections as a conventional course of lower doses lasting several days (20). Patients are likely to be motivated to take a single dose, prescribed at the time they seek advice. During the course of repeated medication, patient motivation may decline, or the patient may decide not to complete the course, because symptoms either have abated or, alternatively, persisted. The effect of compliance with 7-day courses on outcome of treatment for urinary tract infections was studied in patients aged 50 years or older.

The methodology was as follows: The inclusion criterion was microbiologically confirmed urinary tract infection sensitive to cephalexin or trimethoprim. Where there was no preference in terms of the antimicrobial sensitivity of the organism, treatments were allocated randomly. Exclusion criteria were antibacterial treatment already started; pyelonephritis; a history of renal insufficiency; the presence of stones and/or a major anatomical abnormality within the urinary tract; a urinary catheter *in situ;* and a patient living in a residential home where medication is supervised by staff.

Eighty patients consented to assessment of outcome of treatment. Only three dropped out. In the first, the antibacterial was changed because of persistent symptoms. The second vomited after the first dose, and the third patient transferred tablets to another container.

Results showed that prescribing trimethoprim, 200 mg twice daily, was more effective than cephalexin in a dose of 250 mg four times daily (cure rates were 93 and 67%, respectively). The difference between treatments was significant ($p<0.006$). Those cured and not cured were not distinguished by age, gender, genitourinary history, or nature of the infecting organism.

Compliance, as measured by box openings, was worse for cephalexin than for trimethoprim at the 1% level ($p = 0.01$). Figure 11–3A demonstrates this difference. The number of times the container was opened is shown on the vertical axis in (a) the 33 patients who received cephalexin and in (b) the 44 who received trimethoprim. The interrupted horizontal lines indicate the ideal number of openings for each antibacterial. Clearly, compliance was worse in patients receiving cephalexin. The open circles indicate patients who were cured, and the closed, those who were *not* cured. In the case of trimethoprim, only three patients were not cured. For cephalexin, 11 were not cured.

Pill counting gave gross overestimation of the number of compliant patients. Only three of the patients given cephalexin and three given trimethoprim had residual tablets. Given the number of box openings less than the ideal, there should have been a total of 171 residual tablets, but only 55 were found.

Both totality of compliance and an index of consistency as defined above (intervals of 4–6 hr being regarded as ideal in the case of cephalexin) were similar in those cured and not cured by cephalexin. Figure 11–3B illustrates the distribution of dosage intervals in those cured and not cured by cephalexin and in those given trimethoprim. Because only three patients who received trimethoprim were not cured, the corresponding distributions for cured and uncured patients are not shown. It is interesting to note that as expected, intervals on a "four-times-daily" cephalexin dose regimen tended to be less than 6 hr, the commonest interval being 4 hr, while for patients prescribed "twice-daily" trimethoprim the commonest interval was 12 hr.

Totality of compliance as measured by openings correlated with the consistency index in the case of cephalexin ($p<0.05$), but not for trimethoprim (11–13 hr being regarded as ideal).

Two general conclusions may be drawn from this study. Firstly, poor compliance may establish overexacting dosage regimens, which, in turn, may encourage poor compliance. Rigid compliance to a conventional course of cephalexin did not promote cure in this study. Secondly, although counting box openings did overestimate compliance, counting residual tablets overestimated it grossly.

Field Trial of the Pill Box in Patients Receiving Antituberculous Therapy

Poor compliance has been implicated as a cause of failure of antituberculous therapy and of relapses, not only in developing countries but also in developed ones. A reliable objective method of measuring totality and pattern of compliance is a prerequisite to further investigation of these problems.

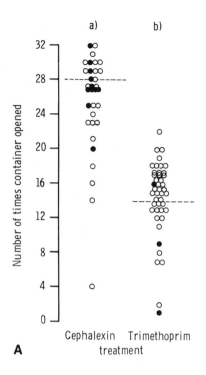

A

FIG. 11–3. A: Number of times the pill box was opened by (a) 33 patients who received cephalexin and (b) 44 who received trimethoprim. *Interrupted lines* indicate the ideal number of openings for each antibacterial course. *Open circles* denote patients in whom the infection was cured, and *closed circles* those in whom it was not. **B:** Percent of total number of intervals between pill box openings to fall within given time limits. *Continuous line* shows the distribution of intervals between openings of boxes containing cephalexin in the 23 patients in whom the infection was cured, and *interrupted line* shows distribution of intervals in ten patients not cured by cephalexin. The *shaded area* shows the distribution of such intervals for 43 patients given trimethoprim. (One patient receiving trimethoprim was excluded because he or she opened the box only once.) (From ref. 2, with permission.)

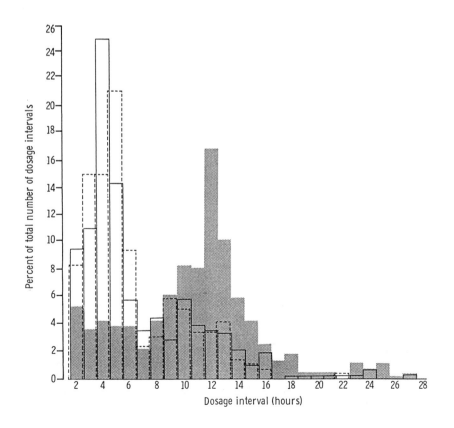

B

In a field trial of our monitored pill box, 23 consecutive adult hospital outpatients receiving the isoniazid/rifampicin combination Rifinah (Merrell Dow Pharmaceutical Ltd., United Kingdom) once daily were studied. In 22 patients the times when the box was opened were recorded successfully for the entire period (an average of 26 days) between successive clinic visits. A broken box was returned by the remaining patient on the follow-up visit.

Only two patients were judged undercompliant by pill counting. These two and seven others opened their boxes fewer than the ideal number of times. In several others, there were more box openings than there were tablets dispensed. It is likely, therefore, that more than nine of the 22 patients failed to remove tablets on the ideal number of occasions.

Figure 11–4 shows a comparison between the compliance of patients studied during the initial 2 months (the so-called intensive phase) of the therapy and those stud-

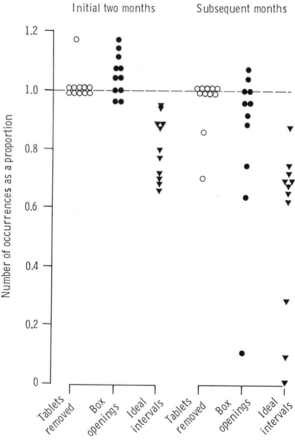

FIG. 11–4. Comparison between compliance of patients studied during the initial 2 months and those studied during subsequent months of Rifinah therapy. Number of tablets removed from monitored box (○) and number of recorded box openings (●) are expressed as a proportion of the number expected were compliance to be perfect. Number of ideal (22–26 hr) intervals (▼) between successive box openings is expressed as a proportion of the total number of intervals. (From ref. 3, with permission.)

ied during subsequent months (the so-called maintenance phase). As described above, the number of tablets removed from the box and the number of recorded openings are expressed as a proportion of the number expected had compliance been perfect. Consistency was expressed as the proportion of the total number of intervals between openings, which were of ideal length (this was regarded as 22–26 hr). Both totality of compliance (as assessed by box openings) and the index of consistency were significantly greater ($p < 0.02$ in each case) in patients studied in the intensive than in the maintenance phase of therapy. It was concluded that patients may have taken the reduction in medication at the end of the intensive phase as signaling cure.

The visual display of recorded data allowed the physician responsible to assimilate at a glance the patient's tablet-taking habits. In routine practice, knowledge by the patient of the presence of the device may act to improve compliance directly, as well as by emphasizing the concern of the health care team. Discussion of the graphical display may prove of value in counseling patients whose compliance is poor.

SUMMARY

Methodology is now available to provide answers to the questions of how much antibacterial therapy is required and for how long (i.e., to define the minimal optimal course with respect to antibacterial agent and disease). Previous lack of such methodology means that many conclusions drawn in clinical trials as to the efficacy of medicines need confirmation. If compliance is poor, both adverse drug reactions and efficacy may be underestimated.

In routine medical practice, considerable monies and professional manpower, not to mention patient time, are currently wasted in modifying the therapy of patients, about whose compliance little or nothing is known, on the assumption that they are compliant. Nowhere is this more pertinent than in the care of the elderly, in which polypharmacy is rife. Selective use of remote monitoring of compliance, using special medication containers, may not only eventually reduce costs of therapy but also curtail suffering of patients. Remote monitoring is likely to be particularly effective when used in conjunction with patient interviews (during which the information yielded by remote monitoring is discussed) and measurement of the medicine, a metabolite, or marker in a biological fluid. Knowledge of whether the patient appears to be compliant and of the timing of the last dose, are, of course, prerequisites to interpretation of assay results for possible dose adjustment.

ACKNOWLEDGMENTS

The authors thank Messrs. J. A. Baker, M. Tate, and V. G. Terry, Department of Bioengineering, CRC, for their invaluable expertise and cooperation in production of the monitored pill boxes, Mr. R. Cheung, Ph.D. student, whose conscientious work made the studies possible, and Mrs. J. Gilbert for preparing the manuscript.

REFERENCES

1. Macdonald ET, Macdonald JB. *Drug treatment in the elderly.* New York: John Wiley & Sons, 1982;218–219.

2. Cheung R, Sullens CM, Seal D., et al. The paradox of using a 7 day antibacterial course to treat urinary tract infections in the community. *Br J Clin Pharmacol* 1988;26:391–398.
3. Cheung R, Dickins J, Nicholson PW, et al. Compliance with anti-tuberculous therapy: a field trial of a pill box with a concealed electronic recording device. *Eur J Clin Pharmacol* 1988;35:401–407.
4. Glick BS. Dropout in an outpatient, double-blind drug study. *Psychosomatics* 1965;6:44–48.
5. Gordis L, Markowitz M. Evaluation of the effectiveness of comprehensive and continuous pediatric care. *Pediatrics* 1971;48:766–776.
6. Luscher TF, Vetter H, Siegenthaler W, Vetter W. Compliance in hypertension: facts and concepts. *J Hypertension* 1985;3(suppl 1):3–9.
7. Porter AM. Drug defaulting in a general practice. *Br Med J* 1969;1:218–222.
8. Bergman AB, Werner RJ. Failure of children to receive penicillin by mouth. *N Engl J Med* 1963;268:1334–1338.
9. Charney E, Bynum R, Eldridge D, et al. How well do patients take oral penicillin? A collaborative study in private practice. *Pediatrics* 1967;40:188–195.
10. Ireland HD. Outpatient chemotherapy for tuberculosis. *Am Rev Resp Dis* 1960;82:378–383.
11. Tuberculosis Chemotherapy Center, Madras. A concurrent comparison of home and sanitorium treatment of pulmonary tuberculosis in South India. *Bull WHO* 1959;21:51–144.
12. East African and British Medical Research Council. Controlled clinical trial of four (6-month) regimens of chemotherapy for treatment of pulmonary tuberculosis. Second report. *Am Rev Resp Dis* 1976;114:471–475.
13. East African and British Medical Research Council. Tuberculosis in Kenya: follow-up of the second (1974) national sampling survey and a comparison with the follow-up data from the first (1964) national sampling survey. *Tubercle* 1979;60:125–149.
14. Dickins J, Cross G, Terry VG, et al. Measurement of compliance with drug therapy in the elderly: a new approach. *Br J Clin Pharmacol* 1986;22:246P.
15. Hulka BS, Kupper LL, Cassel JC, Efird RL, Burdette JA. Medication use and misuse: physician–patient discrepancies. *J Chronic Dis* 1975;28:7–21.
16. Hurd PD, Butkovich SL. Compliance problems and the older patient: assessing functional limitations. *Drug Intell Clin Pharm* 1986;20:228–231.
17. Hermann F. The outpatient prescription label as a source of medication errors. *Am J Hosp Pharm* 1973;30:155–159.
18. Alfredsson LS, Norell SE. Spacing between doses on a thrice-daily regimen. *Br Med J* 1981;282:1036.
19. Kass MA, Meltzer DW, Gordon M, Cooper D, Goldberg J. Compliance with topical pilocarpine treatment. *Am J Ophthalmol* 1986;10:515–523.
20. Stamm WE. Single dose treatment of urinary tract infections: an overview. In: Bailey RR, ed. *Single dose therapy of urinary ract infection.* Sydney: ADIS Press, 1983;98–106.

*Patient Compliance in Medical
Practice and Clinical Trials*
edited by J.A. Cramer and B. Spilker
Raven Press, Ltd., New York © 1991

12

Aerosol Inhaler Monitoring of Asthmatic Medication

Sheldon L. Spector and Helen Mawhinney

Allergy Research Foundation, Los Angeles, California 90025

William Osler remarked that it is more important to know what sort of a patient has a disease than what sort of disease the patient has. Perhaps he had the issue of patient compliance in mind. Certainly when dealing with asthma or other diseases, if a patient does not take the prescribed medications or administers them inappropriately, a favorable outcome is in jeopardy.

Despite increasing attention in the medical literature to the issue of medication compliance, methods of measuring medication usage have had serious drawbacks until recently. For example, it has been shown that the physician's estimate of a patient's compliance is usually grossly inadequate (1). Next, the reporting of medication usage by the patient has been shown to be unreliable (2,3). Biochemical tests, although they are objective, can be inconvenient and expensive and suffer from the major drawback of reflecting medication use only in the period immediately preceding the testing procedure (4). The measurement of residual medication at the end of a study period (e.g., counting the pills remaining in a container) has been shown to suffer from the problem that patients may remove the appropriate number of pills but not necessarily ingest them (5). Finally, the outcome of treatment is sometimes used to assess compliance. This, however, can only be of help where the outcome of treatment can be clearly defined as in the reduction of blood pressure in hypertensive patients on antihypertensive medication (6). There has been a clear need for the continuous and objective measurement of medication usage so that patient compliance can be adequately evaluated.

Until recently the only method available for monitoring compliance with inhaled medication was that of weighing the metered dose inhaler canister. Even if an appropriate amount of medication appeared to have been used, it was impossible to know if the patient had administered the medication correctly during the period of study or even used the medication at all. The advent of technology capable of providing electronic monitoring devices has gone a long way toward achieving the goal of continuous and objective monitoring of medication usage. In this chapter, experience with such a device is described. In addition, Horn et al. (7,8) recently described a biochemical technique for measuring urinary salbutamol (albuterol). Ultimately, this technique combined with an electronic monitoring device may provide an ideal means for determining patient compliance with inhaled bronchodilator medication, ensuring that the medication removed from the metered dose inhaler is actually inhaled by the patient.

In various studies of asthmatic patients, a monitoring device designed for metered dose inhalers called the Nebulizer Chronolog (Fig. 12–1) has been employed. The Nebulizer Chronolog is a small portable device that houses any standard metered dose inhaler canister and fits conveniently into a pocket or purse. Each actuation of the metered dose inhaler triggers a microswitch, and the electronic memory of the Nebulizer Chronolog stores the date and time of each actuation to within 4 min of the actual time of usage. As many as 256 electronic events during a period of several months can be stored at one time. The Nebulizer Chronolog memory is read out by a Chronolog Interpreter, a microprocessor equipped with a printer that produces a record of the date and time of each electronic event stored in the memory unit of the Chronolog.

Unfortunately, studies of patient compliance with aerosolized medication are almost impossible to perform without some degree of awareness on the part of the patient that medication usage is being monitored. It is unlikely that the patient would not be suspicious of the packaging of his or her metered dose inhaler canister within a Nebulizer Chronolog or of biochemical techniques such as measurement of medication levels in blood or urine. More importantly, ethics of medical research require informed consent on the part of the patient before participation in a study. All studies of patient compliance required approval of an Institutional Review Board, which extensively discussed the issue of how much information the patient should be given. The issue was resolved by informing the patient that monitoring would occur but did

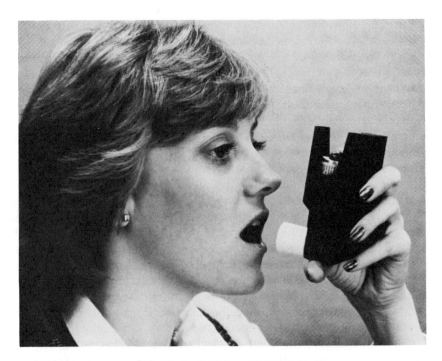

FIG. 12–1. Nebulizer Chronolog.

not give precise details as to how this would be done. It was felt that such a statement was truthful but would interfere to the minimum possible extent with the goal of assessing compliance. It was doubtful if many of the patients guessed the nature of the Nebulizer Chronolog. The majority appeared to assume that the device only recorded the number of activations during the study period and were unaware that it was capable of recording the date and time of each activation.

One study was part of a multicenter clinical trial of an inhaled nonbronchodilator antiasthma medication (i.e., lodoxamide, a cromolyn-like agent). Patients were required to use the inhaler containing lodoxamide or placebo four times daily and to keep a daily diary recording their medication usage. They were also asked to undergo psychological testing. In some instances, this was declined, and if so the patient was not entered into the study. In addition to assessing the efficacy of the medication, the objectives were to determine compliance as measured by the Nebulizer Chronolog and to compare this objective measurement with the subjective reporting of medication usage by the patients. As might be expected, even after recruitment into the study, there were dropouts, including patients who did not fill in their diary forms or refused to complete the psychological testing. Most of these patients had been invited to participate in the clinical trial because they had been thought to be compliant in previous studies. They had also attended the office regularly for follow-up visits during previous studies. Patients who are finally included in a clinical trial are usually those who "appear" most compliant to the investigator and staff. This emphasizes the fact that data derived from most studies probably only represent the proverbial "tip of the iceberg" because the most noncompliant patients either would not have been included in the study or might have been dropped from it because of their failure to comply with its terms.

Traditional studies of compliance have focused primarily on underuse of medication compared with the prescribed dose. In all these studies the definition of compliance has been expanded by classifying medication usage in one of the following four ways (9,10): (a) appropriate usage—the patient takes the medication in a way that conforms satisfactorily to prescribed usage; (b) underusage—the patient fails to take as much medication as prescribed; (c) overusage—the patient takes more medication than prescribed; (d) erratic usage—the patient both overuses and underuses the prescribed medication but at different times. There is an increasing awareness that in a symptomatic disorder such as asthma, overuse of medication needs to be detected. Indeed, because overuse of inhaled bronchodilators may contribute to the increasing frequency of asthma deaths (11), the detection of overuse of medication may be of even greater importance than the detection of underuse. In designating a patient's behavior as noncompliant, this is in no way placing blame on the patient or describing his or her behavior as deviant. Indeed, the term *intelligent noncompliance* has been used to describe the patient who has chosen to stop taking medication either because of adverse reactions or because he or she has determined, by the remission of asthma symptoms, that he or she no longer requires the prescribed medication (12).

The results of this first study were the same as those obtained by other investigators who studied compliance (13). Analysis of 19 patients showed that underusage occurred some time in every patient, the mean rate of underusage being 48%. Approximately half of the patients underused medication at least half of the time. It is impressive that the highest rate of underusage was 96% in a patient who had actually been selected for anticipated compliance with the study. The lowest rate of underusage for a patient was 5%. Overusage would not have been anticipated in a study such as this, in which the medication given did not provide immediate relief of symptoms. Nevertheless, overusage occurred in 13 of 19 patients. This was an overusage range of 0 to 18%, with a mean rate of overusage of 5.3%. Noncompliance occurred on a mean of 53% of days, with a range of 5 to 96%. No patient showed appropriate compliance. The mean compliance rate was less than 50% (i.e., medications were taken by the 19 patients four times per day on an average of 47% of the time).

Younger patients underused the medications more than the older patients. Female patients used the aerosol appropriately a mean of 62% of the time, whereas male patients only used it appropriately a mean of 40% of the time. In fact, 20% of the female patients underused it less than 50% compared with 54% of the male patients. When the diary was compared with the data obtained from the Nebulizer Chronolog, it was found that patients did not tell the truth about their actual usage. Even though patients reported that they had used the aerosol appropriately on an average of 90% of the days studied, the observations recorded revealed appropriate use for an average of only 47% of the study days. Even though male patients underused the aerosols more than female patients, they reported appropriate use more often than female patients. The number of patients studied was too small for full psychological analysis, but the two worst compliers with compliance rates of 4.3% and 11.6%, respectively, failed to complete the psychological tests appropriately, whereas the two best compliers, with compliance rates of 83.5% and 82.5%, respectively, as assessed by the Chronolog, completed all three psychological tests appropriately.

A second study was subsequently carried out (10), which was similar to the first study in that it was a clinical trial of a nonbronchodilator antiasthma medication [i.e., tixocortol pivalate (an aerosolized corticosteroid)] or placebo. This medication was also to be taken on a four-times-a-day schedule, but in contrast to the first study, at a dose of two puffs four times a day. To compare these two studies, a somewhat arbitrary decision was made regarding the issue of "appropriate use." Appropriate use was defined as seven to nine puffs per day. This meant that overuse (i.e., 5 or more puffs in 24 hr in the first study, 10 or more puffs in 24 hr in the second study), and similarly for underuse, represented equivalent percentage deviations from the total prescribed daily dose. Using such definitions, both trials had similar rates of compliance, overuse, and underuse as judged on a day-to-day basis (Table 12–1). In both studies the mean compliance rate was remarkably similar at 37%. This compliance rate was similar to that reported recently by Cramer et al. (14) in a study of antiepileptic medication taken on a four-times-a-day basis in routine clinical circumstances. In this situation they described a compliance rate of 39%. This similarity between the data obtained in the course of the two clinical trials and in routine clinical circumstances was rather surprising. The patients, as previously mentioned, had been selected and to some extent had selected themselves as those anticipated to be more compliant than average. In addition, in a clinical trial, other factors such as unusually frequent follow-up visits, enthusiastic investigators, and payment for participation in the study might be expected to enhance compliance. Some of these aspects may also have been true of the study by Cramer et al. (14), even though the patients were taking their usual medication. In both studies some enhancement of compliance might be expected from the patient's awareness of medication monitoring.

In the context of a clinical trial, the most relevant measure of compliance may be the proportion of days in the study period on which the patient took the study med-

TABLE 12–1. *Comparison of compliance data obtained from subjects participating in clinical trials of lodoxamide and tixocortol pivalate*

| | Lodoxamide trial (Compliance = 4 puffs/day) (n = 19) | Compliance = 8 puffs/day | Tixocortol pivalate trial (n = 15) | | |
			Statistical comparison with lodoxamide	Compliance = 7–9 puffs/day	Statistical comparison with lodoxamide
% Days noncompliance	62.6 (± 21.5)	78.0 (± 16.04)	t = 2.31[a]	62.6 (± 17.2)	t = 0.0046[b]
% Days overuse	23.5 (± 13.0)	22.5 (± 13.6)	t = 0.204[b]	16.6 (± 13.2)	t = 1.62[b]
% Days underuse	38.9 (± 21.1)	55.5 (± 22.6)	t = 2.19[a]	46.0 (± 22.0)	t = 0.95[b]
Puffs/day	4.0 (± 0.86)	7.0 (± 1.26)	t = 8.01[a]		

[a] $p < 0.05$.
[b] Not significant.

ication as directed. A certain level of compliance with medication for the duration of a clinical trial is presumed necessary to establish the efficacy of the medication. For example, evidence is available that at least 80% of most antihypertensive medications must be taken for any benefit to be observed (15). Appropriate use on 75% or more days in the trial was arbitrarily designated as being an acceptable level of compliance for medications such as lodoxamide and tixocortol pivalate. On this basis only one patient could be regarded as truly compliant (Table 12–2). Alternatively, only ten of the 34 patients (1 appropriate user, 3 overusers, and 6 erratic users) would have taken enough medication to allow a valid conclusion about efficacy. Four of these ten patients (3 overusers, 1 erratic user) overused medication on more than 25% of days in the study (i.e., sufficiently frequently to have potentially invalidated any conclusions about adverse reactions).

In practical terms, these low levels of compliance may have significance in both clinical trials and in routine clinical practice. In a clinical trial, a new medication may appear to be ineffective if taken in inadequate dosage by a sufficient number of patients. Conversely, a medication may appear to have an unacceptable frequency of adverse reactions if overuse leads to toxic effects. Toxic effects may be concealed by underuse during clinical trials, only to become apparent during postmarketing surveillance. For these reasons, a task force of the American Academy of Allergy and Immunology has recommended that measures to monitor and enhance compliance be included in the design of trials to evaluate new nonbronchodilator antiasthma medications (16). The full impact of such measures has yet to be deter-

TABLE 12–2. *Numbers and percentages of patients falling into each usage pattern in clinical trials of lodoxamide and tixocortol pivalate*

	Lodoxamide	Tixocortol pivalate	Lodoxamide and tixocortol pivalate
Appropriate use	1 (6%)	0 (0%)	1 (3%)
Underuse	7 (37%)	8 (53%)	15 (44%)
Overuse	2 (11%)	1 (7%)	3 (9%)
Erratic use	9 (47%)	6 (40%)	15 (44%)
Number of patients	19	15	34

mined. In clinical practice the consequence of underuse of medication is most likely to be that of apparent treatment failure. This may lead the physician to suspect the diagnosis and possibly to embark on expensive investigations, which are not genuinely necessary. Apparent treatment failure might also lead the physician to assume that the patient had more severe disease than anticipated and to prescribe more potent medications.

Traditionally, studies of compliance of medication have mainly focused on regularly scheduled medication. The management of a typical asthma patient, however, frequently also includes medication to be taken on an "as-needed" basis. The usual instruction given by the physician to the asthma patient about as-needed medication is to take one to two puffs of medication when required. It is assumed that the patient will use the medication solely to relieve asthma symptoms, increasing his or her medication use with increasing asthma symptoms up to a maximum daily dose defined by the physician. Following these instructions requires a different and more complex decision-making process on the part of the patient than using a regularly scheduled medication. The patient is expected to be able to assess the severity of his or her symptoms and to modify his or her dose accordingly. Under these circumstances, wide variations in medication use relative to the level of airway obstruction would be anticipated.

In a study of as-needed medication requested by inpatients at National Jewish Hospital, Denver, Colorado, only 33% of patients were regarded as having used as-needed medication appropriately, taking more medication on days when airway obstruction was present and less on days when it was not (17). This study was based on the number of days on which as-needed medication was requested relative to morning spirometric measurements. The remaining 67% of patients either overused or underused medication or used medication in an arbitrary fashion relative to airway obstruction. In addition, these authors were able to demonstrate differences in psychological characteristics among these as-needed usage groups (17).

The third study in which the use of inhaled medication using the Nebulizer Chronolog was monitored, an examination was attempted of the real-life situation in which nonhospitalized asthma patients used an inhaled bronchodilator medication, which had been prescribed for use on an as-needed basis (18). The patients were asked to use their usual bronchodilator medication (usually albuterol or metaproterenol) inserted into a Nebulizer Chronolog. They were asked to follow the instructions that they had been given by their physician before participation in the study with the proviso that, consistent with the philosophy on the use of bronchodilator inhalers in asthma, they were asked not to use more than 16 inhalations in 24 hr without consulting a physician. They were asked not to use any other bronchodilator inhaler during the study, but if they did so or used a home nebulizer to report it. To avoid any tendency to underuse medication because of the cost of the medication itself, the medication used in the study was provided free of charge to the patients. The amount of inhaled as-needed medication used daily was related to the level of airway obstruction as determined by peak expiratory flow rates. Analysis was based on the best of three morning peak flow readings. Patients were asked to record the time lapse from the last use of the bronchodilator inhaler, and data were excluded if an inhaler had been used less than 3 hr before the peak flow measurement. The days in the study were characterized as days of no airway obstruction (greater than 80% of the maximum anticipated peak expiratory flow rate), moderate airway obstruction (60 to 80% of the maximum peak expiratory flow rate), and severe obstruction (less than 60% maximum). As in the previous studies, it was a requirement of the Institutional Review Board that patients be informed that their medication use was being monitored. As before, however, the patients were not given precise details as to the functioning of the Nebulizer Chronolog and were not shown either the Chronolog Interpreter or the printouts obtained from it.

Consistent with attempts to determine bronchodilator medication usage in a "real-life situation," appropriate use, overuse, and underuse were defined in simple and logical terms. For example, the use of medication on days with no airway obstruction logically represents overuse, whereas failure to use medication on days with obvious airway obstruction represents underuse. Additional criteria were included to allow for the patients who used acceptable amounts of medication with mild airway obstruction but have either an exaggerated [i.e., exceeding the maximum allowable dosage of more than 16 puffs in 24 hr (overuse)] or an attenuated response to severe obstruction (underuse). It was necessary to include a fourth definition (i.e., that of "arbitrary" use). The patient was regarded as an arbitrary user if he or she tended to use more medication when his or her obstruction was less severe and less medication when it was more severe (i.e., there was no clear relation between the level of airway obstruction and as-needed medication usage).

A total of 47 patients were recruited for the study, but usable data were obtained only from 39. This once again highlights the fact that patients who have been chosen to participate in a study, at least in part because of their apparent willingness to comply with the study, actually failed to do so. Some patients failed to complete the daily diaries recording the peak flow readings or recorded the peak flow data but not the time lapse since the last bronchodilator inhaler use. Other patients recorded the time lapse since their last inhaler use, but there were no corresponding activations of the Nebulizer Chronolog recorded on the Chronolog Interpreter printout for that day (despite the fact that in such instances the Nebulizer Chronolog performed normally when activated repeatedly by one of the investigators). The necessity of combining the characteristic of arbitrariness with the degree of medication use resulted in six as-needed medication usage patterns (Table 12–3). Only one of these, nonarbitrary appropriate use, could be regarded as truly compliant behavior. Of the 39 patients with analyzable data, only 25% fell into this category (i.e., they used their medication as intended by the prescribing physicians). Despite the differences in the study protocols and the means of analysis, this is the same as the 33% appropriate users reported by Kinsman et al. (17) in their group of hospitalized patients with severe asthma. The most common noncompliant patterns observed were nonarbitrary underuse and arbitrary overuse, each making up approximately 25% of the total. These findings confirmed that inappropriate medication use is indeed a prob-

TABLE 12–3. *Usage patterns of as-needed medication in asthma based on daily medication dose versus level of airway obstruction*

Overuse/underuse	Arbitrariness		Total number of patients
	Nonarbitrary	Arbitrary	
Underuser	10 (25.6%)	4 (10.3%)	14 (35.9%)
Appropriate user	10 (25.6%)	2 (5.1%)	12 (30.8%)
Overuser	4 (10.3%)	9 (23.1%)	13 (33.3%)
Total number of patients	24 (61.5%)	15 (38.5%)	39

lem with respect to as-needed medication. The high incidence of overuse is of particular concern in light of the evidence that asthma deaths may result from a delay in the use of corticosteroids because the patient relies on an inhaled bronchodilator (11).

A number of variables were examined that might have influenced the pattern of as-needed medication usage. The six as-needed usage groups did not differ in demographic or clinical variables such as severity of asthma, total medication burden, or the presence of additional chronic disorders. The results of psychological testing were also examined using the Battery of Asthma Illness Behavior as described by Kinsman et al. (19). Briefly this battery provides psychological information at three levels of illness specificity, ranging from general personality (as measured by the Minnesota Multiphasic Personality Inventory) (Table 12–4), through illness-specific attitudes toward asthma and its treatment, to a highly illness-specific level represented by the subjective symptoms reported to occur during asthma attacks. The major psychological difference observed between the groups was in general personality, specifically the Minnesota Multiphasic Personality Inventory variable psychasthenia, which is believed to be indicative of general anxiety (20). The highest psychasthenia scores were characteristic of arbitrary "appropriate" users and the lowest psychasthenia scores of nonarbitrary underusers. If the data for arbitrary "appropriate" and arbitrary underusers were combined and compared with the data for nonarbitrary appropriate and underusers, the difference between arbitrary and nonarbitrary users was more clearly seen, the highest psychasthenia scores being generally characteristic of arbitrary use of as-needed medication. (Arbitrary and nonarbitrary overusers occupied an intermediate position. It is believed that with frequent use of inhaled medication, the distinction between arbitrary and nonarbitrary overuse may be difficult because peak flow data may have underestimated the severity of airway obstruction because of the residual bronchodilator effect persisting for more than 3 hr after the last inhaler use.) A ranking of scores similar to psychasthenia was found for the variable schizophrenia, social introversion, dependency, and inversely, for ego strength. These additional variables have been associated with psychasthenia in the panic-fear personality as described by Dirks et al. (21).

TABLE 12–4. *Mean Minnesota Multiphasic Personality Inventory scores for asthma patients within six as-needed medication usage groups[a]*

Usage groups	Minnesota Multiphasic Personality Inventory scores				
	Psychasthenia	Schizophrenia	Social introversion	Dependency	Ego strength
Arbitrary appropriate use	71.0	68.5	66.0	59.5	44.5
Arbitrary underuse	65.3	73.0	61.3	54.5	42.8
Nonarbitrary overuse	64.3	66.0	61.7	55.3	49.3
Arbitrary overuse	60.9	60.0	60.3	51.1	47.6
Nonarbitrary appropriate use	57.9	58.3	54.3	47.4	52.9
Nonarbitrary underuse	52.4	58.7	57.3	48.6	49.7
p Level	0.004	NS	NS	NS	NS

[a]All values are in *T*-score units. NS, not significant.

The psychasthenia score is said to be the best single Minnesota Multiphasic Personality Inventory indicator of general anxiety (20), whereas high schizophrenia scores may also be characteristic of the agitated, neurotic patient with many anxieties (20). The anxiety measured by both scales is a characterological anxiety occurring as an integral characteristic of the personality and is not merely the result of unhappy circumstances. Because characterological anxiety was found to be a feature of arbitrary use rather than nonarbitrary use, these patients noncompliant as-needed usage patterns may reflect a constant or erratic need to take action (e.g., to reach for their as-needed medication whether or not they are experiencing asthma symptoms). Although the psychological characteristics found to differ between these as-needed usage groups differed from those found by Kinsman et al. (17), in both studies there was evidence that Minnesota Multiphasic Personality Inventory variables that indicate anxiety or panic-fear personality were high in certain noncompliant groups. The finding that noncompliant patients tend to manifest certain psychological characteristics introduces a new aspect to attempts to enhance compliance. For example, with a patient whose arbitrary medication use is related to a high level of characterological anxiety, training in the use of a peak flow meter together with specific guidelines about the peak flow levels at which medication should be used, could help to abolish the arbitrary component of noncompliance.

In the first two studies, which involved the clinical trials of nonbronchodilator medications that would not have given any immediate relief of symptoms, it was surprising to find that almost all the patients overused (or appeared to have overused) their medications at times. Although overuse of a bronchodilator that gives rapid symptomatic relief is easy to understand, overuse of a nonbronchodilator is not. Possibly a patient who had not experienced an improvement in symptoms might overuse such medication in the hope of achieving some benefit. No difference was found between compliance in patients on placebo compared with active medication, nor in patients who did improve clinically compared with those who did not.

Further examination of data from the lodoxamide and tixocortol pivalate trials revealed that some patients appeared to activate the Nebulizer Chronolog repeatedly in rapid succession. That this might have been due to malfunction of the Nebulizer Chronologs was excluded by the fact that the same Chronologs functioned normally when activated by one of the investigators and when issued to other patients. "Multiple simultaneous activations" of the Nebulizer Chronolog, arbitrarily defined as ten or more activations at a single recorded time, suggest a number of possibilities. A panicking patient with severe symptoms might grossly overuse all available asthma medications including those that did not have a direct bronchodilator effect. The number of activations, however, recorded at a single time was often such (the maximum being 61) as to raise the possibility that the Nebulizer Chronolog was being activated without inhalation of the medication. Multiple simultaneous activations of this nature might have been recorded if the Nebulizer Chronolog had been tampered with or if the Chronolog outlet nozzle had become blocked (this was usually apparent at the next follow-up visit, and such data were discarded from the study). It was found that days with multiple simultaneous activations tended to follow underuse days or precede follow-up visits more frequently than might be expected. A similar, although less marked tendency was seen with "simple" overuse days in which multiple simultaneous activations did not appear. These findings imply that patients who failed to comply with the trial, particularly those who underused medication, overused the study medication on other days or activated the Nebulizer Chronolog repeatedly without inhalation. For example, the cooperative patient who inadvertently underused medication on a number of days may have felt it appropriate to overuse medication in a "catch-up" fashion. Alternatively, the noncompliant patient recognizing his or her noncompliance but wishing to persuade the investigator that he or she had complied, either actually overused the study medication or activated the Nebulizer Chronolog repeatedly without inhalation. The motivation for such behavior might have been concern that failure to comply with the clinical trial might jeopardize his or her future relation with the physician or that he or she might not receive the anticipated payment for participation in the trial. This behavior is consistent with the finding that patients who showed multiple simultaneous activations were significantly more noncompliant than patients whose printouts did not demonstrate multiple simultaneous activations. Looked at in another way, those patients who showed multiple simultaneous activations on 2 or more days comprised three of four of the most noncompliant patients in the lodoxamide trial and the three most noncompliant patients in the tixocortol pivalate trial. A particularly strong association was found between multiple simultaneous activations and follow-up visits, more than one-third of such occurrences being observed immediately preceding a follow-up visit. This association (hardly surprising) was much stronger in the tixocortol pivalate trial, which was shorter, with more frequent follow-up visits.

Although the possibility that multiple simultaneous activations (i.e., multiple activations reported at a single date and time on the Chronolog Interpreter printout) were suggestive of patient duplicity that has been previously discussed, analysis of the data obtained from the as-needed medication study caused suspicions about this phenomenon. It was found that in some patients, a large component of the data obtained on the Interpreter printout appeared to consist of activations of the Nebulizer Chronolog at the same date and time. This was initially attributed to malfunction of the Nebulizer Chronolog. This was puzzling because all Nebulizer Chronologs had already been tested by being activated repeatedly by one of the investigators, and they had no other reason to suspect that any might be malfunctioning. In the as-needed medication study, as a cross check for validity of Chronolog data, the investigator had recorded the time of "initialization" of the Nebulizer Chronolog and had triggered the Nebulizer Chronolog three times before issuing it to the patient, and again three times after receiving it back from the patient, recording the dates and times of these triggerings separately. An Interpreter printout became automatically suspect if two of three of these times and dates were incorrect. Investigators were initially alerted to the possible significance of multiple simultaneous activations of the Chronolog when they restudied the printout from one patient in which the dates and times of initialization and of issuing of the Chronolog to the patient were correct on the printout, but the printout concluded with a total of 144 activations of the Chronolog at the same time and date. The activations of the Chronolog by the investigator at the time of return of the Chronolog were missing from the printout. When the data on this printout was compared with the date of the patient's follow-up visit, the investigators realized that these 144 activations had been performed on the morning of a follow-up visit. They further realized that the absence of the three Chronolog activations carried out by the investigator when the Chronolog was returned probably represented the fact that the patient had used up the memory available in the Chronolog (the Chronolog records a total of 256 electronic events).

It was therefore decided to search for other evidence of possible patient duplicity in this study. In addition to the finding of multiple simultaneous activations, the investigators found that a number of patients repeatedly recorded the use of a bronchodilator inhaler a specific number of hours before performance of a peak flow reading, and yet no bronchodilator usage was recorded on the Nebulizer Chronolog (it was assumed in these instances the patient had simply used an alternative metered dose inhaler). It was also found on a few occasions that different peak flow data had been recorded for a single day, suggesting the possibility that some of these data had been fabricated. The investigators used a point system in which they allocated one point for ten or more multiple simultaneous activations on more than 1 day, one point for an inconsistency between the diary and the Chronolog data on more than 5 days, and one point for suspicious peak flow data on more than 1 day. Patients scoring one or more points were suspected of duplicity. Of the 47 patients with data that could be analyzed in this respect, eight were regarded as showing evidence of duplicity. Of these eight patients, five showed evidence of multiple simultaneous activations of the Chronolog. All eight patients had recorded the use of bronchodilator inhaler on their diary sheets without coincidental evidence of activation of the Nebulizer Chronolog, and one patient had suspect peak flow data on 3 separate days. When the data was analyzed to determine which demographic, clinical, or psychological factors might be associated with duplicity, it was found that the only variable by which they differed significantly from the remainder of the patients was that of sex. Male patients were suspected of duplicity significantly more often than female patients. Age did not appear to be a factor. In the clinical trial of Iodoxamide, it was male patients who were significantly more likely to record appropriate usage in their daily diaries despite underuse detected by monitoring.

Investigators also studied this group of patients for evidence of noncompliance with the terms of the study. In this instance also, a point system was used, allocating one point for more than 20% peak flow data missing, two points for more than 40% peak flow data missing, one point for admitting using a nonmonitored inhaler on more than 10 days, one point for failure to complete the psychological tests, and one point for failing to keep follow-up appointments on more than one occasion. Patients who scored three or more points in this system were regarded as being noncompliant with the terms of the study. Of 47 patients whose data could be analyzed in this fashion, a total of ten were regarded as having been noncompliant with the terms of the study. Interestingly, the patients who were suspected of duplicity appeared compliant with the study. In contrast to patient duplicity, it was found that noncompliance correlated most strongly with female sex, but once again age was not a factor. Among the psychological variables, noncompliance correlated with a high ego strength (20), suggesting that overconfidence in their ability to manage their asthma may have contributed to noncompliance with the study.

ASSESSMENT OF THE CLINICAL TRIALS

It is believed that electronic monitoring devices such as the Nebulizer Chronolog and comparable devices monitoring removal of a pill from a container are currently among the best tools available for monitoring patient compliance with medication. Substantially more information can be gained using such tools than using other means of monitoring compliance. For example, it is possible, as has been previously discussed, to distinguish between erratic use of medication and appropriate use. Using electronic monitoring devices, it is possible also to study the way in which medication is taken throughout the day (i.e., whether medicine prescribed on a regular schedule such as four times a day is actually taken in that fashion, or whether the patient modifies the regime to twice a day or even once a day despite taking the total daily prescribed dose).

Electronic monitoring devices are subject to problems of their own. In common with other means of monitoring patient compliance, it is impossible to use such devices without the patient's awareness of the monitoring procedure (even if the Institutional Review Board permitted this type of study). Secondly, the triggering of a metered dose inhaler or the removal of a pill from the container cannot be equated with inhalation of the aerosolized medication or ingestion of the pill. It would be entirely possible for a patient to simulate the use of a regularly scheduled medication to appear totally compliant without actually inhaling or ingesting any medication at all. Unfortunately, patient duplicity can only be suspected in extreme circumstances (e.g., the situation that has been called multiple simultaneous activations). Even this extreme form of duplicity, however, would almost certainly be unrecognized by other means of monitoring compliance. In addition, electronic monitoring devices require periodic battery replacement and are subject to mechanical breakdown, especially if mistreated by the patient. [It was found that one diligent patient washed the Nebulizer Chronolog in the sink, unknowingly causing the component parts to rust. Another dropped the Chronolog in the toilet with the same net effect (i.e., destruction of the Chronolog).] Currently, the optiumum means of monitoring compliance in patients such as asthma patients may be the combination of the continuous use of an electronic monitoring device such as the Nebulizer Chronolog combined with the episodic use of analysis of blood or urine for levels consistent with the therapeutic dose as recorded by the monitoring device. In this context it would be interesting to study patients with the Nebulizer Chronolog and combine this with measurement of urinary salbutamol (albuterol) as recently described by Horn et al. (7,8).

CONCLUSION

In conclusion, these studies raise many issues relating to patient compliance. Despite using a group of patients who might be expected to be better compliers than found in the general population, compliance was poor. Both these studies and those of Cramer et al. (14) of regularly scheduled medication revealed a compliance rate of just more than one-third for medication scheduled to be taken on a four-times-a-day basis. Similarly, both the studies of Cramer et al (14) and those of Kinsman et al (17) showed that with as-needed medication only one-quarter to one-third of the patients could be regarded as appropriately using medication. The major implication of these findings for routine clinical practice is that physicians should anticipate a high rate of noncompliance among their patients. In particular, noncompliance with medication should be considered a major possibility in situations in which a patient apparently fails to respond to appropriate treatment. Although in this situation the patient may admit to noncompliance if challenged on this issue, it is hoped that it will soon be possible for electronic monitoring devices (e.g., the Nebulizer Chronolog) to be available as tools to the practicing physician in such individual circumstances. Also, many clinical trials of medication given at frequent intervals (e.g., four times a day), may have questionable validity. In fact, potentially valuable medications may be discarded because of unrecognized underuse, causing investigators to conclude that they are not effective. If a new study medication is overused, adverse reactions may in fact be related to overuse rather than being a true characteristic of the medication if it were taken as prescribed. It may even be possible to suggest that many medications that have been shown to be efficacious in controlled clinical trials may actually be more effective than actually appreciated from the data obtained from the trials.

Lastly, there is concern about the impact of monitoring compliance in clinical trials, particularly because a means of monitoring compliance is frequently being recommended as a component of clinical trials (16). One might have anticipated that the awareness of monitoring might have enhanced compliance. Indeed, there is the possibility that an even greater degree of underuse of medication would have been found if it had been possible to monitor the patient's medication usage without their awareness. The evidence for patient duplicity in some studies is worrisome because of the degree to which it may have distorted the data obtained. Although the numbers of patients who are strongly suspected of duplicity because of findings such as that of multiple simultaneous activations were relatively small, it may well be that only the proverbial "tip of the iceberg" is being recognized. There is also concern about the distortion of data from clinical trials that may arise from patient duplicity. For example, if as suspected, many days on which overuse of medication was observed in the clinical trial of lodoxamide and tixocortol pivalate would have been appropriate-use days if it had not been for the patient's attempts to comply or to appear to comply with the study. If data from these two trials were to be reanalyzed, assuming that all overuse days would have been appropriate-use days without the patient's awareness of monitoring, data would have been different. The mean rate of medication underusage would have been 39% by comparison with 62.6% in the lodoxamide study and 46% versus 62.6% in the tixocortol pivalate study. Furthermore, in the lodoxamide study, five of 19 patients would have used medication appropriately on more than 75% of the days in the clinical trial by comparison with one of 19. In the tixocortol pivalate trial, four of 15 patients would have used medication on more than 75% of days in the clinical trial instead of no patients. In the light of these findings, although it is believed that monitoring of compliance would be desirable for all clinical trials of new medications, it may not be practical for aerosolized medications until a monitoring device sufficiently small for the patient to be unaware of its incorporation in a metered dose inhaler becomes available. Further discussion of the ethical issue of ideal monitoring of medication usage and what constitutes informed consent would also be appropriate.

Finally, it is believed that lack of patient compliance to a prescribed program may represent one of the most underrecognized problems in clinical medicine today.

REFERENCES

1. Mushlin AI, Appel EA. Diagnosing potential non-compliance. Physicians' ability in a behavioral dimension of medical care. *Arch Intern Med* 1977;137:318–321.
2. Spector SL, Kinsman R, Mawhinney H, et al. Compliance of patients with asthma with an experimental aerosolized medication: implications for controlled clinical trials. *J Allergy Clin Immunol* 1986;77:65–70.

3. Park LC, Lipman RS. A comparison of patient dosage deviation reports with pill counts. *Pharmacologica* 1964;6:299–302.
4. Levy G. Pharmakinetic control and clinical interpretation of steady state of blood levels of drugs. *Clin Pharmacol Ther* 1973;16:130.
5. Roth HP, Caron HS, Hsi BP. Measuring intake of a prescribed medication. A bottle count and a tracer technique compared. *Clin Pharmacol Ther* 1970;2:228–237.
6. Haynes RB, Sackett DL, Taylor DW. Practical management of low compliance with antihypertensive therapy. A guide for the busy practitioner. *Clin Invest Med* 1979;1:175–180.
7. Horn CR, Essex E, Hill P, Cochrane GM. Does urinary salbutamol reflect compliance with inhaled drug regimens by asthmatics. *Respir Med* 1989;83:15–18.
8. Horn CR, Clark TJH, Cochrane GM. Compliance with inhaled therapy and morbidity from asthma. *Respir Med* 1990;84:67–70.
9. Spector SL. Is your asthmatic patient really complying? *Ann Allergy* 1985;55:552–556.
10. Mawhinney H, Spector SL, Kinsman RA, et al. Compliance in clinical trials of two non-bronchodilator anti-asthma medications. (*submitted*)
11. Sly M. Mortality from asthma in children 1979–1984. *Ann Allergy* 1988;60:433–443.
12. Weintraub M. Intelligent non-compliance and capricious compliance. In: Lasagna L, ed. *Patient compliance*. New York: Futura Publishing Company, 1976;39–47.
13. Sackett DL, Snow JC. Magnitude of compliance and non-compliance. In: Haynes RB, Taylor DW, Sackett DL, eds. *Compliance in health care*. Baltimore: Johns Hopkins University Press, 1979;11–22.
14. Cramer JA, Mattson RH, Prevey ML, Scheyer RD, Ouellette VL. How often is medication taken as prescribed? A novel assessment technique. *JAMA* 1989;261:3273–3277.
15. Sackett DL, Haynes RB, Gibson ES, Johnson A. The problem of compliance with antihypertensive therapy. *Pract Cardiol* 1976;2:35–39.
16. Spector SL, Lewis CE, Feldman CH, et al. Compliance factors. In: Bernstein IL, Hargreave FE, Nicklas RA, Reed CE, eds. *Report of the American Academy of Allergy and Immunology Task Force on guidelines for clinical investigation of nonbronchodilator, antiasthmatic drugs. J Allergy Clin Immunol* (suppl) 1986;79:529–533.
17. Kinsman RA, Dirks JF, Dahlen N. Noncompliance to prescribed-as-needed (PRN) medication use in asthma: usage patterns and patient characteristics. *J Psychosom Res* 1980;24:97–107.
18. Mawhinney H, Spector SL, Heitjian D, Kinsman RA, Dirks JH, Pines I. As needed medication use in asthma: usage patterns and patient characteristics. *J Asthma (in press)*.
19. Kinsman RA, Dirks JH, Jones NF. Psychomaintenance of chronic physical illness: clinical assessment of personal styles affecting medical management. In: Milton X, Green X, Meagher X, eds. *Handbook of clinical health psychology*. New York: Plenum, 1982;435–466.
20. Lanyon RI. *A handbook of MMPI profiles*. Minneapolis: University of Minnesota Press, 1968.
21. Dirks JH, Jones NF, Kinsman RA. Panic-fear: a personality dimension related to intractability in asthma. *Psychosom Med* 1977;38:120.

*Patient Compliance in Medical
Practice and Clinical Trials*
edited by J.A. Cramer and B. Spilker
Raven Press, Ltd., New York © 1991

13

Validity of Standard Compliance Measures in Glaucoma Compared with an Electronic Eyedrop Monitor

*,**Mae E. Gordon and **Michael A. Kass

*Division of Biostatistics and **Department of Ophthalmology and Visual Sciences,
Washington University School of Medicine, St. Louis, Missouri 63110

"Glaucoma" is the third leading cause of blindness in the United States and other industrialized countries (1). It is estimated that more than 1 million people in the United States are being treated for glaucoma and that 80,000 individuals are legally blind from the disease. Glaucoma is often referred to as the "sneak thief of vision" because extensive, irreversible damage to the optic nerve can occur before the patient notices any symptoms.

Treatment of glaucoma usually consists of eyedrop medications taken one or more times daily. The eyedrops can produce marked local effects including stinging, burning, and reduced vision and potentially serious adverse systemic reactions such as depression, asthma, tachycardia, and congestive heart failure. The combination of an asymptomatic disease with medical treatments that produce adverse reactions provides a fertile ground for noncompliance to medication regimens. Ophthalmologists and other health professionals have been concerned that patients do not take their antiglaucoma medications as prescribed (2–24). This chapter reviews research to determine if patient compliance to medication regimens can be reliably and cost-effectively ascertained using methods available to the practicing ophthalmologist. These methods include (a) standard clinical measures (e.g., intraocular pressure, pupillary size, and pupillary light reactivity); (b) patient interview; (c) patient medication diary; (d) weighing the amount of medication used between visits; and (e) the physician's educated estimate of the patient's compliance. The validity of each of these methods was evaluated using an electronic eyedrop monitor that resembled a standard medication dispenser. Each method of measuring patient compliance to medication has strengths and weaknesses including cost, convenience, and validity. These studies were undertaken with the hope of identifying valid, cost-effective methods for measuring compliance that could be adopted for use in clinical research studies as well as for routine follow-up care of glaucoma suspects and glaucoma patients.

Patient Sample

Adult patients diagnosed as having either ocular hypertension or glaucoma who were prescribed pilocarpine hydrochloride 0.5 to 10% four times daily to lower intraocular pressure were studied. Table 13–1 lists the demographic characteristics of the study sample. The patients were recruited from the private practices of the full-time faculty of Washington University and the eye clinic of Barnes Hospital by a quota sampling technique. Consecutive patients who satisfied study inclusion criteria were recruited for inclusion into the study (25–27).

The study was conducted with as little perturbation as possible from the usual routine. No patient was treated with pilocarpine solely to measure compliance to pilocarpine. Each patient was given an eyedrop monitor with the appropriate concentration of pilocarpine and was instructed to use the medication as usual. They were requested to use only the pilocarpine as dispensed. Patients were given follow-up appointments for approximately 30 days later and were asked to return the monitors at that time.

Each patient signed a consent form for a questionnaire about glaucoma and its treatment at the time of the return, but the purpose of the electronic eyedrop monitors was not disclosed. This consent procedure was approved by the Institutional Review Board of Washington University Medical School. Data on medication compliance were kept in separate research charts and were not entered in the patient's chart or disclosed to the patient's ophthalmologist.

Electronic Eyedrop Monitor

An unobtrusive electronic eyedrop monitor resembling a commercially available 30-cc bottle of pilocarpine eye drops was developed as previously described (27). The outer shell of the monitor is molded from white, opaque polyethylene. An enclosed inner compartment, which is hidden from sight, contains the electronic components (Fig. 13–1). The monitor can be filled under sterile conditions with any eyedrop medication. The monitor records a medication usage in any 15-min period when two conditions are met: (a) removal of the cap containing a ring magnet, which is sensed by a reed switch inside the bottle, and (b) inversion of the monitor, which is sensed by a mercury switch. Only one medication usage can be recorded in any 15-min period. The monitor can record 6 weeks of data.

TABLE 13–1. *Demographic characteristics of the study sample[a]*

Demographic characteristics	Patients	
	Number	%
Sex		
Male	78	42.4
Female	109	57.6
Race		
Black	74	40.2
White	109	59.2
Other	1	0.5

[a]Mean age ± SD, 67.0 ± 12.1 years; age range, 26–92 years.

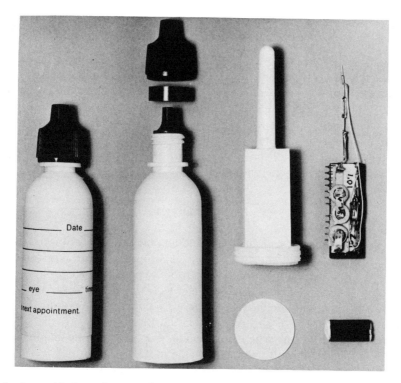

FIG. 13–1. Assembled eyedrop monitor and its components. Note ring magnet in cap and electronic circuit.

On the first visit, the monitor was filled with the patient's usual concentration of pilocarpine, weighed, and dispensed to the patient. On the return visit, the monitor was returned by the patient and weighed by the clinic coordinator. Electronic components were checked by an electronics technician to ensure proper functioning, and the stored information was retrieved using a direct interface to a microcomputer.

The weight of medication used by the patient during the observation period was computed by subtracting the weight of the monitor when it was returned from its weight at the time it was dispensed. Medication compliance as ascertained by the monitor was computed as the percent of the prescribed pilocarpine doses recorded by the monitor (number of doses recorded by the monitor divided by the number of doses prescribed for that period). However, when a patient administered five or more doses in a day, only four doses are computed toward the percent of prescribed doses taken.

On the enrolling visit, the ophthalmologist examining the patient estimated the number of doses of pilocarpine the patient might omit during the next 30 days. In addition, the ophthalmologist was asked how well he or she knew the patient (met today for the first time, slightly, moderately well, very well). To avoid sensitizing the patient to the issue of medication compliance and to elicit an independent assessment of compliance, the ophthalmologist was instructed to make his or her predictions without asking the patient specifically about compliance to the regimen.

Clinical Measures: Intraocular Pressure and Pupillary Reactivity to Light

On the return visit approximately 30 days later, the following clinical measures were completed: (a) intraocular pressure using a calibrated Goldmann tonometer, (b) pupil diameter with a hand ruler, and (c) pupillary reactivity to a hand light, which was graded "no reaction, modest reaction, or brisk reaction." If both eyes were treated with pilocarpine, these measures were averaged for the two eyes. Pilocarpine eyedrops reduce intraocular pressure, constrict the pupil, and reduce or abolish the pupillary light reflex. Each of these clinical responses were compared with the level of compliance measured by the monitor.

Patient Interview

On the return visit, each patient completed an extensive interviewer-administered questionnaire that included questions about eyedrop treatment. The interview was conducted in a private waiting room away from the patient waiting area by an interviewer who was not known to the patient and who was not involved in the patient's care. Questions regarding medication usage were phrased in a nonthreatening manner (e.g., "Most people are not able to take all their drops, . . . the time may be inconvenient or the place may be inconvenient. Can you give me an idea about how many times in the past month you weren't able to take your drops?"). This question provided the estimate of patient self-report of medication compliance. Patients were also asked whether any unusual event (e.g., illness, vacation, changing work hours) had occurred during the past month that could have interfered with their medication regimen.

Patient Diary

Thirty-eight patients were assigned randomly at the time of enrollment to participate in a study to permit simultaneous comparison of medication compliance ascertained by a patient medication diary and an electronic monitor. Patients were instructed to record the time of each pilocarpine administration in a small booklet (daily pilocarpine diary) supplied for this purpose. At the end of the 30-day period, the diary and the monitor were returned and the results compared.

DATA

Monitor

The mean $\pm$ SD period of monitor observation was 29.5 ± 6.4 days (range, 7–42 days). The monitor data indicated that patients administered a mean $\pm$ SD of $76 \pm 24.3\%$ of the prescribed pilocarpine doses (range, 0–100%). Fifty-one patients (27.7%) reported an event (e.g., illness, vacation, changing work hours) that could have altered their daily routine of medication administration. The mean $\pm$ SD rate of compliance in this group was $72 \pm 26.7\%$, which was not significantly lower than the compliance rate in the remainder of the sample ($p = 0.20$, van der Waerden test), suggesting that a change in daily routine does not necessarily interrupt medication use.

Most of the patients in the study had been previously prescribed pilocarpine. The mean duration of pilocarpine treatment was 4.9 years. Twenty-three patients who were initiated on pilocarpine treatment were included in the quota sample. The rate of compliance in this group was $64.7 \pm 33.9\%$, which was substantially lower than in the remainder of the sample ($p = 0.04$, van der Waerden test). Six of the 23 patients initiated on pilocarpine therapy did not take any medication for 10 days or more of the 30-day observation period.

Ninety-seven patients (52.7%) administered extra doses of pilocarpine during the observation period. Although most patients took extra doses infrequently, 13 patients (7.1%) administered extra doses at least 6 days per standard 30-day month. Extra dosing is a concern because of increased potential for local and systemic adverse reactions associated with compression of dose intervals.

Monitor data were scanned to determine whether the patient had administered pilocarpine on the day they returned to the office or clinic. Of the 117 patients for whom this determination could be made, 103 (88%) took a dose of pilocarpine within 8 hr of their return appointment. The rate of compliance in the 24 hr preceding the office or clinic visit was compared with the rate of compliance during the entire observation period. The compliance rate in the 24 hr preceding the return appointment was $87.6 \pm 27\%$ and was significantly higher than the rate during the remainder of the test period ($p < 0.001$, paired t-test).

The rate of compliance, defined as a percentage of prescribed doses taken, does not take the time spacing of doses and therapeutic effectiveness into account. As illustrated in Fig. 13–2, a patient with 100% compliance may not be adequately protected if dose intervals are incorrect. To capture the therapeutic impact of improper dose intervals, an index called therapeutically *uncovered hours* was computed. This index was computed by cumulatively adding the number of hours that exceeded the estimated therapeutic duration of pilocarpine and standardizing the result to a 30-day month. The recommended dose interval for pilocarpine hydrochloride is 6 hr and the duration of therapeutic efficacy is about 8 hr. The dose intervals exceeding the 8-hr therapeutic range were added and standardized to a 30-day month. One hundred thirty patients (71.7%) had 72 uncovered hours or more, 61 (33.1%) were found to have 168 uncovered hours or more (7 days or more), 27 (14.7%) had 336 uncovered hours or more (14 days or more), and 24 (13.0%) had 360 uncovered hours or more (15 days or more, or half of the recording period or more).

Physicians' Educated Judgment

The physicians estimated that patients took $79.4 \pm 15.9\%$ (mean ± SD). Even though physicians' estimates appeared to agree closely with the rate of medication compliance ascertained by the monitor; there was only a modest correlation between the ophthalmologists' estimate of compliance for a given patient and the corresponding monitor data ($r = 0.20$, $p = 0.001$, Kendall tau-b). The accuracy between the physicians' educated judgment and the monitor data was not related to how well the physician knew the patient ($p > 0.05$, Tukey's studentized range test). Ophthalmologists who knew their patients "very well" did no better in judging the patient's com-

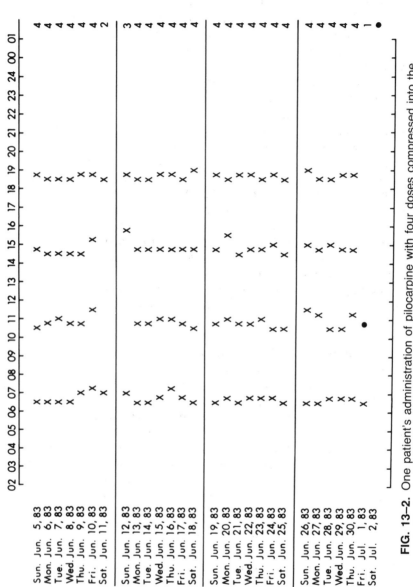

FIG. 13-2. One patient's administration of pilocarpine with four doses compressed into the period between 6:30 AM and 6:30 PM. (*Solid circle*, day of return appointment.)

pliance than ophthalmologists reported meeting their patient for the "first time." The finding that accuracy did not improve with knowledge of the patient and the patient's clinical history suggests that physicians should be cautious about trusting their own "educated" judgment about which patients are noncompliers.

Clinical Measures

Reduction of intraocular pressure is the primary goal of pilocarpine eyedrop therapy. Patients who take their medication as prescribed should have lower intraocular pressure than patients who do not take their medication. However, intraocular pressure as measured on the return visit did not correlate with compliance to pilocarpine regimen as determined by the monitor ($r = 0.024$, $p = 0.64$, Kendall tau-b) (Fig. 13–3). The lack of relation between intraocular pressure and compliance seems attributable to the finding that most patients take a dose within 8 hr of their return appointment.

Similarly, pupillary diameter measured during the return visit did not correlate with compliance to the pilocarpine regimen as measured by the eyedrop monitor ($r = 0.005$, $p = 0.93$, Kendall tau-b).

Pupil reactivity to light was related to compliance as measured by the monitor. One hundred twenty patients who had unreactive pupils (patients with bound or fibrotic pupils were excluded from this analysis) had a mean rate of compliance of $80.5 \pm 19.8\%$, which was substantially different from patients who had reactive pupils who had a mean rate of compliance of $69.4 \pm 27.7\%$. This difference was statistically significant ($p = 0.017$, van der Waerden test).

Patient Report

When interviewed, the patients reported taking a mean $\pm$ SD of $97.1\% \pm$ SD of their prescribed pilocarpine doses. No patient reported taking less than 50% of his

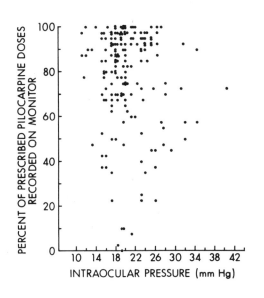

FIG. 13–3. Scatterplot of rate of compliance to pilocarpine eyedrops and intraocular pressure.

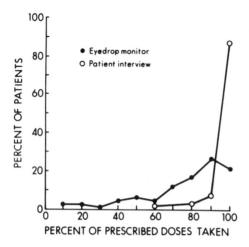

FIG. 13-4. Distribution of medication compliance with pilocarpine eyedrops as reported in patient interviews and recorded by the eyedrop monitor.

or her doses, and only two patients (1.1%) reported taking less than 75% of the prescribed doses (Fig. 13–4). It is often suggested that any patient who admits to missing any medication at all can, with confidence, be considered a noncomplier. However, these data suggest that the patient's admission to missing any doses only slightly improves the odds that the patient is a noncomplier. For patients who reported missing no doses, compliance as measured by the monitor was 79%; for patients who reported missing one to four doses compliance was 78%; and for patients who reported missing five or more doses, compliance was 72%.

Medication Diary

Of the 38 patients randomized to complete a daily medication diary of pilocarpine usage, 32 completed medication diaries (six patients failed to return their daily logs or were lost to follow-up). The mean $\pm$ SD rate of compliance recorded in the daily log was $98.9 \pm 1.8\%$. There was a modest correlation between the daily logs and the eyedrop monitor ($r = 0.25$, $p = 0.084$, Kendall tau-b). Only 29.7% of the doses missed according to the monitor were recorded as missed in the medication diary. Six patients who had compliance rates between 21% and 45% as ascertained by the monitor recorded taking 98% or more of their prescribed medications in their daily logs.

Weight of Medication Used

The weight of pilocarpine medication used by the patient was adjusted for the number of eyes being treated and standardized for a 30-day month. Twenty-one patients forgot to return their monitors by mail and were excluded from this analysis. There was a modest correlation between the weight of pilocarpine used and the rate of compliance computed from the eyedrop monitor ($r = 0.18$, $p = 0.007$, Kendall tau-b) (Fig. 13–5).

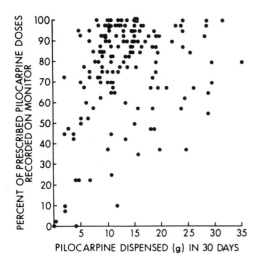

FIG. 13–5. Graph of the rate of compliance with pilocarpine eyedrops and weight of pilocarpine used.

COMMENT

If it were possible to identify patients who fail to comply, physicians might choose alternative forms of therapy including surgery. However, the question remains as to whether poor compliance can be identified, and with what level of accuracy, and at what cost in terms of time, effort, and convenience.

Most physicians and health care workers do not have access to medication monitors capable of yielding objective information in real time. Therefore, judgments about medication compliance must be made using other measures. Physicians rely heavily on standard clinical tests and measures (e.g., blood pressure or blood sugar) as surrogate measures for medication compliance. Such measures entail no additional cost because they are considered part of standard follow-up care. Unfortunately, these results show that any clinical test or measure that reflects the last 24 hours of medication use will substantially overestimate compliance, because medication compliance increases before a return appointment. In this study, intraocular pressure and pupillary diameter measured on a scheduled office visit did not correlate with medication compliance. And pupillary response to light had only a modest correlation with medication compliance. These findings have several important implications for practicing ophthalmologists as well as for clinical research investigators. The measurement of treatment efficacy and disease progression depends on clinical tests and measures performed in the office. If such clinical measures are time-sensitive and reflect medication compliance within the last 24 hours, the level of treatment efficacy attained will be overstated and the physician is likely to have an overly optimistic view of the patient's prognosis.

As an example, ophthalmologists consider elevated intraocular pressure to be a risk factor for the development of visual field damage. However, the evidence for its causal role for the development of visual field damage is sparse. To test the role of intraocular pressure in visual field loss would require a valid measure of intraocular pressure over time, and it is clear that measurements of intraocular pressure made in the office fail to reflect the true level of intraocular pressure over time.

A convenient, low-cost method for ascertaining medication compliance is by simply asking patients about their medication compliance or asking patients to record their medication usage. However, this study found that it was not possible to identify reliably patients with low compliance either by interview or by medication diaries. In this study, an optimal setting for accurate reporting of medication defaulting was provided by interviewing patients away from the waiting room and using an impartial, trained interviewer who was not known to the patient or involved in the patient's care. However, even with these safeguards, it was not possible to identify patients with low compliance using interview techniques.

Many physicians trust their clinical acumen to identify patients who are medication noncompliers. Certainly the physician's "gut feeling" is an important part of the practice of medicine. Unfortunately, there was little correlation between the physician's estimate and the patient's medication compliance as measured by the monitor. The accuracy of the physicians' judgment was no better in the subgroup of patients that the ophthalmologists reported "knowing very well" compared with "met for the first time."

The monitor provides far more detailed information about medication compliance than the patient can possibly be expected to provide. In particular, the patients cannot be expected to recall the pattern of dose intervals, which is likely to be a more important therapeutic indicator than percent number of prescribed doses taken. In these studies some patients with 100% medication compliance compressed the time intervals between doses so greatly that they received therapeutic benefit for only half the day and at the same time increased their risk of adverse reactions. Dose interval data can only be provided by systematic data retrieval mechanisms operating in real time as provided by electronic medication monitoring. None of the conventional methods evaluated in these studies were able to discriminate between patients who were medication compliers and patients who were not. Because of the lack of accuracy of these methods, there is little benefit to be gained from their use. In fact, these methods may provide false security, because noncompliers can seldom be identified.

REFERENCES

1. Vision Research. A national plan: 1983–1987. Report of the Glaucoma Panel. U.S. Department of Health and Human Services, NIH Publication #83-2474.
2. Spaeth GL. Visual loss in a glaucoma clinic. I. Sociologic considerations. *Invest Ophthalmol* 1970;9:73–82.
3. Spaeth GL. Pathogenesis of visual loss in patients with glaucoma. Pathologic and sociologic considerations. *Trans Am Acad Ophthalmol Otolaryngol* 1971;75:296–316.
4. Vincent P. Factors influencing patient non-compliance. A theoretical approach. *Nurs Res* 1971;20:509–516.
5. Vincent P. Patients' viewpoint of glaucoma therapy. *Sight Sav Rev* 1972;4:213–221.
6. Yee RD, Hahn PM, Christensen RE. Medication monitor for ophthalmology. *Am J Ophthalmol* 1974;78:774–778.
7. Bigger JF. A comparison of patient compliance in treated vs untreated ocular hypertension. *Trans Am Acad Ophthalmol Otolaryngol* 1976;81:277–285.
8. Kass MA, Becker B. Compliance to ocular therapy. In: Leopold IH, Burns RP, eds. *Symposium on ocular therapy,* vol 9. New York: John Wiley & Sons, 1976:119–135.
9. Bloch S, Rosenthal AR, Friedman L, Caldarolla P. Patient compliance in glaucoma. *Br J Ophthalmol* 1977;61:531–534.
10. Perkins ES. Blindness from glaucoma and the economics of prevention. *Trans Ophthalmol Soc UK* 1978;98:293–295.
11. Kass MA. Non-compliance to ocular therapy. *Ann Ophthalmol* 1978;10:1244–1245.

12. Worthen DM. Patient compliance and the "usefulness product" of timolol. *Surv Ophthalmol* 1979;23:403–406.
13. Ashburn FS, Goldberg I, Kass MA. Compliance with ocular therapy. *Surv Ophthalmol* 1980; 24:237–248.
14. Davidson SI, Akingbehin T. Compliance in ophthalmology. *Trans Ophthalmol Soc UK* 1980;100: 286–290.
15. Norell SE, Granstrom PA. Self-medication with pilocarpine among outpatients in a glaucoma clinic. *Br J Ophthalmol* 1980;64:134–141.
16. Norell SE, Granstrom PA, Wassen R. A medication monitor and fluorescein technique designed to study medication behaviour. *Acta Ophthalmol* 1980;58:459–467.
17. Norell SE. Monitoring compliance with pilocarpine therapy. *Am J Ophthalmol* 1981;92:727–731.
18. Alfredsson LS, Norell SE. Spacing between doses on a thrice-daily regimen. *Br Med J* 1981;282:1036.
19. Granstrom PA. Glaucoma patients not compliant with their drug therapy. Clinical and behavioral aspects. *Br J Ophthalmol* 1982;66:464–470.
20. Norell SE. Pilocarpine t.i.d.—how is it taken? *Pharmacy Int* April 1982;123–125.
21. Alward PD, Wilensky JT. Determination of acetazolamide compliance in patients with glaucoma. *Arch Ophthalmol* 1981;99:1973–1976.
22. MacKean JM, Elkington AR. Compliance with treatment of patients with chronic open-angle glaucoma. *Br J Ophthalmol* 1983;67:46–49.
23. Kass MA, Meltzer DW, Gordon MO. The compliance factor. In: Drance SM, Neufeld AH, eds. *Applied pharmacology in medical treatment of glaucoma.* New York: Grune and Stratton, 1984;537–568.
24. Granstrom PA. Progression of visual field defects in glaucoma. Relation to compliance with pilocarpine therapy. *Arch Ophthalmol* 1985;103:529–531.
25. Kass MA, Meltzer DW, Gordon M, Cooper D, Goldberg J. Compliance with topical pilocarpine treatment. *Am J Opthalmol* 1986;101:515–523.
26. Kass MA, Gordon M, Meltzer DW. Can ophthalmologists correctly identify patients defaulting from pilocarpine therapy? *Am J Ophthalmol* 1986;101:524–529.
27. Kass MA, Meltzer DW, Gordon M. A miniature compliance monitor for eye drop medication. *Arch Ophthalmol* 1984;102:1550–1554.

Patient Compliance in Medical
Practice and Clinical Trials
edited by J.A. Cramer and B. Spilker
Raven Press, Ltd., New York © 1991

14

Compliance with Treatment of Hyperlipoproteinemia in Medical Practice and Clinical Trials

Wolfgang H.-H. Kruse

University of Heidelberg Krankenhaus Bethanien, 6900 Heidelberg-1,
Federal Republic of Germany

TREATMENT OF HYPERLIPOPROTEINEMIA: PREVENTION OF CORONARY HEART DISEASE

Cardiovascular disease still holds the grim distinction of being the number one cause of death in the United States and western Europe, although the death rates from heart attack and stroke are declining in some countries (1,2). Hypercholesterolemia is a main risk factor for coronary heart disease. Although the detailed pathomechanisms of its causal relation are still the subject of research, the lipid theory of atherogenesis has been well-established (3,4). This concept resulted in therapeutic strategies of primary and secondary prevention by means of various lipid-lowering measures (5,6). However, besides hypercholesterolemia, there are still other risk factors that also have to be taken into account in individual patient counseling and treatment (7,8).

Secondary hyperlipidemia has to be excluded before primary hyperlipoproteinemia is diagnosed and before treatment, particularly with drugs, is initiated (9). In the vast majority of cases in which hypercholesterolemia should be treated, the goal of therapy is to lower low-density lipoprotein–cholesterol levels. There are three genetic syndromes of elevation of low-density lipoprotein cholesterol (10). Familial hypercholesterolemia, familial combined hypercholesterolemia, and nonfamilial polygenic hypercholesterolemia account for most severely hypercholesterolemic patients. Treatment always starts with dietary measures that are sufficient for most individuals with mild or moderate elevations of low-density lipoprotein–cholesterol levels. Dietary measures should be undertaken for at least 2 to 6 months before it is determined whether additional medication is needed. Even when medications are necessary, diet should be maintained. The role of elevated triglyceride levels in atherogenesis is debated. The aim of treating hypertriglyceridemia is to prevent pancreatitis.

The treatment of primary hyperlipoproteinemia with regard to available lipid-lowering drugs has been recently reviewed (11).

Compliance has been defined as the "extent to which person's behaviour (in terms of taking medications, following diets, or executing lifestyle changes) coincides with medical or health advice" (12). Lipid-lowering therapy, when indicated, is to be continued for a lifetime. It has been reported that compliance with prescribed long-term treatment for prevention is likely to decrease over time (13). There is no exception with therapy for hyperlipoproteinemia, as can be readily observed in medical practice.

The maintenance of long-term compliance is difficult, the same as other chronic disease conditions that are asymptomatic. With therapy of hyperlipidemia, as a matter of prevention predominantly, there is a lack of immediate feedback to the patient except occasional blood tests. It is clinical experience that patients avoid having blood tests after periods of heavy eating and drinking. However, it can be assumed that compliance with diet and medicine are likely to increase before blood testings to create low plasma lipid values (toothbrush effect).

COMPLIANCE WITH DIET

Observational and controlled clinical studies revealed secondary failure in hyperlipidemic outpatients caused by poor compliance with dietary recommendations (14–17). Noncompliance with diet is likely to result in prescribing higher doses of lipid-lowering medication (16). Even patients with familial hypercholesterolemia, who are relatively resistant to dietary measures, can be managed adequately in a controlled environment, although plasma cholesterol levels often cannot be normalized. Admission or readmission to a metabolic ward is followed by prompt improvement of disease control, (i.e., decrease in plasma lipid values), which discriminates true nonresponders from noncompliers. However, such "quantitative diet tests" are not feasible for all hyperlipidemic patients. The methods commonly used in assessing compliance with dietary regimens have to be improved; their development is the subject of ongoing research (18).

COMPLIANCE WITH LIPID-LOWERING DRUGS IN MEDICAL PRACTICE

What kind of methods provides information on drug compliance in routine medical practice? Subjective estimates by physicians are inadequate to offer a basis for assessment of patients' intakes of medication (19). For the purpose of routine medical practice, the most simple method, patient interview, may be sufficient in identifying most of the patients who are not compliant. More objective criteria, available to the physician, may be plasma lipid values.

Therapeutic outcome with regard to plasma lipid values was studied in 136 patients with primary hyperlipoproteinemia, consecutively referred to an outpatient lipid clinic (17). Twenty-eight of these patients did not comply with scheduled visits. Diet only had been recommended to one-third of the remaining 108 patients, whereas additional drug therapy had been prescribed to 75 patients. After 1 year, the therapeutic outcome was depressing. Only 30% of the diet group and 25% of the patients on diet and medicines were normalized, and in 36% the metabolic disorder was improved. In total, only 42% of the 136 patients had achieved some therapeutic benefit with regard to their plasma lipid values. However, the clinical outcome may be influenced by other factors besides patient compliance. For example, the degree of cholesterol reduction depends on the severity of the disease, particularly in patients with familial hypercholesterolemia. In some cases, however, plasma lipid values may be appropriate for estimating compliance. Lipid values obtained during a study phase in the metabolic ward compared with those obtained during an outpatient phase were taken as indirect evidence of unchanged patient compliance (20).

Patients' regularity in keeping appointments is another objective criterion. Forty-three patients with heterozygous familial hypercholesterolemia were followed for 5 years after initiating therapy with colestipol (21). Although patients complied with more than 90% of scheduled visits, 30 patients did not comply with the drug regimen.

Objective measures of antacid (bottle count and tracer) and atropin intake (urine test) were made in a study including patients after an acute attack of peptic ulcer (22). Among those patients who completed the program, there was no direct correspondence between regularity of attendance at clinic and the amount of antacid taken. On the one hand, patients' regularity of attendance at the clinic does not seem to provide an index to their medication intake (23). On the other hand, scheduled visits are of extreme importance in the management of patients with hyperlipoproteinemia. This issue, relevant to compliance with dietary recommendations and drug therapy, became evident from several studies.

COUNSELING

Regular counseling by physicians and dieticians improves patients' compliance behavior (16,24). In general, this holds true for compliance with drug therapy (25). Noncompliance, defined as *medication misuse,* was prevalent in outpatients of a teaching hospital (26). Forty-three percent of the 180 patients investigated misused at least one of their medications. In patients treated for circulatory diseases who had the highest prescription–patient ratio of 3.3, the incidence of medication misuse was 53.5%. The factor of physician-provided information about the drug treatment plays an important part in whether the patient will misuse his or her medicine. In patients using their medication correctly, a significantly higher proportion of prescriptions (66%) had been discussed with patients by physicians than in patients who misused their medication (38.6%). There was also evidence, although the numbers were small, that patients who used medications correctly were more likely to follow special diets or vice versa.

Additional medication instruction improved compliance in cardiac and hyperlipoproteinemic outpatients during a 20-day period (27). Compliance was determined by a home interview and pill count. Those hyperlipidemic patients who received additional information made fewer medication errors than the control group.

A comprehensive program of follow-up and reinforcement of patients' knowledge of the disease and the principles of treatment is essential in therapy of hyperlipidemic patients. Special comments concerning patient compliance have become part of the recommendations by the study group of the European Atherosclerosis Society and the U.S. Expert Panel on Detection, Evaluation and Treatment of High Blood Cholesterol in Adults (5,6).

The earlier preventive treatment is initiated, the better should be the result with regard to reduction in risk of coronary heart disease (28). Children with heterozygous familial hypercholesterolemia who were followed for up to 8 years after starting on cholestyramine showed a progressive decrease in compliance with time (29). Only 55% of the patients remained on treatment after 6 years and only 48% after 8 years. Long-term compliance, however, was significantly better in those starting treatment before age 10.

In conclusion, usual sources of information on drug compliance under circumstances of routine medical practice provide, at best, some estimation of the problem.

COMPLIANCE ASSESSMENT IN SELECTED TRIALS ON PRIMARY AND SECONDARY PREVENTION OF CORONARY HEART DISEASE

Compliance measurement in clinical trials seems to be slightly better than in medical practice. In most studies on hyperlipidemic drugs, indirect methods of compliance measurement have been applied. The method most frequently used was pill or packet count (30–35). Three studies are considered in detail to illustrate some methodological problems.

Lipid Research Clinics Coronary Prevention Trial

This was a randomized placebo-controlled trial on cholestyramine, which involved 3,806 patients who were followed for 7 years (32,33). The prescribed dose of cholestyramine was 24 g/day (6 packets). A primary outcome measure was the reduction in coronary risk, defined as the combined risk of death of cardiac origin and nonfatal myocardial infarction. Compliance to medication was estimated from the number of packets (4-g packet of cholestyramine or placebo) returned by participants at bimonthly visits.

Variable intake of cholestyramine was associated with variable percentage reduction in total cholesterol, from -3.9 to -19.0%, and corresponding coronary risk reduction, ranging from 11 up to 39% (34). Mean daily packet count varied from zero to one in about 15%, to at least five packets per day in about 50% of the patients. There was a dose–response relation with cholestyramine. The outcome of the trial, given as average reduction of total and low-density lipoprotein cholesterol and the overall reduction in coronary risk of 19%, was influenced by dilution of drug efficacy caused by noncompliance or partial compliance.

The method of packet count deserves some comment. Overestimating of compliance by pill or bottle count has been demonstrated in studies during which different methods for compliance measurement have been simultaneously used (22,36–40). If compliance is to be related to therapeutic efficacy, problems with tablet count may become even worse, particularly within long-term studies. The relation of percentage decrease in total and low-density lipoprotein cholesterol to compliance was not constant throughout the Lipid Research Clinics study. During the first year, those men who reported an intake of at least 20 g of cholestyramine daily showed mean falls of 23 and 33% in total and low-density lipoprotein–cholesterol levels. The same reported packet count was accompanied, on the average, by only a 17% fall in total and a 27% fall in low-density lipoprotein–cholesterol levels during the seventh year. There is, however, no evidence of diminished lipid-lowering efficacy of resins over time (16,29,31,41).

Cholesterol-Lowering Atherosclerosis Study

To minimize problems with compliance, a prerandomization trial for selection of compliant and responsive patients has been executed in the Cholesterol-Lowering Atherosclerosis Study (35). This placebo-controlled secondary prevention trial was designed to study whether combined therapy with colestipol hydrochloride plus nicotinic acid would produce clinically significant change in coronary, carotid, and femoral atherosclerosis and coronary bypass graft lesions. During a 6-week trial period of colestipol and niacin, patients must have demonstrated sufficient response (at least a 15% reduction in total cholesterol level) to the study medicines to be randomized. Finally, 188 patients were randomized, of whom 162 completed the 2 years of therapy. Every attempt was made to improve compliance with diet by using a computerized pictorial diet record system. During the first 14 days, aspirin and mineral oil were prescribed additionally for the purpose of reducing flushes caused by nicotinic acid and constipation caused by colestipol. The major on-treatment compliance measure used was the change in fasting blood cholesterol level from baseline. Additional compliance measures included the number of missed clinical visits and measurement of a niacin metabolite in 24-hr urine specimens. All analyses were, however, done based on treatment assigned at randomization without regard to compliance. After 2 years of combined drug treatment, there were significant decreases in total and low-density lipoprotein–cholesterol levels, 26 and 43%, respectively, and an increase in high-density lipoprotein–cholesterol level by 37%. Atherosclerosis regression, as indicated by perceptible improvement in overall coronary status, occurred in 16.2% of colestipol-niacin treated versus 2.4% of placebo-treated patients.

Helsinki Heart Study

This primary prevention trial on coronary heart disease investigated the effects of lowering serum total and low-density lipoprotein cholesterol and elevating high-density lipoprotein cholesterol with gemfibrozil in middle-aged men with lipid abnormalities, during a period of 5 years (34). A total of 2,051 men were randomly allocated to receive gemfibrozil 600 mg twice daily, and 2,030 men received placebo capsules. Throughout the study, compliance was estimated by 3-month capsule counts. The proportions of prescribed capsules taken annually in the gemfibrozil group were 85, 85, 84, 84, and 82%. The respective figures for the placebo group were 85, 86, 86, 86, and 83%. Additionally, a cross-sectional measure of compliance was done in 1,739 patients during the last quarter of the third year of follow-up, using digoxin as a marker substance, capsule counting, and a compliance questionnaire (40). Compliance was estimated by measuring the ratio of urinary digoxin to creatinine concentration (42). Digoxin has the advantage of a longer half-life, which makes it less sensitive to the effects of doses immediately before sampling, compared with other markers. A cut-off point for the proportion of unused capsules defining good and poor compliance was set at 25%. The marker was more accurate in measuring poor rather than good compliance but missed a considerable number of poor compliers. Among those patients (64% of the study group) who were classified as good compliers by marker analyses, 11% were poor compliers according to either capsule counting or compliance questionnaire. There were 543 patients (31% of the study group) with poor compliance as measured by at least one method. A total of 990 patients (57% of the study group) were assessed as being good compliers by all three methods. In contrast, annual compliance, determined by capsule counts alone, was 84% in the gemfibrozil and 86% in the placebo group during year 3 of the study. This study demonstrates methodological problems of compliance measurement, which have been previously discussed (43). Standard methods such as pill count do not provide information on the distribution of doses. A continuous compliance measurement would provide much more detailed information on patients' medication intake behavior.

CONTINUOUS MEDICATION MONITORING: A NEW DIMENSION OF COMPLIANCE ASSESSMENT

Previous attempts to use automatic devices as medication monitors were not feasible because of technical problems such as unusual appearance of the medication containers and their limited memory capacity (44–46). Progress in microelectronic technology facilitated the design of a convenient unobtrusive system with sufficiently enlarged data storage capacity.

The Medication Event Monitoring System (Aprex Corporation, Fremont, California) is an adaptation of a United States standard polypropylene vial. Within its child-proof closure is a microelectronic circuit for recording day and time of each opening and closing. Data are retrieved by connecting the medication container to a microcomputer communication port. Openings of the medication container are recorded as presumptive doses. Compliance data are obtained as listings of the date and time of individual container openings and closings, the duration of openings, and the time since the previous opening. From the time pattern of openings, information is yielded about patients' compliance to the prescribed daily drug regimen. Compliance is defined as openings recorded during the period divided by prescribed number of doses during the period multiplied by 100 and expressed in percent.

Medication behavior in outpatients on long-term treatment for chronic diseases, mainly cardiovascular, including hyperlipoproteinemia, was observed by means of continuous medication monitoring for up to more than 100 days (47). The monitoring showed marked inter- and intraindividual variations of compliance with different medicines, ranging from 43 up to 120%. Deviations from prescribed drug regimens were mostly due to omission of doses (23% of the prescribed doses) and less frequently caused by the use of extra doses (5.5% of the prescribed doses). In total, 403 days (32%) of the 1,259 monitored days were covered by partial or no intake of medication.

No other method of compliance assessment but continuous medication monitoring provides information on different patterns of noncompliance or can visualize the dynamics of drug intake behavior. One pattern of noncompliance recently described is patient-initiated drug holidays (48). These are defined as multiday drug-free periods when prescribed doses are consistently omitted. The occurrence of patient-initiated drug holidays seems to be prevalent; this pattern of noncompliance was observed in 50% of the patients studied (47). Mean compliance with lipid-lowering drugs was 84%, as evaluated by continuous medication monitoring in routine medical practice. It has been reiterated by investigators that patients with severe familial hypercholesterolemia participating in clinical trials were highly motivated and highly compliant with drug treatment. However, there is virtually no reason to believe that patients' medication intake behavior during clinical trials is principally different from that of patients under routine medical care.

RESULTS OF CLINICAL TRIALS WITH TWO HMG-CoA-REDUCTASE INHIBITORS, SIMVASTATIN AND LOVASTATIN

The HMG-CoA-reductase inhibitors are highly effective cholesterol-lowering agents. They have become a promising breakthrough in the treatment of severe hypercholesterolemia (49,50).

Compliance with simvastatin and lovastatin was evaluated in clinical trials by means of medication monitoring (Medication Event Monitoring System). Twelve patients with heterozygous familial hypercholesterolemia were prescribed simvastatin 20 mg once daily to be taken with the evening meal for 8 weeks (51). Mean total and low-density lipoprotein cholesterol decreased significantly from 377.2 mg/dl to 299.9 mg/dl and from 314.2 mg/dl to 241.4 mg/dl, respectively. However, wide variations of therapeutic response were measured in individual patients. Percentage reduction in low-density lipoprotein cholesterol from baseline values ranged from -8.7 to -50.1% (Fig. 14–1). Compliance data were available in 11 patients. The mean compliance was 82.6%, ranging from 33 to 114%. Variable degrees of drug compliance corresponded to variable therapeutic response. A clear dose–response relation with simvastatin was evident ($r = 0.790$, $p < 0.05$). Drug efficacy was confounded by partial compliance ($<75\%$) in four of 11 patients (Fig. 14–2).

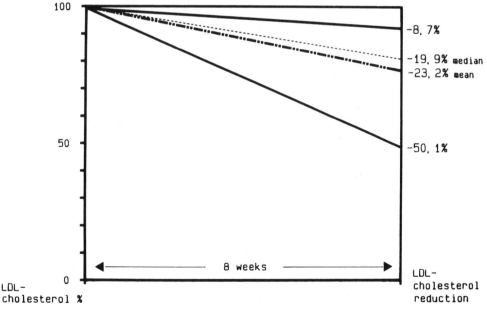

FIG. 14–1. Variability of low-density lipoprotein (LDL)–cholesterol reduction in 12 patients with familial hypercholesterolemia prescribed simvastatin 20 mg once daily for 8 weeks.

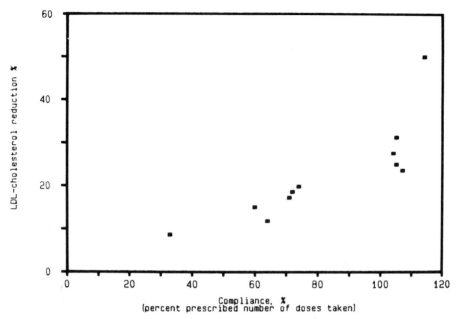

FIG. 14–2. Dose response with simvastatin 20 mg once daily in 11 patients with familial hypercholesterolemia. LDL, low-density lipoprotein.

Four different patterns of noncompliance were revealed by continuous monitoring, missed doses, patient-initiated drug holidays, extra doses, and deviations from the prescribed time of drug intake. Compliance with the prescribed time of drug intake was defined by opening events that occurred within an interval from 5 PM until midnight. The cutpoint of 5 PM was fixed as the earliest time of the evening meal. On average, 68% of container openings fell within this interval (range, 12.5 to 100%). Thus, complete patients' compliance even with a simple dosage regimen, as in taking one tablet with the evening meal, cannot be assumed.

Findings comparable to these were also revealed by medication event monitoring in the trial described next.

Twenty patients with heterozygous familial hypercholesterolemia completed a placebo-controlled study on lovastatin (38). Each patient received sequential 4-week periods of treatment with the following:

1. placebo
2. one 20-mg lovastatin tablet per day
3. two 20-mg lovastatin tablets per day
4. four 20-mg lovastatin tablets per day

all administered with the evening meal. Compliance was assessed by tablet count and by medication event monitoring. Returned unused tablets were counted at the end of each 4-week treatment period. Compliance by medication event monitoring was based on 16 weeks (112 days) of continuous monitoring in each patient, with the contents of the monitored drug container changed every 28 days, as noted above. Mean low-density lipoprotein cholesterol was lowered from baseline by 20, 29.5, and 36% with 20, 40, and 80 mg of lovastatin once daily.

Mean compliance by tablet count throughout the study (16 weeks) was 101.2% (range, 94 to 107%) compared with 84.4% compliance (range, 25 to 100%), as assessed by continuous medication monitoring.

Attenuated drug response was particularly due to frequent drug holidays, which were observed in 30% of the patients. On average, 79% of doses were used after 5 PM while patients were to take 20 mg of lovastatin. Again, there was a wide range from 12 to 100%. Deviations from the prescribed timing of drug intake were found in 40% of the patients. Furthermore, 80% of the patients deviated from the once-daily dosage regimen while they were to take two or four tablets.

PERSPECTIVES

Preliminary experience with continuous medication monitoring is promising with regard to several issues of the compliance problem. The system cannot prove dosage from ingestion and thus is not a perfect method, but neither are any of the other methods mentioned. However, its advantage is that it offers much more detailed information on patients' medication intake behavior, especially dose timing. This information could be used in medical practice for the purpose of patient counseling. Including patients in discussions during long-term treatment is the core of the compliance counseling process (52). Compliance data, provided by continuous monitoring, could be used as feedback with regard to patients' plasma cholesterol levels (5). It would then be possible to evaluate whether detailed therapeutic recommendations are accepted and acted on by patients. Furthermore, it would be of interest to evaluate different programs for improving patients' compliance (53), including the adjusting of drug regimens to patients' schedules (5). For example, flexible timing of doses by patients themselves may be appropriate with lipid-lowering drugs such as fibrates and HMG-CoA-reductase inhibitors.

For sustained release formulations of fibrates, once-daily dosage is recommended in the evening. It is assumed that this time schedule optimizes drug efficacy, according to the concept that the rate-limiting enzyme in cholesterol biosynthesis (HMG-CoA reductase) has its maximum activity during the night (54). However, the evening administration of bezafibrate retard was not superior in lowering low-density lipoprotein–cholesterol levels compared with the morning administration (55). The once-daily evening dosage of lovastatin was slightly more effective in low-density lipoprotein–cholesterol reduction than in once-daily morning dosage. However, the difference did not reach statistical significance (56). Therefore, it appears that patients' strict compliance with the evening schedule does not seem to be of major importance. The optimal timing of drug intake should be further investigated.

What are the implications of these data for drug trials? There is no doubt that patient compliance is an essential determinant of the outcome of drug trials, provided the prescribed drug regimen under investigation is effective (57). Compliance data may be of great value for the interpretation of drug trials (58). Medication event monitoring has the potential of increasing the amount of information on the relation between dose and response.

Deviations from prescribed drug regimens can be considered as "trials" or natural "experiments" executed by patients themselves, willingly or not (59–61). By dividing patients into compliers and noncompliers according to certain arbitrarily fixed cutpoints (e.g., number of medication returned, positive test of marker), information about the range of compliance or partial compliance and its relation to drug response is lost. The classification of compliers or noncompliers should be based on the level of compliance required to achieve the therapeutic response. Continuous medication monitoring is likely to comply with these requirements.

Principally, it has the potential to discriminate between patients' failure (partial or noncompliance) as one reason and drug failure (ineffectiveness) as another reason for the failure of drug therapy.

Patient compliance during clinical trials may be controlled by excluding noncompliers at entry. However, there are good reasons for taking compliance observations into account in the trial data analysis (51,58,62). The application of adequate compliance measurements is a prerequisite, however.

This information, compliance data, may also facilitate the interpretation of adverse drug reactions, of which most are dose-related. Data on the relation of adverse reactions with patients' medication intake behavior are still scarce and controversial (63).

Compliance measurement is only the first step. More research is needed to answer arising questions concerning the reasons for imperfect compliance. By this, even greater value could be achieved from clinical trials. Therefore, trial protocols should include well-controlled procedures for elucidating the reasons for partial compliance (64).

REFERENCES

1. American Heart Association. *1988 heart facts*. Dallas: American Heart Association, 1988.
2. Uemura K, Pisa Z. Recent trends in cardiovascular mortality in 27 industrialised countries. *World Health Stat Q* 1985;321:676–680.
3. Ross R. The pathogenesis of atherosclerosis: an update. *N Engl J Med* 1980;314:488–500.
4. Simons LA. Interrelations of lipids and lipoproteins with coronary artery disease mortality in 19 countries. *Am J Cardiol* 1986;57:5G–10G.
5. Expert Panel. Report of the National Cholesterol Education Program Expert Panel on Detection, Evaluation, and Treatment of High Blood Cholesterol in Adults. *Arch Intern Med* 1988;148:36–69.
6. European Atherosclerosis Society Study Group. The recognition and management of hyperlipidaemia in adults: a policy statement of the European Atherosclerosis Society. *Eur Heart J* 1988;9:571–600.
7. Castelli WP. Epidemiology of coronary heart disease: the Framingham Study. *Am J Med* 1984;76(suppl 2A):4–12.
8. Taylor WC, Pass ThM, Shepard DS, Komaroff AL. Cholesterol reduction and life expectancy. A model incorporating multiple risk factors. *Am Intern Med* 1987;106:605–614.
9. La Rosa J. Secondary hyperlipoproteinemia. In: Rifkind BM, Levy RI, eds. *Hyperlipidemia: diagnosis and therapy*. New York: Grune and Stratton, 1977;205–261.
10. Goldstein JL, Schrott HG, Hazzard WR, Bierman ER, Molidsky AG. Hyperlipidemia in coronary heart disease. II: Genetic analysis of lipid levels in 176 families and delineation of a new inherited disorder, combined hyperlipidemia. *J Clin Invest* 1973;52:1544–1568.
11. Illingworth DR. An overview of lipid-lowering drugs. *Drugs* 1988;36(suppl 3):63–71.
12. Haynes RB. Introduction. In: Haynes RB, Taylor DW, Sackett DL, eds. *Compliance in health care*. Baltimore, London: The Johns Hopkins University Press, 1979; 1–7.
13. Sackett DL, Snow J. The magnitude of compliance and noncompliance. In: Haynes RB, Taylor JW, Sackett DL, eds. *Compliance in health care*. Baltimore, London: The Johns Hopkins University Press, 1979;11–22.
14. Brown MB, Meredith AP, Page IH. Serum cholesterol reduction in patients; response, adherence and rebound measured by a quantitative diet test. *Am J Med* 1962;33:753–762.
15. Lewis LA, Brown HB, Page IH. Ten years' dietary treatment of primary hyperlipidemia. *Geriatrics* 1970;25:64–81.
16. Witters LA, Shulman RS, Krauss RM, Levy RI. Therapeutic failure in familial type II hyperlipoproteinemia. *Metabolism* 1976;25:1017–1026.

17. Schlierf G, Nikolaus TH, Oster P, Kruse W. Management of hyperlipoproteinemia—clinical aspects. In: Widhalm K, Naito HK, eds. *Recent aspects of diagnosis and treatment of lipoprotein disorders. Impact on prevention of atherosclerotic diseases.* New York: Alan R. Liss, 1988;197–203.
18. Lee-Han H, McGuire V, Boyd NF. A review of the methods used by studies of dietary measurement. *J Clin Epidemiol* 1989;42:269–279.
19. Caron HS, Roth HP. Patients' cooperation with a medical regimen: difficulties in identifying the noncooperator. *JAMA* 1968;203:922–926.
20. Malloy MJ, Kane JP, Kunitake ST, Tun P. Complementary of colestipol, niacin, and lovastatin in treatment of severe familial hypercholesterolemia. *Arch Intern Med* 1987;107:616–623.
21. Kruse W, Kohlmeier M, Nikolaus TH, Vogel G, Schlierf G. Langzeitbehandlung mit Colestipol. Compliance—Ein ungelöstes Problem. *Münch Med Wschr* 1989;131:407–409.
22. Roth HP, Caron HS, Hsi BP. Measuring intake of a prescribed medication: a bottle count and a tracer technique compared. *Clin Pharmacol Ther* 1970;11:228–237.
23. Roth HP, Caron HS, Hsi BP. Estimating a patient's cooperation with his regimen. *Am J Med Sci* 1971;262:269–273.
24. Gotto AM, De Bakey ME, Foreyt JP, Scott LW, Thornby JI. Dietary treatment of type IV hyperlipoproteinemia. *JAMA* 1977;237:1212–1215.
25. Green LW. Educational strategies to improve compliance with therapeutic and preventive regimens: the recent evidence. In: Haynes RB, Taylor DW, Sackett DL, eds. *Compliance in health care.* Baltimore, London: The Johns Hopkins University Press, 1979;157–173.
26. Latiolais CJ, Berry CC. Misuse of prescription medications by outpatients. *Drug Intell Clin Pharm* 1969;3:270–277.
27. Chubb M, Winship W III. The pharmacist's role in preventing medication errors made by cardiac and hyperlipoproteinemic outpatients. *Drug Intell Clin Pharm* 1974;8:430–436.
28. Slack J. Risks of ischaemic heart disease in familial hyperlipoproteinaemic states. *Lancet* 1969;II:1380–1382.
29. West RJ, Lloyd JK. Long-term follow-up of children with familial hypercholesterolaemia treated with cholestyramine. *Lancet* 1980;II:873–875.
30. Coronary Drug Project Research Group. The Coronary Drug Project: design, methods, and baseline results. *Circulation* 1973;47,48(suppl 1):1–179.
31. Kuo PT, Hayase K, Kostis JB, Moreyra AE. Use of combined diet and colestipol in long-term (7–7 1/2 years) treatment of patients with type II hyperlipoproteinemia. *Circulation* 1979;59:199–211.
32. Lipid Research Clinics Program. The Lipid Research Clinics Coronary Primary Prevention Trial results. I. Reduction in incidence of coronary heart disease. *JAMA* 1984;251:351–364.
33. Lipid Research Clinics Program. The Lipid Research Clinics Coronary Primary Prevention Trial results. II. The relationship of reduction in incidence of coronary heart disease to cholesterol lowering. *JAMA* 1984;251:365–374.
34. Frick MH, Elo O, Haapa K, et al. Helsinki Heart Study: Primary-prevention trial with gemfibrozil in middle-aged men with dyslipidemia. *N Engl J Med* 1987;317:1237–1245.
35. Blankenhorn DH, Nessim SA, Johnson RL, Sanmarco ME, Azen SP, Cashin-Hemphill L. Beneficial effects of combined colestipol-niacin therapy on coronary atherosclerosis and coronary venous bypass grafts. *JAMA* 1987;257:3233–3240.
36. Cramer JA, Mattson RH, Prevey ML, Scheyer RD, Quelette VL. How often is medication taken as prescribed? A novel assessment technique. *JAMA* 1989;261:3273–3277.
37. Feely M, Kumar S, Tindall H, Pullar T. Assessing compliance: is return tablet count worthwhile? *Br J Clin Pharmacol* 1988;25:641P–642P.
38. Kruse W, Nikolaus TH, Weber E, Schlierf G. Lovastatin in patients with heterozygous familial hypercholesterolaemia—a placebo-controlled study with special regard to patients' compliance. *Eur J Clin Pharmacol (in press).*
39. Pullar T, Kumar S, Tindale H, Feely M. Time to stop counting the tablets? *Clin Pharmacol Ther* 1989;46:163–168.
40. Mäenpää H, Manninen V, Heinonen OP. Comparison of the digoxin marker with capsule counting and compliance questionnaire methods for measuring compliance to medication in a clinical trial. *Eur Heart J* 1987;8:39–43.
41. Dorr AE, Gundersen K, Schneider JC Jr, Spencer TW, Martin WB. Colestipol hydrochloride in hypercholesterolaemic patients—effects on serum cholesterol and mortality. *J Chron Dis* 1978;31:5–14.
42. Mäenpää H, Javela K, Pikkarainen J, Mälkönen M, Heinonen OP, Manninen V. Minimal doses of digoxin: a new marker for compliance to medication. *Eur Heart J* 1987;8(suppl I):31–37.
43. Norell SE. Methods in assessing drug compliance. *Acta Med Scand* 1983;213:35–40.
44. Moulding T. Proposal for a time-recording pill dispenser as a method for studying and supervising the self-administration of drugs. *Am Rev Respir Dis* 1962;85:754–757.
45. Moulding T, Onstad GD, Sbarbaro JA. Supervision of outpatient drug therapy with the medication monitor. *Arch Intern Med* 1970;73:559–564.

46. Norell SE, Granström PA, Wassen R. A medication monitor and fluorescein technique designed to study medication behaviour. *Acta Ophthalmol* 1980;58:459–467.
47. Kruse W, Weber E. Dynamics of drug regimen compliance—its assessment by microprocessor-based monitoring. *Eur J Clin Pharmacol* 1990;38:561–565.
48. Urquhart J, Chevalley C. Impact of unrecognized dosing errors on the cost and effectiveness of pharmaceuticals. *Drug Inf J* 1988;22:363–378.
49. Grundy SM. HMG-CoA reductase inhibitors for treatment of hyperlipoproteinemia. *N Engl J Med* 1988;319:24–33.
50. Henwood JM, Heel RC. Lovastatin A preliminary review of its pharmacologic properties and therapeutic use in hyperlipidaemia. *Drugs* 1988;36:429–454.
51. Kruse W, Schlierf G, Weber E. Continuous compliance monitoring—its utility for the interpretation of drug trials. *Eur J Clin Pharmacol* 1989;36(suppl A):289.
52. Cramer JA. Practical strategies for compliance. *VA Practitioner* 1988;5:109–119.
53. Norell SE. Improving medication compliance: a randomised clinical trial. *Br Med J* 1979;2:1031–1033.
54. Parker TS, McNamara DJ, Brown C, et al. Mevalonic acid in human plasma: relationship of concentration and circadian rhythm to cholesterol synthesis rates in man. *Proc Natl Acad Sci USA* 1982;79:3037–3041.
55. Hanefeld M. Timing of intake of lipid lowering drugs: is that of importance? *Klin Wochenschr* 1989;67:511–512.
56. Illingworth DR. Comparative efficacy of once versus twice daily mevinolin in the therapy of familial hypercholesterolemia. *Clin Pharmacol Ther* 1986;40:338–343.
57. Feinstein AR. Biostatistical problems in "compliance bias." *Clin Pharmacol Ther* 1974;16:846–857.
58. Joyce CRB. Patient co-operation and the sensitivity of clinical trials. *J Chron Dis* 1962;15:1025–1036.
59. Guayatt G, Sackett DL, Taylor DW, Chong J, Roberts R, Pugsley S. Determining optimal therapy—randomized trials in individualized patients. *N Engl J Med* 1986;314:889–892.
60. Weintraub M. Intelligent and capricious non-compliance. In: Lasagna L, ed. *Compliance*. Mt. Kisco, New York: Futura Publishing Company, 1976;35.
61. Weintraub M. A different view of patient compliance in the elderly. In: Vestal RE, ed. *Drug treatment in the elderly*. Sidney, Auckland, Bristol, Boston, Hong Kong, Tokyo: ADIS Health Science Press, 1984;43–50.
62. Coats AJS, Adamopoulos S, Meyer TE, Conway J, Sleight P. Effects of physical training in chronic heart failure. *Lancet* 1990;335:63–66.
63. Haynes RB. Determinants of compliance: the disease and the mechanisms of treatment. In: Haynes RB, Taylor DW, Sackett DL, eds. *Compliance in health care*. Baltimore, London: The Johns Hopkins University Press, 1979;49–77.
64. Kruse W, Schlierf G, Weber E. Monitoring compliance in clinical trials. *Lancet* 1990;335:803–804.

Patient Compliance in Medical
Practice and Clinical Trials
edited by J.A. Cramer and B. Spilker
Raven Press, Ltd., New York © 1991

15

Clinical Correlates of Antidepressant Compliance

Frederick W. Engstrom

Mental Health Department, Park Nicollet Medical Center,
Minneapolis, Minnesota 55416

Psychiatry affords two windows with which to view the field of compliance research. First, as practitioners of one branch of medicine, psychiatrists can investigate factors that enhance compliance and that detract from compliance, and they can then look at strategies that improve compliance. In this regard, psychiatry offers the same perspectives that other branches of medicine do, albeit with different illnesses and different treatments. Second, as practitioners of psychological treatments and as trained observers of psychological phenomena, psychiatrists can be particularly attuned to the psychological nuances of compliance issues in all areas of medicine. Psychiatrists may be in a unique position to discuss with patients the psychological aspects of their treatment, and in particular, they can make psychological observations about compliance. It should be noted, however, that no firm data imply that psychiatrists are any more successful at enhancing compliance than are any other physicians. The field of compliance research within psychiatry is in its infancy because of the poor methodology of the past. Definitive methods have not been available to measure compliance until recently. Without such methodology, physicians have not had good data, and without good compliance data, the physician cannot always make well-informed treatment decisions.

REVIEW OF THE LITERATURE CONCERNING COMPLIANCE WITH PSYCHIATRIC TREATMENT

One South African study on compliance (1) was notable for its careful 2-year follow-up, its excellent methodology, and its large (406) patient cohort. The patient sample consisted of those on phenothiazines and/or lithium and thus presumably included those with bipolar disorder, schizophrenia, and other psychotic disorders. Compliance was measured by pill count, medication refill records, urine tests for metabolites, serum levels of patients on lithium, and by interviews with reliable family members. Compliance was defined as the percent of the total prescribed doses that were actually taken. The results indicated that 51% of men and 41% of women were noncompliant, with black and colored patients having poorer compliance than white patients. Results were similar for lithium and phenothiazines. Socioeconomic status did not seem to be an important factor. Intramuscular medication seemed to lead to slightly better compliance. Patients younger than age 30 were less compliant than older patients. The authors concluded that the main reasons for noncompliance were active resistance to taking medication, adverse reactions, and nonattendance at clinics.

Another uncontrolled compliance study (2) involved 26 adult men who were treated with lithium at an outpatient Veterans Administration clinic in California. When these patients exhibited either a worsening of their psychiatric condition or other behavioral indicators of noncompliance, serum levels of lithium were taken. Sometimes patients were forewarned about upcoming serum lithium levels (standard). At other times, unannounced (spot) levels were drawn. Seventeen patients showed unexplained symptoms of mania. Four of these 17 had normal spot levels and normal standard test levels. Four of them had low standard levels and thus did not need to have spot levels drawn. Nine of the 17 had normal standard test levels but low spot levels. In addition to the 17 patients with unexplained mania, three patients had an attitude that suggested noncompliance. All three of these patients had normal standard test levels, but two of three had low spot test levels. Overall it can be concluded that of the 15 patients who had low serum levels and thus who were probably noncompliant with the medicine, only four were detected by standard preannounced lithium levels and the other 11 of them were detected only when they were evaluated with unannounced spot serum lithium levels. Interviewing the 11 surreptitious noncompliers revealed that eight of them took lithium sporadically but always resumed it before planned blood drawings. The other three patients took no lithium at all except for active preloading to deceive the staff. Further questioning revealed that four of the patients believed that they were normal and did not need medicine, three of them did not like the adverse reactions, and four simply did not bother to take it. Subsequent interventions were aimed at the 11 noncompliant patients, and eventually six of them were able to become compliant (as measured by subsequent spot checks) to an effective regimen.

Another study (3) involved 48 outpatients on lithium who were studied for 12 months. Compliance was measured by serum levels and by measuring the attendance at scheduled appointments, with 75% attendance used as the cutoff point for defining compliance. One patient was noncompliant by both measures and 11 more were noncompliant by one of the two measures. There was a correlation between noncompliance and relapse, including a relation between noncompliance and hospitalization. As part of the study, patients were administered the Standardized Compliance Questionnaire developed by Sackett. This questionnaire was based on the Health Belief Model. Importantly, neither the items rated on that questionnaire nor demographic variables accounted for the variation to any extent. In particular, patients' perception of the efficacy of the treatment, seriousness of the illness, relative costs and benefits of the illness, diagnostic subgroups, mood state, reported adverse reactions, age, sex, and educational background all failed to predict which patients would be noncompliant.

One study in Kenya (4) of 100 adult patients discharged from the psychiatric hospital on antidepressants or neuroleptics were interviewed 3 months after discharge, and then a relative was interviewed. Through this crude method a 55% noncompliance rate without specific criteria was revealed.

One study (5) involved psychiatric inpatients who refused to take medicine. All patients who refused to take medicine during a 3-month period of time were interviewed. One group of patients had paranoia and responded to stress by refusing to do whatever was requested of them, including taking medicine. A second group also seemed to have a high degree of psychiatric symptomatology, although their distinguishing characteristic was their statement that it was their legal right to refuse medicine. A third group represented patients with reasons for refusing medicine that varied with the individual situation. Some had transient delusional reasons, some had adverse reactions, and some used drug refusal as a manipulative pattern. Only five of 72 episodes of refusing medicine seriously impaired patient care, and most episodes of drug refusal were self-limited. Adverse reactions to the medicine played only a small role in accounting for drug refusal.

Patients who were discharged from a psychiatric hospital in Toronto were enrolled in a controlled study (6) at the time of discharge. The experimental group received nine weekly lectures to educate them about their medicine. Compliance was measured by pill count and urine samples. Only nine of 35 controls and 23 of 32 experimentals submitted to the pill count, and only 20 of 35 controls and 18 of 32 experimentals gave a urine sample at follow-up. Groups did not match well at baseline. Questionnaires at baseline and at follow-up revealed that experimentals became less frightened of adverse reactions and were less fearful of addiction than were controls. Twelve other items rated on the questionnaire revealed no advantage for the experimental group. Experimentals received more contact from health professionals than did controls. Overall, the patients given education had higher rates of compliance.

A fascinating study (7) of outpatients from the lithium clinic at University of California at Los Angeles tried to validate a hypothesis for compliance termed the Theory of Reasoned Action. Forty-eight patients were surveyed, of whom 54% said that they took medicine exactly as prescribed, 15% did not take it at all, and 31% had periodic lapses. The researchers concluded that normative beliefs were the most potent factors in determining whether patients intended to take pills and that patients' intent determined compliance. The most powerful normative belief was whether the patient's physician thought that the patient should take the medicine. Other normative beliefs that contributed to compliance were the encouragement of families, friends, and lithium experts. The authors stated that "if the self-report differed greatly from the 'true' compliance rate, then the model discussed in this paper was not tested adequately."

Another study (8) involved 30 psychiatric outpatients taking neuroleptic medication who were enrolled in a program for those with repeated psychiatric hospitalizations and failure to remain involved with outpatient treatment. After patients were provided extensive information and an educational program, careful measurement revealed that their knowledge base improved. They had four sessions at 1-month intervals, and compliance was assessed at each session. First, patients gave verbal reports to the psychiatrists. Second, patients gave verbal reports to case managers during therapy sessions. Third, monthly pill counts were made. There was a high degree of correlation between the three methods of assessing compliance. Despite the education, no improvement in compliance was noted. Furthermore, there was no correlation between knowledge gain, decreased adverse reaction reporting, and improved compliance. Two previous papers (9,10) had also shown no correlation between forewarning of the occurrence of adverse reactions and subsequent discontinuation of psychotropic medication.

Firm conclusions are lacking from this review of the psychiatric literature. The conclusions mimic the weak methodologies employed in the studies reviewed:

1. No reliable predictors of compliance or noncompliance were revealed for patients with psychiatric illness. Demographic data, health beliefs, and perceptions of illness did not predict compliance.
2. Rates of noncompliance varied widely with the populations studied.
3. When compliance was measured directly by spot drug serum concentration testing, the rate of noncompliance was much higher than revealed by other methods. The spot checks of lithium levels were particularly revealing.
4. It is not clear that education helps to improve compliance with psychotropic medicine.
5. Noncompliance is associated with poor outcome in severely ill psychiatric outpatients. The line of causality is unclear: Does worsening psychiatric condition cause noncompliance or does noncompliance cause the relapse?
6. In short, studies are needed in which the patient's compliance is known and in which the patient is accountable to the physician for that information.

EXPERIENCES WITH A COMPLIANCE MONITORING DEVICE IN AN OUTPATIENT PSYCHIATRIC PRACTICE

Method

Twenty-seven outpatients who were prescribed antidepressant drugs were given a standard medication container of the type routinely used by retail pharmacies to dispense prescription medicines, fitted with a specially designed cap that incorporated microcircuitry capable of recording times and dates of cap opening and closing (Medication Event Monitor System, Aprex, Fremont, California). Encoded data for the opening and closing of pill bottles were collected by connecting the Medication Event Monitoring System cap via a communication cable to a personal computer, loading onto a floppy disk, and sending to Aprex for statistical analysis. Thus, by design the medication event monitoring data were not available to the physician at the time of the patient visits, and judgments of clinical status were made before receipt of analyzed compliance data.

In the interpretation of the medication event data, opening and closing times recurring within 15 min of one another were ignored, by policy, as being indicative of difficulties in opening or reclosing the childproof cap. Unscheduled openings and closings in excess of the prescribed daily number (and these were rare events) were ignored for the purposes of this study, which exclusively focused on omissions of doses.

All patients were diagnosed as having major depression by criteria in DSM III-R. Some of the patients were prescribed antidepressants for the first time, whereas others already had been stabilized on antidepressants and were taking them either as a continuation of their treatment or to prevent recurrence of depression.

Patients were prescribed a variety of antidepressants: desipramine, trazodone, nortriptyline, fluoxetine, doxepin, amitriptyline, imipramine, and phenelzine. Ten patients took medicine once a day, 15 patients took it twice daily, three patients took it thrice daily, and one patient took it four times daily.

Clinical status was judged on clinical grounds alone, and the observer was blinded to the results of the compliance measurements. Thus, this was an observational study to collect information about compliance in normal clinical practice.

Results

The study made the physician more attentive to compliance problems than he previously had been. He asked more questions about compliance than usual. Three patients expressed the view that knowing their dosing was being monitored helped them follow the regimen more faithfully.

Had compliance data been immediately available during the patient's visit, certain treatment decisions would have changed. For example, one seriously depressed patient had missed eight doses but had only reported missing one or two. In retrospect, it seems she was too confused to remember correctly. She was hospitalized a few days after this visit because of her worsening condition. Had the compliance data been available, the hospitalization might have either been averted or expedited; in either case, her care would have changed had the data showing the many missed doses been immediately available. Three other poorly compliant patients were later confronted with this fact during therapy sessions when the data became available. One decided to drop out of treatment, because he recognized that his motivation for improving was marginal; the other two patients subsequently improved clinically. Compliance was no longer being monitored so the reasons for the improvement were unclear.

Overall, irrespective of compliance, 21 of 27 patients (78%) improved clinically or stayed improved if previously they had been stabilized. Of the three patients who took less than 80% of their prescribed doses, none improved. Of those who took 80 to 89% of their doses, three of four improved. Of those who took at least 90% of their prescribed doses, 18 of 20 improved.

Overall, in the entire group, 16% of all prescribed doses were omitted. None of the seven patients who took less than 90% of prescribed doses volunteered that they were poorly compliant.

THE FUTURE OF COMPLIANCE RESEARCH

The results of the experiences are intriguing. The discussion that follows presumes that the methodology reported can be used in many settings and, in particular, that the Medication Event Monitoring System monitor can be placed in the physician's office and can give immediate information. Thus the psychological and behavioral issues underlying compliance can be elucidated now that a much sturdier method of measuring compliance is available.

Measuring and Assessing Degrees of Compliance

With such methodology, one can evaluate which patients are noncompliant and which are compliant. By using continuous monitoring of compliance, one can measure the effects of

1. Different diagnoses. It is often assumed that manic and schizophrenic patients are poorly compliant and that depressed and anxious patients are more compliant.

2. Different severity of illnesses. It is often assumed that more severely depressed, psychotic, anxious, or manic patients are less compliant than are patients who are less severely ill, even if they have the same diagnosis. By measuring the relation between illness severity and compliance, one can also help determine which patients need close monitoring or hospitalization if they are to receive full benefit from their medicine.
3. Different medicines. Controlled studies have not shown statistical differences of efficacy when comparing antidepressants. Yet clinical experience indicates that such differences exist. In the past it was difficult to prove differential effectiveness because of the confounding effects of poor compliance and the difficulty measuring the compliance. A sturdy method of measuring compliance should make it possible to compare efficacy of antidepressants when the medicine is taken as directed. Such knowledge is particularly helpful when dispensing medicines in controlled situations (e.g., hospitals).
4. Different regimens. Folk wisdom suggests that more complex regimens cause lower compliance, but the careful study of that belief is lacking.
5. Different organizational aspects of health care. Many studies (9) suggest that organizational factors influence compliance:
   • nature of the referral process
   • continuity of care
   • personalized care
   • scheduling of appointments
   • length of referral times
   • length of waiting time
   • on-site treatment
   • increased patient supervision
   • good links between inpatient and outpatient services
   • positive staff attitude
Careful methodologies could look at the relative importance of these.

Compliance Monitoring and Therapeutics

A second area for research involves the effect of compliance monitoring on therapeutics in the outpatient setting. The following questions could be addressed:

1. Does a patient who knows he or she is being monitored for compliance have better compliance to the medication regimen than the patient who is not being monitored?
2. Will physicians who measure compliance discuss adverse reactions and other issues related to compliance more often than physicians who do not measure compliance? Will measuring compliance lead to a different therapeutic interaction, in which compliance is discussed in more detail and with more honesty? Will discussions about compliance lead to discussions about the following factors?
   • disagreement about the diagnosis
   • denial about the illness
   • forgetfulness
   • disagreement about the severity of the condition
   • anger at the physician

- anger at the medicine
- unhappiness with the treatment plan in general

3. Will information about compliance help physicians to make more confident decisions about treatment? With objective data on compliance such as that provided by Medication Event Monitoring System monitors, it could be easier to decide whether to change medicines, change the dose, or continue the regimen as is, with or without adding strong encouragement for good compliance. Monitoring could make it easier to decide if a patient can comply at all as an outpatient—a major issue with those who are delusional, delirious, or demented.

4. Which strategies improve compliance? It should be possible to determine which strategies best address certain causes of noncompliance. When forgetfulness is a factor, the relative efficacy of memory aids and the recruitment of family members can be assessed. When denial or anger are issues, the usefulness of different psychological interventions can be measured. When adverse reactions and the prescribing regimens confound compliance, the efficacy of various changes in the medication regimen can be assessed.

5. With this above data, it should be possible to measure whether improving compliance really improves outcome.

6. Finally, the costs of both measuring compliance and trying to improve compliance can be compared with any potential savings realized by avoiding hospitalization; eliminating unnecessary procedures, physician visits, or medication changes; or hastening the treatment response.

Compliance Monitoring and Psychiatric Research

Continuous monitoring of compliance could be particularly important in psychiatric research, as the following considerations suggest:

1. When new antidepressants or other psychotropic agents are tested, an accurate measure of compliance could be used, with placebo control data, to show the relation between dosage actually taken and both efficacy and adverse reactions. In this way, data from noncompliant patients are included in the analysis but interpreted, whenever possible, as effects related to low or zero dosage. Furthermore, a more accurate picture could emerge as to the adverse reactions experienced by those patients taking the full dose. The effective dosage level could be detected more readily, based on the lowest dosage *actually taken* that is consistent with satisfactory efficacy.

2. Microelectronic monitoring of compliance could help in better understanding the comparative efficacies of two antidepressants or neuroleptics with substantially different adverse reaction profiles. For example, when comparing a tricyclic antidepressant with a monoamine oxidase inhibitor, fluoxetine or bupropion, one would expect different rates of compliance because they have different adverse reaction profiles. Understanding a medicine's pharmacologic effectiveness (i.e., its effects when taken correctly) is one dimension of efficacy but quite different than its use-effectiveness (i.e., its range of effects in a representative group of variably compliant patients). However, both are important. With differential compliance measured reliably, one could also get a better idea about both practical and theoretical differences in efficacy and how those interrelate in various clinical and social conditions.

3. Research comparing psychotherapy with antidepressants could be improved by reliable measurements of compliance with prescribed drug regimens. In such studies, the effect of antidepressants may be underestimated by unwittingly averaging data from noncompliant patients together with data from compliant patients. Focus on measuring noncompliance with the one mode of treatment naturally focuses attention on the parallel problem in the other. Dropouts and noncompliers with both modalities of treatment should be analyzed comparably.

REFERENCES

1. Gillis LS, Trollip D, Jakoet A, Holden T. Noncompliance with psychotropic medication. *SAMJ* 1987;72:602–606.
2. Schwarcz G, Silbergeld S. Serum lithium spot checks to evaluate medication compliance. *J Clin Psychopharmacol* 1983;6:356–358.
3. Connelly CE, Davenport YB, Nurnberger JI. Adherence to treatment regimen in a lithium carbonate clinic. *Arch Gen Psychiatry* 1982;39:585–588.
4. Okonji MMO, Dhadphale M. Treatment compliance among psychiatric outpatients in Kenya. *Acta Psychiatr Scand* 1987;75:240–242.
5. Appelbaum PS, Gutheil TG. Drug refusal: a study of psychiatric inpatients. *Am J Psychiatry* 1980;137:340–346.
6. Seltzer A, Roncari I, Garfinkel P. Effect on patient education on medication compliance. *Can J Pyschiatry* 1980;25:638–645.
7. Cochran SD, Gitlin MJ. Attitudinal correlates of lithium compliance in bipolar affective disorders. *J Nerve Ment Dis* 1988;176:457–464.
8. Brown CS, Wright RG, Christensen DB. Association between type of medication instruction and patients' knowledge, side effects, and compliance. *Hosp Community Psychiatry* 1987;38:55–60.
9. Myers ED, Calvert EJ. The effect of forewarning on the occurrence of side effects and discontinuance of medication in patients on dothiepin. *J Int Med Res* 1976;4:237–240.
10. Myers ED, Calvert EJ. The effect of forewarning on the occurrence of side effects and discontinuance of medication in patients on amitriptyline. *Br J Psychiatry* 1973;122:461–464.
11. Meichenbaum D, Turk DC. *Facilitating treatment adherence*. New York: Plenum Press, 1987.

*Patient Compliance in Medical
Practice and Clinical Trials*
edited by J.A. Cramer and B. Spilker
Raven Press, Ltd., New York © 1991

16

Oral Contraceptive Compliance and Its Role in the Effectiveness of the Method

Linda S. Potter

Family Health International, Research Triangle Park, North Carolina 27709

More than 63 million women around the world take oral contraceptives, colloquially known as "the Pill." In the United States, one of every four sexually active women of reproductive age uses oral contraceptives, adding up to more than 13 million users in this country alone.

Yet, despite the volume of use in the 30 years since oral contraceptives were introduced, little attention has been paid to oral contraceptive compliance and its role in the effectiveness of oral contraceptives.

DEFINITIONS OF ORAL CONTRACEPTIVE EFFECTIVENESS/COMPLIANCE

To examine the effectiveness of oral contraceptives in preventing pregnancy and the role of compliance in oral contraceptive effectiveness, the terms *effectiveness* and *compliance* are defined:

1. *Effectiveness* of a contraceptive method is "the reduction its use brings to the risk or probability of conception when no method is used" (1).
2. *Use-effectiveness rate* is "the percentage of women not experiencing a contraceptive failure, pregnancy or conception, by duration of use" (2). Data on use-effectiveness are usually presented as failure rates (i.e., as the percentage of women who do experience conception or pregnancy while using oral contraceptives.[1]
3. *Oral contraceptive compliance* is defined as "the use of a contraceptive method in a consistent and ongoing manner for the prevention of pregnancy" (4). As with other medications, this definition does not imply that poor compliance is necessarily the fault of the user. It also does not assume that the clinician, pharmacist, and/or manufacturer have provided the user with complete or correct information about the pharmaceutical prescription for use.

---

[1]A 3% failure rate for the pill is compared with a 7% overall failure rate for contraception in general (3).

EFFECTIVENESS OF ORAL CONTRACEPTIVES

Method-Effectiveness

When used exactly as prescribed, oral contraceptives have the lowest failure rates of any reversible form of contraception available in the United States. The lowest expected first-year failure rates, if oral contraceptives are taken correctly, are between 0.1 and 1% for the combined estrogen-progestin pills (5–7).

Use-Effectiveness

Despite the low method failure rates, oral contraceptive failure rates are much higher in the general population than in clinical trials. Effectiveness in actual use has varied dramatically from study to study, with reports varying from the usually cited 3%, based primarily on clinical trials data, to as high as 16 to 20% in some surveys of the combined pill (8–22) (see Table 16–1).

The 1982 United States National Survey of Family Growth found typical first year failure rates to be 2.9% for married women of reproductive age in the United States but 5.7% for single women, when standardized and adjusted for age, contraceptive intention, race, parity, income, and underreporting of abortions (5). Underreporting of abortions may inflate use-effectiveness rates in many studies.

Failures During Use Versus Because of Discontinuation

As many as 60% of new oral contraceptive users discontinue use before the end of the first year, most within the first 6 months. Pregnancies that occur after discontinuation are not dealt with in this chapter because, as Trussell & Kost (7) stated, "It is preferable to measure separately continuation and failure during use, because they are both of interest and are behaviorally and analytically distinct." This also means that a woman who has missed several pills in sequence is defined as a continuing (if poorly compliant) user as long as she describes herself as such.

FACTORS AFFECTING COMPLIANCE/EFFECTIVENESS

Three groups of factors have been shown to affect oral contraceptive compliance and its relation to adverse reactions and continuation. Those factors include personal characteristics of the user, method-related factors, and service-system characteristics (see Fig. 16–1).

User Characteristics

Sociodemographic characteristics clearly affect oral contraceptive use. Older women, those with more children, and those who want no more children tend to have the lowest failure rates in the United States and in developing countries (5,7,15). Lower failure rates among older women may be due to greater motivation to not become pregnant, or as one study found, one reason for the greater use-effec-

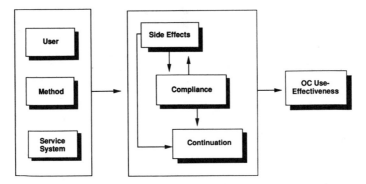

FIG. 16–1. Conceptual model of oral contraceptive use.

tiveness of oral contraceptives in older women is that they had sexual intercourse less often than younger women (5).

Higher education is associated with a better understanding of the rules of oral contraceptive use but may or may not be associated with more effective use (15). Correct use may also be affected by the amount of social support received, especially from the husband (23) but also from providers (24,25). Psychosocial characteristics are dealt with most often in studies of adolescents (12,17,25–27).

One of the strongest predictors of oral contraceptive compliance is simply correct knowledge of *how* to take the pill. Five oral contraceptive compliance studies (12,13,19,21,28) that examined levels of user knowledge found real gaps. For example, Potter et al. (19) found that less than 30% of the 500 women studied in Colombia knew the correct length of time to wait between pill packets (21- or 28-day), a fact verified by the calendar data collected in that study. The 1988 Demographic Health Survey in Egypt found less than 12% of a national sample of 1,258 pill users interviewed knew how long to wait between packets (29). Similar problems have been found with knowledge of what to do when more than one pill is missed. Even in developed countries, several studies have confirmed that poor knowledge contributes to poor compliance (12,13,21,28) (see Table 16–1).

Method-Related Factors

Menstrual irregularities and other adverse reactions are the most frequent reasons given by patients for discontinuing the pill. These include nausea, vomiting, dizziness, and headaches, as well as spotting or breakthrough bleeding (16,22,30–36). Metson (37) and Wheble et al. (38) found that the fear of adverse reactions also could be used to predict discontinuation.

There are almost no data on the relation between adverse reactions and noncompliance. This is because adverse reactions and menstrual irregularities can be either the cause or the effect of missed pills, making it difficult to tease out the sequence of the problem. For example, nausea after starting oral contraceptives may lead to sporadic use, which in turn may provoke breakthrough bleeding. Only four studies report on the association between adverse reactions and compliance. One found no relation (17,18) and three found a clear relation (12,19,22). Breakthrough bleeding is a particularly common adverse reaction of missed pills and is sometimes confusing

TABLE 16–1. *Literature that measures oral contraceptive compliance*

Study	N/Time	Site	Method of measuring compliance	Definition of compliance	Compliance rate	Comments
Cobb et al. 1966 (9)	45/15 months	Lahore, Pakistan (rural, poor)	Monthly home visits with spot checks of pill bottles (all started each month on 1st day of new moon) (P)[a]	Regular (none missed, none extra) Took all pills in each cycle but irregularly Omitted 1 pill in any cycle Omitted 2 or more pills in any cycle	53% 4% 9% 33%	Reinforcement effect of monthly visits increased compliance "Prohibitively expensive for natural program" 5 became pregnant 9.5/100 woman-years
DuRant et al. 1984 Jay et al. 1984 (11,25,26)	56/1 year	Atlanta, Georgia (14–19 yr old) (low-income teen clinic)	Self-report Pill count Urinary fluorescence for riboflavin Appointment compliance Avoidance of pregnancy (P) (NOTE: self-report found to be 90% accurate based on riboflavin measure)	Did not miss 3 or more contraceptive pills during month + positive urine + kept appointment + not pregnant	Guttman scale	Noncompliance associated with multiple partners, previous abortions, low self-esteem, fear of pregnancy. Peer counselors more effective than nurses 3 pregnancies in 1st 3 months
Emans et al. 1987 (12)	209/1 year	Boston, Massachusetts (13–19 yr olds) I—Teen clinic = 61 II—Family planning clinic = 99 III—Private practice = 49	Data collected by the examining physician at 3 months, 12 months Does not define how measured (P)	Returned for scheduled visit and either took pill as directed or stopped because no longer needed oral contraceptives	I = 48% (3 mo) II = 65% III = 84% I = 34% (12 mo) II = Missing III = 55%	At long-term follow-up, site was only predictor of compliance; few read written instructions at Site I (10 pregnancies, all at Site I: inner-city teen clinic)
Finlay and Scott 1986 (13)	161/3 months	Glasgow, Scotland (16–35 yr old) (middle-class private practice)	Questionnaire given during a clinic visit (R)[a]	Followed manufacturer's instructions Missed pill in last 3 months Transition error (all on 21-day pills)	28% 27% 32%	Only 26% would use condom if missed pill; 35% believed it harms body not to menstruate No pregnancies
Goldstuck et al. 1987 (28)	216/3 months	Johannesburg, South Africa (family planning clinic, teens 18 years)	Questionnaire given during a clinic visit (based on Finlay & Scott's) (R)	Took correctly cycle to cycle Missed at least 1 pill in last 3 months Transition error (all on 28-day pills)	93% 31% 7%	Only 25% would use back-up if missed a pill; regular time = half as likely to miss; no relation between length of oral contraceptive use and compliance No mention of pregnancy
Hamilton and Hoogland 1989 (41)	30/2 cycles	Maastricht, The Netherlands	Experimental noncompliance (P) I—intact pill pack II—day 1 placebo III—day 2 placebo	Blinded incorrect dosing on 1st or 2nd day of 2nd cycle (groups II and III)	N/A	Studied evidence of follicular activity at beginning of 2nd cycle: I—25%; II—33%; III—11% Concluded that escape ovulation is most likely if pill for day 1 is missed (group II)

198

Reference	Sample/duration	Location/population	Method (study type)	Compliance measure	%	Findings
Laurie and Korba 1972 (16)	2173/10 cycles	United States and Puerto Rico (15–49 yr old) (8 sites)	Clinical trial of microdose norgesterol (P)	No tablet omitted per cycle	86%	17% discontinued use due to adverse reactions; 37 pregnancies
Neel et al. 1985, 1987 (17,18)	55 teens/4 months	Stanford, California Adolescent clinics = 22 College health service = 34	1) Serum levels of norethindrone 2) Urinary florescence for riboflavin 3) Self-report and absence of pregnancy (P) (based on DuRant et al.)	Remained in study 4 months, had positive urine	48% clinic group 70% college group	Positive self-concept, high autonomy associated with compliance; compliance *not* associated with adverse reactions; 3 pregnancies
Potter et al. 1988 (19)	341/4 months	Magdalena, Colombia Rural primary health care service	2-week calendar data collected in home interviews (P)	No pills missed; Missed 1 pill, took 2 next day; Ran out; Missed 1 or more pills in 2 weeks; Transition error (in 2 weeks)	41% 1% 6% 25% 27%	Home delivery of oral contraceptives; both users and providers had poor knowledge of oral contraceptive use; 7 pregnancies
Preston 1974 (20)	3,974/7 cycles	15 sites, United States	Daily record of pills taken or missed (P)	Number of missed pills per cycle by dose	6.5–16% of patients missed pills	Compared effectiveness of 6 hormonal formulations, 0.16–4.13 pregnancies per 100 women-years depending on dose
Rovinsky 1964 (21)	235/9.5 cycles	New York, New York (15–44) (poor, urban) Hospital family planning clinic	Daily calendar data in clinical trial of low-dose pill (P)	Patient followed instructions (to take 1 pill a day)	97%	41% discontinued; 8 who had difficulty understanding directions were removed from study; No pregnancies during study
Scher et al. 1982 (22)	101/26 months	Boston, Massachusetts (14–25 yr old) Hospital adolescent clinic	Structured interview Compliance measure not described (P)	Continued oral contraceptive without interruption, stopped while abstaining from intercourse, substituted other method; Had unprotected intercourse at some point after starting the pill	62% 38%	Compliance linked to parental involvement, satisfaction with visit, few adverse reactions, satisfaction, method, age; 66% discontinued; 19 pregnancies
Seaton 1985 (50)	175/3–4 months	Matlab, Bangladesh (rural, poor)	Fortnightly home visits recorded: date of visit, number of unopened cycles in a clients possession, number of pills removed from current cycle, number of new cycles provided (P)	One oral contraceptive pill consumed for each day during interval between monthly observations	Over- or undertook on avg. about 8 pills/cycle 13% missed average of 1 pill or less/cycle	Noncompliance may be higher: if same number of pills overtaken and undertaken, they cancel each other out; No mention of pregnancy

[a] P, prospective study; R, retrospective study.

to the user, who may think she has started her menses or that something more serious is wrong.

Breakthrough ovulation is more dangerous, but invisible, to the user. Oral contraceptives work primarily by preventing ovulation, and failing to take pills can cause ovulation to occur. If unprotected coitus occurs when a woman has omitted her pills, pregnancy can result.[2] Breakthrough ovulation is most likely to occur if a pill is missed either at the beginning or end of the 21-day hormonal cycle, extending the hormone-free period beyond seven days (35,39–42). Otherwise, as Fraser and Jansen (39) point out, a women apparently has to miss three or more pills in a cycle to increase her risk of pregnancy significantly.

Variations in Oral Contraceptives

Oral contraceptives can no longer be viewed as homogeneous. For example, three major types and 42 brands of the pill are on the market in the United States (43). Some of these brands are also packaged in both 21- and 28-day packages, the latter including a fourth week with seven placebo (or iron) pills to allow uninterrupted use.

Lower Doses of Hormones

"Combined" oral contraceptives contain estrogens and progestins. The earliest oral contraceptives contained as much as 150 mg of estrogen and 10 mg of progestin. This was at least three times the current dose of the estrogens and more than five times the progestin level of today's "low-dose" formulations (36). Although the higher doses of hormones in the early versions caused more adverse reactions, they did have the virtue that a woman could forget to take a pill for one or two days and still not become pregnant (44,45).

The lower dose oral contraceptives have the same method-effectiveness rates as the higher doses. At the same time, they have greatly reduced the most serious adverse reactions or risks of oral contraceptives, from cardiovascular complications and certain cancers to headaches, dizziness, nausea, and fatigue. However, there is less margin for error with the new, lower dose oral contraceptives, which require careful compliance to avoid both breakthrough bleeding and ovulation (6,20,37,39–42,46).

Triphasics are combined (estrogen and progestin) oral contraceptives packaged with 1 week each of three different levels of hormones to simulate the body's own hormonal fluctuations. The triphasics were introduced in 1979 and are now the most frequently prescribed type of oral contraceptive for first-time pill users in the United States. Almost 70% of all new users are prescribed triphasics. In fact, a single brand of triphasics, Ortho 7/7/7, was the method of choice for new users of 60% of practitioners in one national survey (47). The triphasics have less progestin than other combined oral contraceptives. Hence they have fewer effects on blood pressure and

---

[2]Whether missing two pills can lead to breakthrough ovulation may depend on the specific hormonal combination being used (35). Missing pills in the second half of the cycle is most likely to lead to breakthrough bleeding (35,39). Although their recommendations for how to compensate for missed pills do not always agree completely, the three clearest and/or most comprehensive sources of information in the literature are Fraser and Jansen (39), Guillebaud (40), and Hatcher et al. (6).

other metabolic processes and fewer of the other adverse reactions related to the progestins (e.g., fatigue or oily skin and acne).

Although the triphasics have the fewest adverse reactions overall, they have a higher incidence of breakthrough bleeding and breakthrough ovulation than combined pills (6,41). These problems often result from missed pills. If more than two contraceptive pills are missed, an alternative method of contraception is usually recommended by the treating physician for the remainder of the cycle. Another problem with the triphasics is the fact that each month's packet contains three colors of pills (or four in 28-day packets), one color for each hormonal combination. This can be confusing to new users. If they take them out of sequence, this will increase the chance of breakthrough ovulation or bleeding. It is not clear yet whether triphasics are less effective than low-dose monophasic oral contraceptives in practice (48,49).

The progestin-only, or "mini-pills," have been available since 1973. They are recommended for women with headaches or hypertension and for breastfeeding women. They contain no estrogens but demand particularly scrupulous compliance for effective protection. Not only is a consistent time of day important when taking these oral contraceptives, but a back-up method (such as a condom) must be used every time one or more pills are missed. Even with perfect compliance, the efficacy of the mini-pills is not as high as the efficacy of the combined pills (6). Moreover, including data from breastfeeding women would tend to inflate effectiveness rates of the mini-pills artificially because the fertility of nursing mothers is already lower.

Variations in Packaging

Packaging of oral contraceptives has also changed during the past 30 years. The first oral contraceptives were dispensed as loose tablets in bottles, and some Chinese formulations are still distributed this way. However, in the rest of the world, the familiar 21-tablet blister pack is the version most often used. Each cycle of 21-day pills is followed by a 7-day pill-free week, then initiation of the next packet. The 28-day packet includes seven additional placebo or iron tablets. These 28-day packets were designed specifically to make compliance easier by allowing uninterrupted use. Nevertheless, in most of the world, 21-day packets are more common.

In addition, some oral contraceptives are sold in rectangular packets, whereas others are sold in circular ones; some have special containers or cases; and some are more clearly labeled with the days of the week and other compliance aids than others.

Rates of compliance with the oral contraceptive regimen of one pill each day for 21 days, followed by the 7-day pill-free week, or the 28-day continuous cycles with the seven placebo or iron pills, vary from almost perfect in some clinical trials (41,42) to as low as 3.4% in one study of abortion clinic patients (38).

Service System Characteristics

Service system characteristics are the third contributor to how well women take the pill. Accessibility of services and availability of oral contraceptives, having a choice of methods, information provided on methods, education about correct use of oral contraceptives, their adverse reactions, and how to deal with them are all important factors (8–10,23–25,50). The quality of services varies more in developing countries, making the impact more obvious (10,19).

MEASURING COMPLIANCE

Oral contraceptive compliance has rarely been studied directly. In fact, in an exhaustive literature search, only 13 studies from six countries were found that had collected quantitative data on compliance as defined in this chapter (see Table 16–1). Four of those studies were clinical trials (16,20,21,41). The others were population-based studies; most studied adolescents, and three were done in developing countries (9,19,50).

Criteria for noncompliance in these studies varied greatly, from missing one pill in 3 months (13,28) to three pills in 1 month (11,25,26). Medication compliance can be measured both by direct and indirect methods (51,52). Daily pill compliance in the 13 oral contraceptive studies was measured primarily by indirect methods: (a) pill counts (9,11,50); (b) daily calendars (16,19,21); and (c) questionnaires only (13,22,28). The study in Colombia (19) asked for the reason for *each* missed day, essential to improving correct use and ultimately use-effectiveness. Clinical trial studies generally rely entirely on self-report, using diary cards or retrospective interviews (16,20,21). As Pearson (51) pointed out, the manner in which this is done is important. "Better to ask 'Were you able to take your tablets?' than 'Did you take your tablets?'" (p. 788).

Only three series of studies of oral contraceptive use have used *direct* methods (i.e., urine checks for riboflavin levels in riboflavin-containing oral contraceptive tablets) (11,18). Hamilton and Hoogland (41) used ultrasonographic scanning of ovarian activity in women who were given placebo pills for the first or second day of each new cycle.

A device recently developed by the Aprex Corporation for Ortho Pharmaceuticals promises to provide the first precise, unobtrusive measurement of oral contraceptive compliance. A battery-powered Medication Event Monitoring System fits in the base of Ortho's "Dialpak" contraceptive dispenser (Fig. 16–2). A microprocessor linked to an optical sensor digitally records the exact time and date each individual pill is removed from the Dialpak. The data are then transferred to a computer for plotting a calendar of compliance, showing exactly when pills were missed, if and when they were made up, and how many days pills were omitted between cycles.

Used in conjunction with diary cards and personal interviews, other important information about specific error patterns can be gained from such a device, including why particular pills were missed, timing of missed pills in relation to coitus and adverse reactions, and whether back-up methods were used when needed.

FINDINGS OF ORAL CONTRACEPTIVE COMPLIANCE STUDIES

The findings of this small group of studies are not encouraging (Table 16–1). The rates of compliance in the 13 studies reporting daily oral contraceptive use are for varying lengths of time, making them hard to compare. However, the clinical trials (16,20,21) had the highest rates of compliance. The trend is then toward poorer compliance as one progresses through the studies of adults in developed countries, then teens, then inner city teens, and finally, women in developing countries, who had the poorest compliance.

It should be noted that compliance standards generally become looser as compliance rates become poorer. Thus, the real differences between best and worst com-

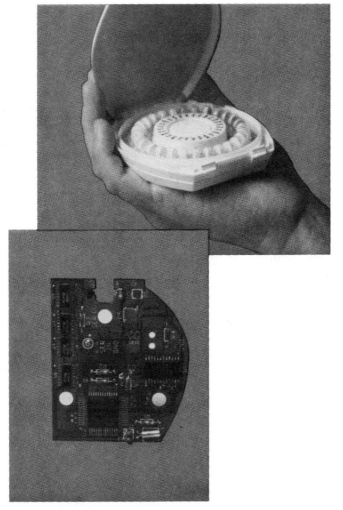

FIG. 16–2. The battery-powered Medication Event Monitoring System microprocessor will be fitted into the bottom of the Dialpak contraceptive dispensers to record when each pill is dispensed. This will enable researchers to determine OC use-effectiveness.

pliers are even greater than first appears. The same pattern applies to pregnancy rates (failure rates), except with less tidy results depending on the size and length of the study. Those rates range roughly from 0 to 16% (9,11–13,16–22) (see Table 16–1).

SPECIAL COMPLIANCE ISSUES OF ORAL CONTRACEPTIVES VERSUS OTHER MEDICATIONS

Each type of medication has its own idiosyncrasies of use. What are some of the issues that affect correct use of oral contraceptives? First, a healthy woman must comply with the daily medical regimen for months or years at a time, whether her intent is to delay or to prevent further pregnancies and whether she is consistently sexually active or not (27,53). She must put up with adverse reactions of varying intensity and know which are dangerous. She must know how long to wait between pill cycles, know when to use a back-up method, have it available, and actually use it. She must have confidence in the pill's effectiveness and safety, despite negative reports in the press, most recently about breast cancer, that fan fears and misconceptions (38,54,55).

The effectiveness of the method depends on correct daily use, frequency of coitus, the hormonal combination and dose being taken, and when during the monthly cycle the pills are missed. The effectiveness of the method also can be diminished by interactions with other medications (e.g., antibiotics), severe vomiting, or diarrhea (6,36,39).

WHAT TO DO ABOUT POOR COMPLIANCE

It is clear, even from this small body of data, that pill compliance is a problem wherever oral contraceptives are used. Based on these limited findings about users' incorrect or insufficient knowledge and use of the pill, the first step to increase oral contraceptive compliance is to be sure users do, in fact, know how to take their oral contraceptives correctly.

This means providing new oral contraceptive users with (a) easily understandable written materials, (b) careful oral instructions, and (c) clearly labeled pill packets, preferably in 28-day cycles to reduce transition errors (28) (Table 16–2). Illiterate users may require pictorial as well as written instructions. If women are on 21-day cycles, it means having them start their first pill packet on day 1 or 2 of menstruation so that there is no confusion later as to when to start the next pack.

They should be encouraged to buy several packs of pills at a time to be sure they do not run out. They should also be provided with a back-up method (e.g., condoms or foam) when they are given their first packet of pills, then taught when and how to use them. They should know that the most hazardous times to miss pills are at

TABLE 16–2. *Recommendations to improve compliance and thereby use-effectiveness of oral contraceptives*

Be sure that pill packets clearly indicate the type of pill (combination, triphasic, progestin-only), the number of pills in the packet, and how long to wait between packets.

Provide information verbally and in writing before a new user initiates her first pack of oral contraceptives.

Be sure that users (and providers) know at least three things about correct oral contraceptive use before initiating use:
the number of days to wait between pill packets;
how and when to use a back-up method;
which adverse reactions are transient (less than 3 months) and minor, and which require medical attention.

Help users establish a regular time each day to take the pill.

Provide back-up methods (e.g., condoms) to all new oral contraceptive users, with instructions on when and how to use them.

Monitor the knowledge and actual pill-taking patterns of oral contraceptive users regularly to be sure they understand the above points and are taking the oral contraceptives correctly.

Monitor the knowledge of oral contraceptive providers regularly.

Provide at least two packets of pills at a time so that users are less likely to run out.

Help an oral contraceptive user who has difficulty remembering to take oral contraceptives or other serious problems to switch to another method.

the beginning and the end of a cycle, next is missing two or more pills during the first half of the cycle. Users also need to establish a regular time to take their contraceptive pill each day. Providers must themselves be highly knowledgeable about correct oral contraceptive use; then repeatedly monitor users' knowledge and pill-taking habits as well as adverse reactions until clients are correct, consistent, and satisfied users or have switched to another contraceptive method.

CONCLUSION

No medicine can work well if it is improperly used. To maintain the same level of use-effectiveness, the modern, refined low dose oral contraceptives require stricter compliance than the older high dose pills. In the future, more precise measurements of use-effectiveness are needed. Studies must take unreported abortions and coital frequency into account and report data on subgroups of women, especially single as well as married women, because half of single United States women of reproductive age are taking oral contraceptives (5).

Also more must be known about actual day-by-day compliance; not only how many days are missed each month, but when and why, what type and dosage of oral contraceptive was being used, and if a back-up method was used when pills were omitted.

Compliance should be objectively measured. Special dispensers such as the computerized Dialpak (Fig. 16–1) (56) could add important information about specific error patterns, in conjunction with diary cards and personal interviews about why those pills were missed, when they were missed in relation to coitus, and whether back-up methods were used. Interest in medical compliance research is increasing. Many more studies on oral contraceptive compliance are needed if the use-effectiveness of the pill is to be improved.

ACKNOWLEDGMENTS

The author especially would like to acknowledge Malcolm Potts, Gary Grubb, and Markus Steiner, who coauthored the paper on which much of this chapter is based, and to thank Nancy Williamson, Ian Fraser, John Guillebaud, Laneta Dorflinger, and Inder Sharma, who reviewed one version or the other, as well as Cindy Visness and Brenda Gómez, who helped with the preparation of this chapter. This work was funded under a cooperative agreement between Family Health International and the U.S. Agency for International Development's Office of Population Research.

REFERENCES

1. Schirm AL, Trussell J, Menken J, Grady WR. Contraceptive failure in the United States: the impact of social, economic and demographic factors. *Fam Plann Perspect* 1982;14:68–75.
2. Tietze C, Lewit S. Statistical evaluation of contraceptive methods: use-effectiveness and extended use-effectiveness. *Demography* 1968;5:931.
3. Vaughan B, Trussell J, Menken J, Jones EF. Contraceptive failure among married women in the United States, 1970–1973. *Fam Plann Perspect* 1977;9:251–258.
4. Jay MS, DuRant RH, Litt IF. Female adolescents' compliance with contraceptive regimens. *Pediatr Clin North Am* 1989;36:731–745.
5. Grady WR, Hayward MD, Yagi J. Contraceptive failure in the United States: estimates from the 1982 National Survey of Family Growth *Fam Plann Perspect* 1986;18:200–209.

6. Hatcher RA, Guest F, Stewart F, et al. *Contraceptive technology, 1988–89,* 14th revised ed. New York: Irvington Publishers, 1988.
7. Trussell J, Kost K. Contraceptive failure in the United States: a critical review of the literature. *Stud Fam Plann* 1987;18:237–283.
8. Choudhury AY, Laing J, Khan AR, Clark S. *Use-effectiveness of oral pills and condoms.* Dhaka, Bangladesh: Program for the Introduction and Adaptation of Contraceptive Technology, 1986.
9. Cobb JC, Farhat S, Shah NA, Ameen SI, Harper P. Oral contraceptive program synchronized with moon phase. *Fertil Steril* 1966;17:559–567.
10. DeClerque J, Tsui A. *Contraceptive discontinuation in Egypt.* Research Report No. 4. Chapel Hill: Carolina Population Center, November 1984.
11. DuRant R, Jay M, Linden C, Shoffitt T, Litt I. Influence of psychosocial-factors on adolescent compliance with oral contraceptives. *J Adolesc Health Care* 1984;5:1–6.
12. Emans SJ, Grace E, Woods ER, Smith DE, Klein K, Merola J. Adolescents' compliance with the use of oral contraceptives. *JAMA* 1987;257:3377–3381.
13. Finlay IG, Scott MG. Patterns of pill taking in an inner city practice. *Br Med J* 1986;293:601–602.
14. Goldman N, Pebley R, Westoff C, Paul L. Contraceptive failure rates in Latin America. *Int Fam Plann Perspect* 1983;18:50–57.
15. Laing JE. Continuation and effectiveness of oral contraceptive practice. *Stud Fam Plann* 1985;16:138–153.
16. Laurie RE, Korba VD. Fertility control with continuous microdose Norgestrel. *J Reprod Med* 1972;8:165–168.
17. Neel E, Jay S, Litt I. The relationship of self-concept and autonomy to oral contraceptive compliance among adolescent females. *J Adolesc Health Care* 1985;6:445–447.
18. Neel E, Litt I, Jay S. Side effects and compliance with low- and conventional-dose oral contraceptives among adolescents. *J Adolesc Health Care* 1987;8:327–329.
19. Potter L, Wright S, Berrio D, Suarez P, Pinedo R, Castañeda Z. Oral contraceptive compliance in rural Colombia: knowledge of users and providers. *Int Fam Plann Perspect* 1988;14:27–31.
20. Preston SN. A report of the correlation between the pregnancy rates of low estrogen formulations and pill-taking habits of females studied. *J Reprod Med* 1974;13:76–77.
21. Rovinsky JJ. Clinical effectiveness of a low-dose progestin-estrogen combination. *Obstet Gynecol* 1964;23:840–850.
22. Scher PW, Emans SJ, Grace EM. Factors associated with compliance to oral contraceptive use in an adolescent population. *J Adolesc Health Care* 1983;3:120–123.
23. Phillips JF. Continued use of contraception among Philippine family planning acceptors: a multivariate analysis. *Stud Fam Plann* 1978;9:182–192.
24. Einhorn R, Sear AM, Perez E, Cabrera E. Contraceptive method continuation according to type of provider. *Am J Public Health* 1977;67:1157–1164.
25. Jay MS, DuRant RH, Litt IF. Effect of peer counselors on adolescent compliance in use of oral contraceptives. *Pediatrics* 1984;73:126–131.
26. Jay MS, Litt IF, DuRant RH. Compliance with therapeutic regimens. *J Adolesc Health Care* 1984;5:124–136.
27. Winokur D. *An organizational and behavioral analysis of the contraceptive compliance process.* Ann Arbor: University Microfilms International, 1985.
28. Goldstuck ND, Hammar E, Butchard A. Use and misuse of oral contraceptives by adolescents attending a free-standing clinic. *Adv Contracept* 1987;3:335–339.
29. Sayed HAA, Way AA. *Egypt demographic health survey 1988.* Egypt National Population Council and Institute for Resource Development, Columbia, Maryland. September 1989.
30. Bailey J, Keller K. Post family planning acceptance experience in the Caribbean: St. Kitts-Nevis and St. Vincent. *Stud Fam Plann* 1982;13:44–58.
31. Basnayake S, Higgins J, Miller P, Rodgers S, Kelly SE. Early symptoms and discontinuation among users of oral contraceptives in Sri Lanka. *Stud Fam Plann* 1984;15:285–290.
32. Bhatia S, Kim Y. Oral contraception in Bangladesh. *Stud Fam Plann* 1984;15:233–241.
33. Janowitz B, Kane T, Arruda J, Covington D, Morris L. Side effects and discontinuation of oral contraceptive use in southern Brazil. *J Biosoc Sci* 1986;18:261–271.
34. Nair N, Smith L. Reasons for not using contraceptives: an international comparison. *Stud Fam Plann* 1984;15:84–92.
35. Wang E, Shi S, Cekan SZ, Landgren B-M, Diczfalusy E. Hormonal consequences of "missing the Pill." *Contraception* 1982;26:545–566.
36. Wharton C, Blackburn MS. Lower-dose pills. *Popul Rep* Series A, No. 7. November 1988.
37. Metson D. Lessons from an audit of unplanned pregnancies. *Br Med J* 1988;297:295–296.
38. Wheble AM, Street P, Wheble SM. Contraception: failure in practice. *Br J Fam Plann* 1987;13:40–45.
39. Fraser I, Jansen R. Why do inadvertent pregnancies occur in oral contraceptive users? Effectiveness of oral contraceptive regimens and interfering factors. *Contraception* 1983;27:531–551.
40. Guillebaud J. Missed pills—what advice should we give? *Br J Fam Plann* 1981;7:41–44.

41. Hamilton CJCM, Hoogland HJ. Longitudinal ultrasonographic study of the ovarian suppressive activity of a low-dose triphasic oral contraceptive during correct and incorrect pill intake. *Am J Obstet Gynecol* 1989;161:1159–1162.
42. Molloy BG, Coulson KA, Lee JM, Watters JK. "Missed pill" conception: fact or fiction? *Br Med J* 1985;290:1474–1475.
43. Piper JM, Kennedy DL. Oral contraceptives in the United States: trends in content and potency. *Int J Epidemiol* 1987;16:215–221.
44. Pincus G. *The control of fertility*. New York: Academic Press, 1965.
45. Potts M, Diggory P. *Textbook of contraceptive practice,* 2nd ed. London: Cambridge University Press, 1983.
46. Edgren R. Bleeding patterns with low-dose, monophasic oral contraceptives. *Conception* 1989;40:285–297.
47. Robertson EM, ed. Orthonovum 7/7/7 is first choice for 60% of CTU survey respondents. *Contracept Tech Update* 1987;8:109–114.
48. Ketting E. The relative reliability of oral contraceptives: findings of an epidemiological study. *Contraception* 1988;37:343–348.
49. Waldron T. How effective are low-dose triphasics when pills are missed? *Contracept Tech Update* 1988;9:117–120.
50. Seaton B. Noncompliance among oral contraceptive acceptors in rural Bangladesh. *Stud Fam Plann* 1985;16:52–59.
51. Pearson RM. Who is taking their tablets? *Br Med J* 1982;285:757–758.
52. Spilker B. *Guide to clinical studies and developing protocols*. New York: Raven Press, 1984.
53. Whelan E. Compliance with contraceptive regimens. *Stud Fam Plann* 1974;5:349–351.
54. Perceptions of the Pill Survey Group. Women's perceptions of the safety of the pill: a survey in eight developing countries. *J Biosoc Sci* 1987;19:313–321.
55. Thapa S, Salgado M, Fortney J, Grubb G, De Silva V. Women's perception of the pill's potential risks in Sri Lanka. *Asian Pac Pop J* 1987;2:39–56.
56. Cramer JA, Mattson RH, Prevey ML, Scheyer RD, Ouellett VL. How often is medication taken as prescribed? A novel assessment technique. *JAMA* 1989;261:3273–3277.

*Patient Compliance in Medical
Practice and Clinical Trials*
edited by J.A. Cramer and B. Spilker
Raven Press, Ltd., New York © 1991

17

Compliance to Diabetes Regimens

Conceptualization, Complexity, and Determinants

Russell E. Glasgow

Oregon Research Institute, Eugene, Oregon 97401

Compliance to diabetes regimens presents an extraordinarily complex challenge to patients, providers, and researchers. This complexity is illustrated by the multiple and disparate ways in which the issue has been approached. Measures of diabetes compliance have ranged from observations of skill in performing technical tasks (e.g., application of drops of blood to reagent pads; drawing insulin into a syringe) to frequency and timing of recommended actions (e.g., number and scheduling of meals/snacks and exercise sessions) and self-adjustment of insulin administration. Many professionals use the term *compliance* to refer to one or more of the array of diabetes management activities performed by patients, but several researchers prefer concepts such as self-care (1–3) or self-management (4,5). To provide continuity with other chapters, the term *compliance* has been used to connote the constellation of self-care behaviors that patients must do on a daily basis to manage their diabetes.

Three facts are necessary to understand about diabetes regimen compliance. First, diabetes compliance is not a unitary construct, but includes several important dimensions of diabetes self-care activities. These dimensions include (a) dietary behavior, (b) exercise, (c) medication taking, (d) glucose monitoring, (e) safety/preventive actions (e.g., carrying a supply of sugar; checking's one's feet), and (f) appropriate integration and timing of all these activities. To complicate matters further, it has generally been found that compliance to a given aspect of the diabetes regimen (e.g., diet) is not highly correlated with compliance to other aspects of the regimen (6–9). There even appear to be different dimensions within some regimen areas (e.g., diet) (10). One of the premier assessment studies of diabetes compliance discusses 13 different aspects of self-care among children and adolescents with type I (insulin-dependent) diabetes and concludes that the five different dimensions of diabetes compliance are exercise, insulin injection, diet type, frequency (of eating and glucose testing), and diet amount (8).

The second important conceptual issue is that diabetes patients often have not received explicit regimen prescriptions in several of these areas (2,11). It is impossible to calculate a compliance score if there is no standard or specific criteria against which to compare the patient's behavior (1,12). This failure to provide regimen prescriptions seems to occur for two reasons. In some cases, no set prescription exists—as exemplified by programs attempting to teach insulin self-adjustment skills. The appropriate "prescription" is to be determined by the patient and may repeatedly change (13). For other regimen areas, because of concerns about patients' limited ability to follow recommendations, health care providers do not provide specific recommendations. Particularly for many older type II (noninsulin-dependent) patients, providers simply give general statements such as "eat less, loss weight, and try to get more exercise."

Diabetes is not a single disease but a heterogeneous collection of disorders having in common disruption of glucose metabolism (14–16). For example, the tasks, issues, and influences on compliance for a 13-year-old insulin-dependent adolescent are quite different than those of an overweight 70-year-old noninsulin-dependent grandmother. Partially because of these differences and partially because of differences in the type of physician (endocrinologist versus family practitioner) who treats these patients and treatment trends in different communities, the regimen prescriptions that diabetes patients receive vary considerably in complexity as well as in relative emphasis on different regimen areas. Therefore, it will be necessary to refer to the patient subgroup and the type of regimen task when discussing findings. The next section discusses compliance rates, followed by a presentation of a model of diabetes self-management and the factors related to compliance.

COMPLIANCE TO DIFFERENT ASPECTS OF DIABETES REGIMENS

It has been known for more than 20 years that patient compliance to diabetes regimens is generally poor, especially to dietary recommendations. Classical studies of adult patients by Watkins et al. (17) and the discussion of dietary compliance failures by West (18) first pointed out the tremendous difficulties in complying with diabetes regimens. It would be desirable to create a matrix-like table summarizing compliance rates by regimen areas (e.g., medication taking, diet, glucose testing, exercise) and patient subgroups (e.g., type I adolescents, type I adults, type II adults, and mixed types). However, review of the literature revealed a number of surprises that precluded this possibility. First, very few studies reported actual compliance rates for either adolescents or type II adults. Although it is commonly assumed, with some empirical support (8,19), that adolescents are particularly nonadherent, the vast majority of psychosocial studies of adolescents with diabetes focus on glycemic control, omitting measurement or discussion of compliance. In the case of type II adults, there are several studies of compliance, but they have usually presented data on predictors of compliance without reporting actual compliance rates. When reported, data were often expressed as absolute levels of self-care (e.g., number of calories consumed, number of times glucose was tested) or as standardized scores for a composite index of compliance. It was not possible to translate these data into compliance rates. These problems resulted in seven of the eight cells of the regimen area by subgroup matrix for these subgroups being blank or only containing data from a single study.

The one subgroup for which there are a reasonable number of data points is adults with unspecified or mixed types of diabetes. Here, however, additional problems emerge. Compliance rates varied widely across studies, but compliance seemed to be primarily determined by the type of measurement (e.g., self-report versus record keeping versus objective index) and definition of compliance. For example, Irvine

(20) reported that a sample of adult patients with mixed types of diabetes self-reported following their diet on average more than 4 of the last 7 days, whereas Watkins et al. (17), using interview and observational methods, found that only 25% of adult patients were judged to have meals and "reasonable spacing" of meals judged acceptable. Possibly most important, Cerkoney and Hart (21) reported that only 7% of a sample of insulin-treated adult patients complied with all aspects of the diabetes regimen considered essential for good diabetes control.

It is difficult to make conclusive statements about compliance with various diabetes regimen tasks because of the lack of standard methods of assessing compliance and the problem of comparing measures such as timing and regularity of insulin injections to amount of calories consumed. Still, studies that have assessed regimen compliance across two or more aspects of the diabetes regimen have fairly consistently concluded that compliance is better to "medical" aspects of the regimen (e.g., medication taking and especially insulin injections) than to life-style aspects of the regimen (e.g., diet and exercise) (6,9,20,22–24). In particular, long-term compliance with diet is consistently seen as the most difficult aspect of the diabetes regimen (6,22,23,25).

One regimen area in which technological advances have allowed more objective determination of self-care levels is blood glucose testing. Several studies have compared patient self-reports of number of glucose tests with number of tests registered on glucose monitors with built-in memories. When patients are unaware of the memory capability of the meter, these studies have found overreporting of the number of tests conducted by as much as 50%, especially among type I adolescent patients (26). The general conclusion is that patient glucose testing records are often inaccurate (26–29), but there is debate about whether patients alter their records to present a more positive picture of their compliance and glycemic control status (26–28). Such findings call into question the results of studies relying solely on patient self-reports of compliance. Blood glucose monitoring studies also point out the inadvisability of considering compliance to a single regimen area in isolation. Several studies have found that simply increasing the frequency of blood glucose monitoring is of negligible benefit—if the results are not used to adjust insulin administration or to modify other regimen behaviors (13,27,29).

FACTORS RELATED TO DIABETES COMPLIANCE

Figure 17–1 illustrates a working model of diabetes compliance. Compliance, or self-management, is represented in the center of the figure. To its left and above are factors that influence compliance (patient–health care provider interactions, psychological variables, environmental factors), and to the right are consequences or outcomes of diabetes compliance and biological factors affecting health outcomes. The factors within each box are discussed in more detail below, but a few general comments about the model are needed by way of introduction.

The model, which is adapted from the work of Anderson (30) and our own previous conceptualizations of diabetes self-care (1,31,32), places primary emphasis on "the cycle of care" (30) involving patient–provider interactions, compliance, and health outcomes. In this cycle, the relations among these three factors in the triangle are considered the most direct influences on the other two factors. These "primary" relations are denoted by solid arrows, and the dynamic or cylical nature of the in-

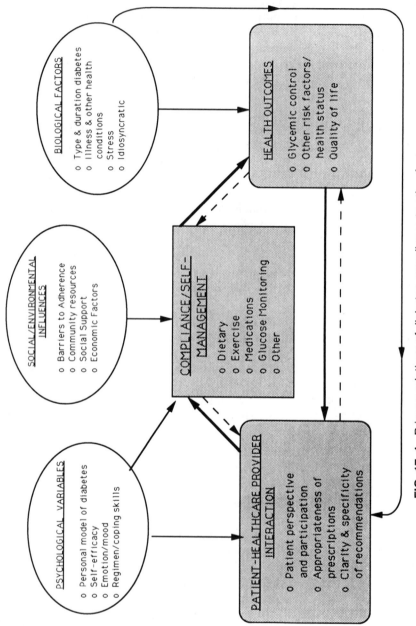

FIG. 17–1. Primary relations of diabetes compliance to other factors.

teractions is indicated by the triangle of solid arrows. These relations are not unidirectional, however, as often portrayed. The reciprocal, although secondary influences of these factors on each other are indicated by dashed lines and arrows.

There are also other factors that influence patient–provider interactions, compliance, and health outcomes. The most important such factors are illustrated in the upper half of Fig. 17–1. As can be seen, psychological variables (e.g., personal model of diabetes, self-efficacy) are hypothesized to influence patient–provider interactions and to have direct effects on compliance. Social-environmental factors are also seen as influencing diabetes compliance. Biological factors significantly influence a variety of health outcomes and thus moderate the effect of compliance on health outcomes. Finally, biological factors are also seen to affect patient–provider interactions (especially regimen prescriptions).

This model is not totally comprehensive, and other variables could be included and many additional paths could be drawn. One could certainly draw arrows from every circle or box to every other factor as many recent causal models seem to do. To communicate more clearly, however, each factor has been restricted to having no more than two arrows, representing the primary influence(s) of that factor. Pathways have also been restricted to those influencing one or more of the three factors involved in the cycle of care relation (30). The resulting model conveys the multifactorial nature and complexity of diabetes compliance and illustrates the most important relations without becoming overwhelming.

The list of the various regimen areas under diabetes compliance in Fig. 17–1 is to remind the reader that there are several relatively independent dimensions to diabetes self-management. It should also be noted that the factors influencing these various dimensions may also differ (22,32). At present, not enough comparative research has been conducted to evaluate this latter issue adequately. Another general point about factors related to diabetes compliance concerns their level of specificity. Although general measures of constructs such as social support, self-efficacy, and community resources are appealing because of their potential for use across disease areas (e.g., hypertension, asthma, renal dialysis), studies that have compared diabetes-specific predictor variables with more general measures have found the diabetes-specific variables to be stronger predictors (7,33). With these caveats, each of the five major factors shown in Fig. 17–1 is discussed as influencing diabetes compliance or related health outcomes.

Patient–Health Care Provider Interactions

These encounters are seen as the most proximal influence on diabetes self-management. At the most basic level, if patients are not given regimen prescriptions, they are unlikely to comply. If they are not given appropriate recommendations, even perfect compliance will fail to produce beneficial outcomes. Related issues involve the clarity and specificity of recommendations. Ley (34) and other researchers (35) found that patients frequently do not recall recommendations and are less likely to do so when recommendations are vague, complex, or delivered in a threatening manner.

A final important patient–provider issue is the level of patient participation and understanding of the patient's perspective on compliance issues. Greenfield et al. (36) found patient participation to be causally related to improvements in blood glu-

cose control and reductions in functional limitations. Rost (37) found patient partic-
ipation during examinations to be highly correlated to medication compliance ($r = 0.85$) among a sample of adult patients. Understanding of the patient's perspective
can aid in tailoring regimen prescriptions. It can also provide clues for how to mo-
tivate different patients to comply.

Psychological Variables

At least two important factors are relevant to compliance from the patient's perspective: their personal model of diabetes, and their perceived self-efficacy for being
able to perform various regimen tasks. Personal models of illness (38,39) refer to
patients' cognitive representations of their disease and include such things as beliefs
and emotions about the cause, symptoms, course, treatment, and consequences of
their disease. Dimensions of personal models have been found to predict dietary and
exercise self-care among type II patients (40). Patient views of regimen tasks, especially those regarding reasons for noncompliance, have been found to differ significantly from those of providers (11,23,41), and this incongruence may be a major
factor determining noncompliance (38,39,41). Patients' self-efficacy or expectations
regarding their ability to perform specific tasks (42) have been found to be strong
prospective predictors of compliance for both type I and type II diabetes (31,43) and
for many other health behaviors (44).

The emotional state or mood of the patient is also seen as affecting compliance.
At clinically significant levels, depression has been found to be related to substantially reduced involvement in many different kinds of activities (45). The effect of
depression, as well as more moderate mood levels, on diabetes self-care (46) is worthy of further investigation.

The final psychological variable listed in Fig. 17–1 is regimen and coping skills.
Regimen skills refer to patients' ability to translate recommendations into the many
motor (e.g., correctly mixing and injecting insulin; operating glucose monitors) and
decisional skills (e.g., selecting food portions consistent with dietary recommendations). If patients do not possess these skills or can only perform them with great
difficulty, it is unlikely that they will be able to manage their diabetes appropriately.
Having this behavioral repertoire of skills is viewed as a necessary but by no means
sufficient condition for good diabetes self-management. A basic level of such skills
is critical for successful compliance, as illustrated by the difficulties of older patients
with dementia. These skills are included in Fig. 17–1, rather than patient knowledge,
because it is this behavioral application of knowledge, rather than general abstract
knowledge about diabetes (e.g., how insulin works), that influences compliance.
There have been many reports of nonsignificant and, at times, even inverse relations
between general knowledge and diabetes compliance (17,31).

Coping or problem-solving skills refer to patients' ability to adapt creatively to and
overcome the many challenges and barriers to compliance (47,48). Diabetes-specific
problem-solving skills have recently been found to be almost as strong a predictor
of glucose monitoring and exercise self-care among adult type II patients as a combination of several other psychosocial predictor variables (49).

Because of the general lack of relation between demographic factors and compliance, such factors are not included in Fig. 17–1. For example, although intuitively
appealing, educational level is seldom found to predict compliance. Age is the one

demographic factor that is somewhat consistently related to diabetes compliance. This relation varies across subgroups, however. Among type I children, age appears to be inversely related to compliance (8,19,50), whereas among adult patients age is often positively associated with reported compliance (20,43).

Social/Environmental Influences

The array of obstacles or challenges to compliance faced by patients has been termed *barriers to compliance* (16,51). Like beauty, to some extent, barriers are in the eye of the beholder, and they can include both intrapersonal (e.g., negative self-statements) and environmental factors. Barriers are considered here, however, because they consist largely of competing demands, social pressures, scheduling, financial, and other environmental factors. The extent of barriers has been found to predict regimen compliance among both type I (28,51) and type II patients (32,74), as well as mixed groups (52).

Resources to combat compliance barriers come from community organizations and services, social support from family and peers, and financial (especially health care insurance) sources. Community resources include services provided by various public (welfare, county health departments, senior citizen centers) and voluntary health organizations (e.g., American Diabetes Association, American Heart Association), as well as hospital and community health programs (e.g., diabetes education and support groups, visiting nurse programs, and mall walking clubs). The awareness, cost, and accessibility of these resources can significantly influence levels of diabetes compliance in the community. Finally, the way these organizations and activities, as well as related health issues, are covered in the media provides a supportive or nonsupportive context for compliance behaviors.

Many of these activities also provide a less tangible but equally important resource: social support. The opportunity to interact with peers experiencing similar life circumstances can be an important stimulus for compliance, especially in areas such as diet and exercise (53). The level of social support provided by family members for diabetes compliance has been found to predict compliance in several regimen tasks for adolescent type I patients (33,50), adult type II patients (7,54), and mixed groups (55). Among adolescents with type I diabetes, several aspects of the family environment including marital adjustment, family cohesion, and parental support of diabetes treatment have been found to relate to compliance (33,50).

These relations are complex, however, and it may be that there are certain types of social support or certain conditions under which social support is more or less important (56). For example, Heitzmann and Kaplan (57) found smaller social networks to be more satisfactory for male patients but larger networks to be more satisfactory for female patients, and Uzoma and Feldman (43) found different dimensions of social support to be related to insulin compliance for black adult male and female patients. In addition, Hanson et al. (73) found that associations between family relations and health outcomes for adolescent patients with diabetes were much stronger for patients with shorter rather than longer durations of diabetes.

Finally, financial contingencies and economic incentives/disincentives must certainly affect levels of diabetes compliance, especially among poorer patients. The cost to the patient of medications, injection equipment, glucose monitoring machines, and supplies, perceived cost of nutritious foods, and availability of free or low-cost fitness facilities and equipment would all be expected to influence compliance behaviors. The extent of third-party coverage/reimbursement for diabetes education activities is another prime example of a financial factor that affects both patient compliance and the willingness of providers to devote time to compliance teaching.

Much more research needs to be focused on environmental and societal level contextual factors potentially related to compliance. To date, there has been an excessive number of studies on intrapersonal variables and other patient characteristics and far too little research on interpersonal barriers and community/health care resource factors related to compliance.

Biological Factors and Diabetes Outcomes

As shown in Fig. 17–1, biological factors influence health outcomes and moderate the relation between diabetes compliance and outcome. In particular, the type and duration of diabetes may moderate the extent to which biomedical (e.g., insulin compliance) or life-style (e.g., eating and physical activity) factors are more strongly related to glycemic control (15). Other factors such as illness, stressful life events, shifting metabolic needs, and drug interactions can also affect blood glucose levels (58,59). Failure to consider such issues, to separate patients into type I versus type II in analyses, or to control for changes in medication may be partially responsible for the modest relations often observed in compliance–glycemic control studies (9,15,17,20). However, even studies that have controlled for type of diabetes as well as duration, gender, and other potential confounding variables have not consistently observed significant relations between diabetes compliance and glycemic control (6,7,40).

These findings underline the tremendous heterogeneity of diabetes and lead to two conclusions. The first is that diabetes compliance is clearly not the same thing as diabetes control, and investigators should no longer use glycemic control as an index of compliance. Second, many biological variables, other health conditions, and idiosyncratic factors influence compliance–control relations. More research effort should be devoted to identifying subgroups of patients for whom compliance is strongly related to diabetes control. For example, there may be some patients whose glucose levels are responsive to dietary factors, whereas others are not (60).

A final point concerning the relation of health outcomes to diabetes compliance is that this relation is reciprocal. That is, improvements in glycemic control and/or other risk factors (e.g., lower blood pressure, cholesterol levels, or weight) may reinforce compliance efforts (35). Conversely, negative outcomes such as a worsening or no effect on glycemic control despite concerted efforts to improve compliance can discourage further efforts to comply. The impact of compliance on patient quality of life may be either positive or negative, and if the latter (e.g., reduced range of social activities, continued sacrifice of preferred foods, unacceptable time or monetary costs), this may lead to reduced long-term compliance.

Future Research Recommendations

The research reviewed in this section has identified some potentially important factors related to diabetes compliance, but these studies have not contributed as much to our understanding and enhancement of compliance as would be expected given the volume of studies. There are several reasons for this. First, the majority of studies have used cross-sectional or retrospective designs. To have predictive significance and to begin to separate cause and effect (e.g., does compliance affect health beliefs, vice versa, or both?), prospective studies are needed. Second, most investigators have developed their own idiosyncratic measures of compliance and have often made suboptimal choices (e.g., relying solely on global self-reports and/ or failing to address compliance to different components of the regimen) (4). Greater use of methods such as those of Johnson et al. (8) involving reports of specific regimen behaviors at different points in time and standardized self-report measures such as the Diabetes Education Profile (15) would advance the field.

Most investigators have focused on a fairly narrowly defined set of predictor variables, rather than a more conceptually driven or comprehensive set of measures. As shown in Fig. 17–1, diabetes compliance is influenced by multiple factors, making it difficult to attribute observed relations solely to any given factor. Also, factors associated with compliance may vary across regimen area or patient subgroup, but these issues are seldom considered. Multivariate analytic procedures (e.g., hierarchical multiple regression and structural equation modeling) have been developed to deal with these complexities and to assess the relative importance of various factors but are not often used by diabetes researchers (61,62).

There is also a clear need to expand the range of outcome variables assessed (see Fig. 17–1). Research to date has relied far too extensively on glycemic control as the sole index of health outcome. A recent study predicting diabetes survival by Davis et al. (63) found that social impact factors are important predictors of survival and that these factors, along with other outcomes such as renal function and cigarette smoking, were stronger predictors of mortality than were glycosylated hemoglobin levels.

Finally, there has simply been too much correlational research and not enough intervention research or attempts to modify predictor variables to improve compliance. Research on interventions to improve diabetes compliance is discussed next.

EFFORTS TO INCREASE COMPLIANCE

There are few experimental tests of interventions to increase diabetes compliance. Although there have been many reports of diabetes education programs, these studies have major limitations (64). Most of these studies report on improvements in patient knowledge and glycemic control, but far fewer report measures of patient compliance. A recent meta-analysis of patient education for diabetes concluded that the mean effect size for compliance was less than those for knowledge and physical outcomes (65). Of 93 diabetes education studies reviewed, only 28 included compliance measures, and most of those relied exclusively on self-reports of compliance. Because of the small numbers of patients often involved in these studies and the use of nonrandomized or pre–post designs without control conditions, it is difficult to attribute changes observed to the intervention being evaluated. A few of the more comprehensive controlled trials of interventions to improve diabetes compliance are presented, followed by recommendations of ways to improve compliance.

Mazzuca et al. (3) studied a sample of 532 adult patients who were predominantly female (79%), black (72%), and had type II diabetes (95%). Patients were randomly assigned to comprehensive patient education or routine education, and 275 completed the treatment and follow-up, with rates of attrition and characteristics of patients who dropped out either being comparable across conditions or working against detection of treatment effects. The experimental intervention contained a number of exemplary features such as modules tailored to patient needs, negotiation of compliance goals between patients and instructors with written copies given to both parties at each session, and follow-up telephone contact 2 and 6 weeks after completion of each module. Patients received an average of 2-1/2 instructional modules, averaging 90 min per module, and 76% of the experimental patients also received the diet and activity module, requiring an additional 5 hr of instruction. Follow-up results 6 to 14 months after intervention revealed significantly greater improvement in both self-care skills (e.g., glucose testing and insulin-taking procedures) and compliance (e.g., reduced caloric intake) for comprehensive education patients. The comprehensive education condition was also found to produce superior improvements in glycemic control and other risk factors (e.g., blood pressure).

The long-term results of a controlled evaluation of a weight loss intervention for 53 type II adults by Wing et al. (66) were less encouraging. They randomized patients to a behavioral weight loss and exercise program, nutrition education, or a usual care condition. The behavioral program included self-monitoring of caloric intake and exercise, goal setting, rearranging one's environment to support healthier eating, and contracting for weight loss. Weight losses at the conclusion of the 16-week program were significantly greater for the behavioral intervention (mean = 6.4 kg) than either of the comparison conditions (3.9 and 2.9 kg), as were increases in exercise. However, there were no significant between-groups differences in food consumption, and at a 1-year follow-up, weight loss differences were no longer significant. This study points out the difficulty of producing long-term changes in life-style behaviors among diabetic patients. Other research by this group suggests that obese patients with diabetes may have an even more difficult time losing weight than other obese patients (67).

A final controlled trial that should provide valuable information on the long-term results of interventions to improve diabetes compliance is the Diabetes Control and Complications Trial (68). Results of this multicenter trial comparing a comprehensive intervention to control tightly glucose levels among type I patients with a usual care condition are not yet available. The trial will report on the impact of the intervention on quality of life (69) as well as numerous other health outcomes in addition to glycemic control.

Future Research Needs

One problem with the above interventions is that they do not report on the percent or representativeness of eligible patients who participated. The only exception is a single sentence in the Mazzuca et al. (3) report, stating that 532 (30%) of approximately 1,800 diabetes patients agreed to participate (about half of whom later dropped out). This criticism also applies to the majority of other diabetes education studies. Given that interventions that appear effective (70) are generally intensive, time-consuming, and in some cases, relatively expensive (64), it is unlikely that a high percentage of patients participate. A recent study found that only a minority of type II patients older than 60 years of age were willing to participate in a diabetes self-care program (71). This was disappointing given that the program was specifically designed for these patients, attempted to overcome several major barriers to participation, was offered without charge, and was heavily promoted. This study also reviewed diabetes education studies reported in the 1988 and 1989 issues of *Diabetes Care* and *The Diabetes Educator* and concluded that there has been little attention to how to reach a large percentage of diabetes patients. Only five of 19 studies reported on the percent of patients approached who ended up participating. Further, in four of these studies, the patients approached to participate were a self-selected group who were participating in other diabetes education activities. Only one of the 19 studies reported on characteristics of participants versus nonparticipants.

One of the few examples of how to develop interventions that can reach a large percentage of patients is a study by Anderson et al. (47). They evaluated a problem-solving training program for type I adolescent patients and their parents (separate group meetings for parents and adolescents) consisting of five modules during an 18-month period. Although the total intervention time was considerable, the intervention was integrated into standard office visits every 3 to 4 months. The problem-solving interventions improved self-care (e.g., use of glucose monitoring to adjust exercise and insulin) and prevented deterioration in glycemic control more than a usual care condition. This study also has a number of positive methodological features including data on participation (70 of 92 eligible families participated) and is a good example of how to develop disseminable intervention procedures (e.g., brief telephone follow-up calls by the clinic nurse between visits). We need more such reports on interventions that are feasible into routine office care.

If we are to reach more people, efforts will almost surely need to employ community-based and public health approaches (2,72). Hallmarks of such approaches are the mobilization and integration of multiple influences and community sectors (e.g., health care providers, media, voluntary and other organizations, citizen groups). This approach is in contrast to the more intensive clinical approach typically found in diabetes care. The goal is also different—to produce modest changes in entire populations rather than major changes in selected patients.

The most comprehensive assessment of diabetes care practices and patient self-care in communities has been conducted by researchers at the University of Michigan Diabetes Research and Training Center (2). This conceptually driven study assessed the structure (e.g., accessibility of hospital, physician, and community services), process (e.g., level of patient involvement, individualization of educational plans), and outcomes of diabetes care (e.g., levels of self-care, metabolic outcomes). The study employed representative sampling procedures to select eight communities in Michigan, 61 primary care physicians, and 428 adult patients of these physicians to be assessed in 1981 and again in 1985. Only one-third of hospitals in smaller communities studied compared with 80% in larger communities offered formalized diabetes education programs. Concerning patient–physician interaction, 79% of physicians but only 47% of patients perceived that the physician encouraged the patient about the way he or she was taking care of his or her health; only 29% of patients (27% of type I and 30% of type II patients) reported being told to exercise on a regular basis. Finally, three-quarters of all patients felt they could take better care of their diabetes, and only 21% of type I and 16% of type II patients felt that they were always able to follow their meal plan closely.

How to Increase Compliance

Recommendations for ways to use the factors illustrated in Fig. 17–1 to facilitate patient self-care are outlined in Table 17–1. There are several ways that patient–health care provider interactions can be used to improve compliance (59). Several of these actions were embodied in the Greenfield et al. (36) study previously mentioned. The most basic recommendation is simply to listen to the patient to understand his or her perspective on the relevant compliance task(s). Specific, written regimen recommendations should be given, making a copy for both the patient and provider. For example, rather than advising the patient to "get more exercise," a recommendation should be made for a specific type, frequency, and intensity of exercise after understanding the patient's attitudes, preferences, and concerns about exercise. It is also important to tailor recommendations to the patient's life-style and type of diabetes, with particular attention to not trying to change too much at a single visit. In general, having a goal of modifying one regimen activity at a time is best. Possibly most important, follow-up contact (e.g., a phone call or repeat visit) should be made in the near future. On returning home, patients often remember questions they forgot to ask or find they did not understand directions.

Understanding the degree to which the patient's environment will be supportive or nonsupportive of attempts to change compliance behaviors is important. More specifically, anticipated barriers to compliance should be discussed and lists of likely barriers presented (51,74) to patients. This discussion should include cost and financial reimbursement issues. Specific referrals to community resources offering services relevant to the compliance behaviors being addressed should be made. It may be possible to make referral phone calls while the patient is in the office. If not, written information on recommended services or organizations and how to contact them should be provided. If the patient has supportive family members or friends whom they would like to help them achieve regimen recommendations, plans can be made for their involvement. Referral to organizations that focus on compliance be-

TABLE 17–1. *Recommended actions to increase diabetes compliance through different channels*

Channels	Recommended actions
Patient–health care provider interaction	Listen to the patient; understand his or her perspective on compliance behavior(s)
	Make specific recommendations tailored to patient life-styles; keep recommended changes simple and provide a copy for both parties
	Follow-up recommendations with a brief contact in the near future
Social/environmental influences	Identify likely compliance barriers, including financial limitations
	Refer patients to community organizations and resources offering related programs
	Incorporate supportive family members and friends in ways desired by the patient
Psychological variables	Elicit and frame recommendations in ways consistent with the patient's model of diabetes
	Probe the patient's self-efficacy; design supports or gradual approximations to promote compliance as needed
	Ensure that patients have strong problem-solving skills and/or specific plans for coping with likely compliance barriers
Health outcomes	Provide feedback on changes in glycemic control and other health outcomes
	Assess the impact of compliance on the patient's quality of life; reinforce or modify regimen as appropriate

haviors with which the patient is struggling (e.g., mall walking groups, Weight Watchers, or diabetes support groups) should also be considered.

One of the most important reasons to listen to the patient is to elicit his or her personal model of diabetes, especially regarding the role and importance of different regimen activities. In general, efforts should be made to frame recommendations in ways consistent with the patient's model. In cases in which the patient's model is clearly maladaptive or vastly incongruent with the provider's, attempts to modify the patient's model or to discuss a change in providers may be warranted. Another important patient variable to consider is self-efficacy. Often this can be assessed by a simple direct question such as "Being honest and not trying to please me, how confident are you that you'll be able to carry out the (*regimen activity*) as we've just discussed until our next visit?" Positive answers to such questions are indicative of successful compliance. Negative or uncertain responses should be probed, and ways to provide support and/or graduated success experiences should be developed (44). It may be less practical to teach problem-solving or coping skills during routine office visits, but office staff can work with patients (47) or provide homework assignments to develop specific plans for dealing with likely barriers to compliance.

Finally, as shown in Table 17-1, health outcomes can be used to reinforce compliance. If improvements in glycemic control or other health outcomes (blood pressure, cholesterol, weight) are observed associated with changes in compliance, this should be explicitly discussed with the patient (61). If the patient has complied but improvements are not observed in health outcomes, possible reasons should be explored. Adjustments in regimen prescriptions may need to be made, and the patient should actively participate in making such decisions (36,37). The impact of regimen changes on the patient's quality of life should also be addressed. Often patients will experience improvements in mood, self-confidence, friendship patterns, etc., on making behavior changes. These effects should be noted and used to reinforce compliance. However, if compliance has adversely affected the patient's quality of life, this will need to be addressed—possibly through refinements in the regimen to achieve long-term maintenance.

CONCLUSIONS

In summary, diabetes self-management is a complex multiple determined task, of which dietary compliance is often the most difficult component. Interventions to improve compliance need to focus on actively involving the patient and also on his or her social environment and interactions with the health care team. Given the heterogeneity of patients with diabetes, it is critical to take into account patients' type of diabetes and other health conditions, as well as their personal model of diabetes. Useful beginnings have been made in identifying factors that facilitate or impede diabetes self-care. However, much more needs to be done to develop intervention procedures capable of reaching large numbers of patients and feasible to use in routine care.

ACKNOWLEDGMENTS

Research for this chapter was supported by grant DK 35524 from the National Institute of Diabetes, Digestive and Kidney Diseases. Appreciation is expressed to Dr. Cindy Hanson for helpful comments on an earlier draft of the manuscript.

REFERENCES

1. Glasgow RE, Wilson WW, McCaul KD. Regimen adherence: a problematic construct in diabetes research. *Diabetes Care* 1985;8:300–301.
2. Hiss RG, ed. *Diabetes in communities.* Ann Arbor, MI: Univeristy of Michigan, 1986.
3. Mazzuca SA, Moorman NH, Wheeler M, et al. The diabetes education study: a controlled trial of the effects of diabetes patient education. *Diabetes Care* 1986;9:1–10.
4. Goodall TA, Halford WK. Self-management of diabetes mellitus: a critical review. *Health Psych (in press).*
5. Wing R, Epstein LH, Nowalk MP, Lamparski DM. Behavioral self-regulation in the treatment of patients with diabetes mellitus. *Psychol Bull* 1986;99:78–89.
6. Glasgow RE, McCaul KD, Schafer LC. Self-care behaviors and glycemic control in type I diabetes. *J Chronic Dis* 1987;40:399–412.
7. Wilson W, Ary DV, Biglan A, Glasgow RE, Toobert DJ, Campbell DR. Psychosocial predictors of self-care behaviors (compliance) and glycemic control in non-insulin-dependent diabetes mellitus. *Diabetes Care* 1986;9:614–622.
8. Johnson SB, Silverstein J, Rosenbloom AR, Carter R, Cunningham W. Assessing daily management in childhood diabetes. *Health Psych* 1986;5:545–564.
9. Orme CM, Binik YM. Consistency of adherence across regimen demands. *Health Psych* 1989;8:27–43.
10. Webb KL, Dobson AJ, O'Connell DL, et al. Dietary compliance among insulin-dependent diabetics. *J Chronic Dis* 1984;37:633–643.
11. D'Eramo-Melkus GA, Demas P. Patient perceptions of diabetes treatment goals. *Diabetes Educator* 1989;15:440–443.
12. Haynes RB, Taylor DW, Sackett DL, eds. *Compliance in health care.* Baltimore: Johns Hopkins Press, 1979.
13. Marrero DG, Kronz KK, Golden MP, Wright JC, Orr DP, Fineberg NS. Clinical evaluation of computer-assisted self-monitoring of blood glucose system. *Diabetes Care* 1989;12:345–350.
14. Cox DJ, Gonder-Frederick L, Pohl S, Pennebaker JW. Diabetes. In: Holroyd KA, Creer TL, eds. *Self-management of chronic diseases.* New York: Academic, 1986;305–346.
15. Davis WK, Hess GE, Van Harrison R, Hiss RG. Psychosocial adjustment to and control of diabetes mellitus: differences by disease type and treatment. *Health Psych* 1987;6:1–14.
16. Sims DF. Barriers to adherence. *Diabetes Care* 1979;2:524–525.
17. Watkins JD, Williams TF, Martin DA, Hogan MD, Anderson E. A study of diabetic patients at home. *Am J Public Health* 1967;57:452–459.
18. West KM. Diet therapy of diabetes: an analysis of failure. *Ann Intern Med* 1973;79:425.
19. Jacobson AM, Hauser ST, Wolfsdorf JI, et al. Psychologic predictors of compliance in children with recent onset of diabetes mellitus. *J Pediatr* 1987;110:805–811.
20. Irvine A. Self care behaviors in a rural population with diabetes. *Patient Education Counseling* 1989;13:3–13.
21. Cerkoney KAB, Hart LK. The relationship between the health belief model and compliance of persons with IDDM. *Diabetes Care* 1980;3:594–598.
22. Ary DV, Toobert D, Wilson W, Glasgow RE. A patient perspective on factors contributing to nonadherence to diabetes regimens. *Diabetes Care* 1986;9:168–172.
23. House WC, Pendleton L, Parker L. Patients' versus physicians' attributions of reasons for diabetic patients' noncompliance with diet. *Diabetes Care* 1986;9:434.
24. Linn MW, Linn BS, Skyler JS, Edelstein J, Sandifer R. Predicting compliance with medical regimens in type II diabetic patients. *(Unpublished manuscript,* 1989, Miami VA Med Ctr).
25. Lorenz RA, Christensen NK, Pichert JW. Diet-related knowledge, skill, and adherence among children with insulin-dependent diabetes mellitus. *Pediatrics* 1985;75:872–876.
26. Wilson DP, Endres RK. Compliance with blood glucose monitoring in children with type 1 diabetes mellitus. *J Pediatr* 1986;108:1022–1024.
27. Mazze RS, Pasmantier R, Murphy JA, Shamoon H. Self-monitoring of capillary blood glucose: changing the performance of individuals with diabetes. *Diabetes Care* 1985;8:207–213.
28. Gonder-Frederick LA, Julian DM, Cox DJ, Clarke WL, Carter WR. Self-measurement of blood glucose: accuracy of self-reported data and adherence to recommended regimen. *Diabetes Care* 1988;11:579–585.
29. Davidson MB. Futility of self-monitoring of blood glucose without algorithms for adjusting insulin doses. *Diabetes Care* 1986;9:209–210.
30. Anderson LA. Health-care communication and selected psychosocial correlates of adherence in diabetes management. *Diabetes Care* 1990;13:66–76.
31. McCaul KD, Glasgow RE, Schafer LC. Diabetes regimen behaviors: predicting adherence. *Med Care* 1987;25:868–881.
32. Glasgow RE, Toobert DJ, Riddle M, Donnelly J, Mitchell DL, Calder D. Diabetes-specific social

learning variables and self-care behaviors among persons with type II diabetes. *Health Psych* 1989;8:285–303.

33. Schafer LC, Glasgow RE, McCaul KD, Dreher M. Adherence to IDDM regimens: relationship to psychosocial variables and metabolic control. *Diabetes Care* 1983;6:493–498.
34. Ley P. Psychological studies of doctor–patient communication. In: Rachman S, ed. *Contributions to medical psychology,* vol 1. Oxford: Pergamon Press, 1977;9–42.
35. Mazzuca SA, Weinberger M, Kurpius DJ, Froehle TC, Heister M. Clinician communication associated with diabetic patients' comprehension of their therapeutic regimen. *Diabetes Care* 1983;6:347–350.
36. Greenfield S, Kaplan SH, Ware JE, Yano EM, Frank HJL. Patients' participation in medical care: effects on blood sugar control and quality of life in diabetes. *J Gen Intern Med* 1988;3: 448–457.
37. Rost K. The influence of patient participation on satisfaction and compliance. *Diabetes Educator* 1989;15:139–143.
38. Anderson RM, Nowacek G, Richards F. Influencing the personal meaning of diabetes: research and practice. *Diabetes Educator* 1988;14:297–302.
39. Leventhal H, Nerenz DR. The assessment of illness cognition. In: Karoly P, ed. *Measurement strategies in health.* New York: Wiley & Sons, 1985;517–554.
40. Hampson SE, Glasgow RE, Toobert DJ. Personal models of diabetes and their relations to self-care activities. *Health Psych* 1990;9:632–646.
41. Starfield B, Wray C, Hess K, Gross R, Birk PS, Loguff BC. The influence of practitioner–patient agreement on the outcome of care. *Am J Public Health* 1981;71:127–131.
42. Bandura A. Self-efficacy: toward a unifying theory of behavioral change. *Psychol Rev* 1977; 84:191–215.
43. Uzoma CU, Feldman RH. Psychosocial factors influencing inner city black diabetic patients' adherence with insulin. *Health Ed* 1989;20:29–32.
44. Bandura A. *Social foundations of thought and action: a social cognitive theory.* Englewood Cliffs, NJ: Prentice Hall, 1986.
45. Lewinsohn PM, Hoberman H, Teri L, Hautzinger M. An integrative theory of depression. In: Reiss S, Bootzin R, eds. *Theoretical issues in behavior therapy.* New York: Academic Press, 1985;331–359.
46. Lustmann PJ, Griffith LS, Clouse RE. Depression in adults with diabetes: results of 5-year follow-up study. *Diabetes Care* 1988;11:605–612.
47. Anderson BJ, Wolf FM, Burkhart MT, Cornell RG, Bacon GE. Effects of peer-group intervention on metabolic control of adolescents with IDDM: randomized outpatient study. *Diabetes Care* 1989;12:179–183.
48. Hanson CL, Cigrant JA, Harris MA, Carle DL, Relyea G, Burghen GA. Coping styles in youths with insulin-dependent diabetes mellitus. *J Consult Clin Psychol* 1989;57:644–651.
49. Toobert DJ, Glasgow R. Problem solving and diabetes self-care. *J Behav Med (in press).*
50. Hanson CL, Henggeler SW, Burghen GA. Model of associations between psychosocial variables and health-outcome measures of adolescents with IDDM. *Diabetes Care* 1987;10:752–758.
51. Glasgow RE, McCaul KD, Schafer LC. Barriers to regimen adherence among persons with insulin-dependent diabetes. *J Behav Med* 1986;9:65–77.
52. Harris R, Linn MW, Skyler JS, Sandifer R. Development of the diabetes health belief scale. *Diabetes Educator* 1987;13:292–297.
53. Wilson W, Pratt C. The impact of diabetes education and peer support upon weight and glycemic control of elderly persons with noninsulin-dependent diabetes mellitus (NIDDM). *Am J Public Health* 1987;77:634–635.
54. Glasgow RE, Toobert DJ. Social environment and regimen adherence among Type II diabetic patients. *Diabetes Care* 1988;11:377–386.
55. Heiby EM, Gafarian CT, McCann SC. Situational and behavioral correlates of compliance to a diabetic regimen. *J Compliance Health Care* 1989;4:101–116.
56. Heitzmann CA, Kaplan RM. Assessment of methods for measuring social support. *Health Psych* 1988;7:75–109.
57. Heitzmann CA, Kaplan RM. Interaction between sex and social support in the control of type II diabetes mellitus. *J Consult Clin Psychol* 1984;52:1087–1089.
58. Harris R, Linn MW. Health beliefs, compliance, and control of diabetes mellitus. *South Med J* 1985;78:162–166.
59. Sanson-Fisher RW, Campbell EM, Redman S, Hennrikus DJ. Patient–provider interactions and patient outcomes. *Diabetes Educator* 1989;15:134–138.
60. Wing RR, Epstein LH, Nowalk MP, Scott N. Self-regulation in the treatment of type II diabetes. *Behav Ther* 1988;19:11–23.
61. Brownlee-Duffeck M, Peterson L, Simonds JF, Goldstein D, Kilo C, Hoette S. The role of health beliefs in the regimen adherence and metabolic control of adolescents and adults with diabetes mellitus. *J Consult Clin Psychol* 1987;2:139–144.

62. Peyrot M, McMurry JF. Psychosocial factors in diabetes control: adjustment of insulin-treated adults. *Psychosom Med* 1985;47:542–557.
63. Davis WK, Hess GE, Hiss RG. Psychosocial correlates of survival in diabetes. *Diabetes Care* 1988;11:538–545.
64. Kaplan RM, Davis WK. Evaluating the costs and benefits of outpatient diabetes education and nutrition counseling. *Diabetes Care* 1986;9:81–86.
65. Padgett D, Mumford E, Hynes M, Carter R. Meta-analysis of the effects of educational and psychosocial interventions on management of diabetes mellitus. *J Clin Epidemiol* 1988;41:1007–1030.
66. Wing RR, Epstein LH, Nowalk MP, Koeske R, Hagg S. Behavior change, weight loss and physiological improvements in type II diabetic patients. *J Consult Clin Psychol* 1985;53:111–122.
67. Wing RR, Marcus, MD, Epstein LH, Salata R. Type II diabetic subjects lose less weight than their overweight nondiabetic spouses. *Diabetes Care* 1987;10:563–566.
68. Diabetes Control and Complications Trial Research Group. Reliability and validity of a diabetes quality-of-life measure for the diabetes control and complications trial (DCCT). *Diabetes Care* 1988;11:725–732.
69. Diabetes Control and Complications Trial Research Group. The Diabetes Control and Complications Trial (DCCT): design and methodologic considerations for the feasibility phase. *Diabetes* 1986;35:530–545.
70. Rubin RB, Peyrot M, Saudek CD. Effect of diabetes education on self-care, metabolic control, and emotional well-being. *Diabetes Care* 1989;12:673–679.
71. Glasgow RE, Toobert DJ, Hampson SE. Participation in outpatient diabetes education programs: how representative are participants? (*submitted*).
72. Winett RA, King AC, Altman DG. *Health psychology and public health*. New York: Pergamon Press, 1989.
73. Hanson CL, Henggeler SW, Harris MA, Burghen GA, Moore M. Family system variables and the health status of adolescents with insulin-dependent diabetes mellitus. *Health Psych* 1989;8:239–263.
74. Irvine AA, Saunders JT, Blank M, Carter W. Validation of scale measuring environmental barriers to diabetes regimen adherence. *Diabetes Care* 1990;13:705–711.

*Patient Compliance in Medical
Practice and Clinical Trials*
edited by J.A. Cramer and B. Spilker
Raven Press, Ltd., New York © 1991

18

Developing More Clinically Meaningful Definitions of Medication Compliance

Seth A. Eisen

*Washington University Medical Service, St. Louis Veterans Affairs Medical Center,
St. Louis, Missouri 63106*

The primary goals for defining medication compliance are, firstly, to describe patient medication-taking behavior ("the extent to which a person's behavior . . . coincides with medical . . . advice") (1) and, secondly, to explain the relation between medication prescribing and clinical outcome (e.g., how dosing intervals affect the control of hypertension). This chapter addresses the latter goal (i.e., how to develop more meaningful definitions of medication compliance, which will assist health care providers treat specific illnesses with specific medications). Although the focus is on compliance definitions as applied to groups of patients, the concepts are also useful for interpreting the clinical responses of individual patients.

Definitions of compliance used in the literature have been constrained by the characteristics of available measuring methods. Patient self-report and pill counts have been used most commonly to measure compliance. However, frequency of obtaining medication refills, blood levels of the medication, of another medication mixed with the medication, or of a biologic parameter affected by the medication, and physiologic changes induced by the medication have also been used (2). The limitation on all of these measuring methods is that they provide little or no information about the date and time of medication ingestion.

In recent years, electronic devices have become available that represent a major advance toward solving this problem, since they collect detailed data about the timing of dose removal. A reasssessment of the best approach to defining compliance, based on these innovative measuring instruments, is therefore warranted.

COMPONENTS OF A COMPREHENSIVE COMPLIANCE DEFINITION

Ideally, satisfactory compliance is defined on the basis of knowledge about the pharmacokinetics of the medication being studied (3) and the relation between pharmacokinetics and the optimal clinical response of the disease being treated. For example, knowledge about the biological half-life of medications is necessary to develop a recommendation about optimal dosing intervals. Generally, the length of the half-life is directly related to the recommended interval between doses. However, for some drugs and disease states, intermittent periods of "subtherapeutic" drug levels are necessary to enhance the patient's clinical course. For example, the optimal treatment of angina with nitrates may require periods of absent drug levels to prevent tachyphylaxis (4), and the treatment of rheumatoid arthritis with methotrexate requires regular medication-free intervals of several days to minimize the risk of adverse drug reactions (5). In addition, for some disease states, periods of subtherapeutic drug levels may have no measurable adverse consequences. For example, the omission of occasional doses of medication in the treatment of moderate hypertension or seizure disorder may not alter the morbidity or mortality associated with these diseases.

CURRENT DEFINITIONS OF SATISFACTORY COMPLIANCE

Typical research studies define adequate compliance using inexact measurement methods and without reference to clinical outcome. For example, after correlating digoxin blood levels with the medication-taking pattern of a cholesterol-lowering agent to which small amounts of digoxin had been added (6), the Helsinki Heart Study defined good compliance by pill count as 85% and by patient report (using a complex formula that included patient-reported pause in drug intake, change in dose, and dose omissions) as 94%. The pill count cut-off point that distinguished good from poor compliers was then arbitrarily defined as 75% (7). Similarly, the Systolic Hypertension in the Elderly Program defined compliance with treatment with chlorthalidone as having removed at least 80% of the prescribed number of pills. The lack of correlation at the annual follow-up visit between compliance and systolic blood pressure control suggests that the definition of compliance used in the study is not meaningful (8). Studies that define compliance on the basis of blood lithium levels being within a "therapeutic window" must be interpreted cautiously because no prospective data are available that correlate serum concentration with clinical response (9).

Some research studies using conventional measurement methods have attempted to determine the level of compliance associated with optimal clinical outcome. Sackett et al. (10) examined the effect of treating hypertension at the work site on satisfactory compliance, defined as having removed 80% or more of prescribed medications. The authors note that the "appropriateness of the 80 percent value as a lower limit for designating patients as 'compliant' was supported by a regression analysis which showed that it was only above this level of compliance that diastolic blood pressure fell systematically."

Defining underuse of antihypertensive agents as the ratio of lack-of-antihypertensive-drug days (quantitated from pharmacy refill frequency) to the total number of days in the study, patients with poorer compliance were more likely to be hospitalized than patients with better compliance (11). Similarly, in a study that analyzed the effectiveness of an intervention program in improving the control of hypertension, level of patient compliance, defined as whether the patient filled his or her prescription(s) within a 7-day period before or after his or her 30-day supply of medication was due to be exhausted, correlated with blood pressure control (12).

By identifying noncompliance on the basis of at least one "subtherapeutic" plasma level of anticonvulsant medications during the study period and by refilling of at least one prescription more than 1 week later than expected, Peterson et al. (13) demonstrated that improvement in these two parameters was associated with a decrease in seizure frequency.

Using a "compliance score" derived from clinic attendance, alcohol intake, expected effects of the patients' medications on heart rate or biochemical parameters, and the patients' admission and/or practitioner's assessment of medication noncompliance, systolic and diastolic blood pressures of compliant patients were determined to be significantly lower than that of noncompliant patients (14).

In summary, although some research studies have correlated compliance with outcome, no attempt has been made to study the relation in detail, in part because of the relatively crude measures of compliance that have been available.

ELECTRONIC MONITORING DATA CONFIRMS THAT STANDARD COMPLIANCE MEASURES PROVIDE LITTLE INSIGHT INTO MEDICATION-TAKING PATTERNS

Electronic medication monitors are now available that provide data on the date and time of medication removal of aerosolized (15), liquid (16–18), and pill-type medications [using either cylindrical containers (19) or blister pack pill dispensers (20)]. The following is a brief overview of the blister pack monitoring device. A more thorough description has been published (20). Two clear plastic blister sheets, each containing 21 blisters, are filled with the patient's medications. A self-adhering paper, with loops of conductive "wires" in the same pattern as the blisters, is then placed over the open face of each of the sheets of blisters to form blister packs. The packs are connected to electronic components and placed inside an easily opened plastic case (Fig. 18–1). Every 15 min the battery-operated electronic memory sends an impulse through each loop of conductive material. If a dose of medication has been removed (i.e., if the paper covering a blister was torn), the electrical impulse fails to return to the electronic memory, and the 15-min interval during which this occurred is recorded. After the patient returns the compliance monitor, the data are collected with a microcomputer, and a computer file is generated that contains the date and time at which each dose was removed from each blister. Analyses can proceed using any one of several standard statistical software packages.

Data obtained using the blister pack monitor (21,22) have complemented data derived from other electronic monitors (15,19,23,24) in demonstrating that the correlation between traditional methods of measuring compliance and the date and time of medication removal is poor. For example, research with the blister pack device has revealed that on a three-times-daily regimen of antihypertensive medications, patients removed 84% of their total prescribed doses but removed the prescribed number of doses on only 59% of days (21).

Similarly, in a study examining the effect of an intervention on medication compliance with lithium among psychiatric outpatients, the level of compliance was found to be dependent on the compliance measure examined. For example, at one point during the study, 49% of all patients stated that they did not omit any doses during the preceding 2 weeks, 82% of prescribed lithium refills were obtained, 67% of patients had therapeutic lithium blood levels, 90% of prescribed medications were removed from pill containers, and compliance measured with electronic blister pack monitors was 83% (22).

Thus, patient compliance estimates, derived from data provided by different mea-

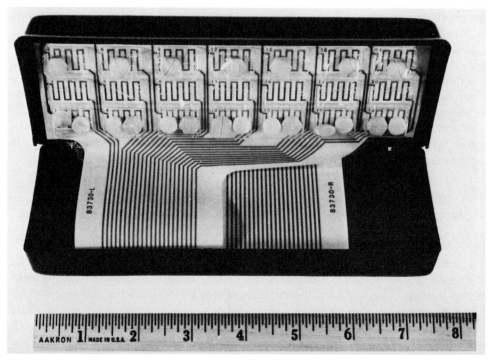

FIG. 18–1. Blister pack compliance monitor, with the case open. The two blister packs are folded into the case's top. Wire-like loops of conductive material can be seen behind the medication-containing blisters. (From ref. 3, with permission.)

suring instruments, consist of multiple discrete assessments, which are not necessarily closely related to one another. The problem is to determine which measure and definition of compliance correlate best with the clinical goals of treatment.

USEFULNESS OF ELECTRONIC MONITOR DATA TO DEFINE SATISFACTORY COMPLIANCE

In an investigation of the relation between medication-taking patterns and blood pressure control in hypertensive outpatients being treated with once-daily doses of hydrochlorothiazide or chlorthalidone, compliance (based on 88 months of blister pack monitoring data) was calculated using five definitions that employed progressively more narrow time windows within which patients had to remove medication doses (25). Compliance estimates varied substantially among definitions. Although each definition was associated with a reduction in diastolic blood pressure, the highest significance was observed with the simple pill count performed in the month preceding blood pressure measurement. This demonstrates that (a) the higher the proportion of prescribed doses taken during an entire month, the lower the blood pressure, and (b) blood pressure is relatively independent of the precise time of medication ingestion. Additional analyses indicated that patients who took their medications irregularly but nonetheless took a high proportion of their doses had a significantly lower blood pressure than patients who missed doses and did not "catch up" to their schedule. These conclusions are consistent with pharmacokinetic data that demonstrates that the therapeutic half-life of hydrochlorothiazide and chlorthalidone (several days) (26) is considerably longer than the prescribed dosing interval (once daily). Consequently, blood pressure control with these two medications is relatively independent of the precise time interval between doses.

Thus, it appears that pill count is a clinically useful indicator of compliance in the treatment of hypertension with long-acting medicines such as hydrochlorothiazide or chlorthalidone. Furthermore, there does not appear to be a specific level of compliance above which compliance can be considered to be "satisfactory," because the greater the proportion of prescribed doses of these medications that are ingested the lower the diastolic blood pressure. Of course, conclusions on the use of long-acting thiazide diuretics in the treatment of hypertension do not necessarily apply to other medications or illnesses. It would be of interest to determine whether results with other medications with long half-lives [e.g., phenobarbital (half-life between 75 and 120 hr)] (3) are similar.

AN APPROACH TO DEFINING SATISFACTORY COMPLIANCE WHEN DATA ARE INCOMPLETE

The preceding discussion demonstrates that with appropriate pharmacokinetic information, knowledge of the medication-taking patterns of the patient population being assessed, and clinical outcome data, specific recommendations can be made about monitoring methods that will satisfactorily assess compliance and about prescribing regimens that will maximize overall health. In practice, however, pharmacokinetic information is typically derived from patients with characteristics that do not match the population being studied, compliance data are not definitive, and correlations of compliance with clinical outcome is incomplete. In this situation, decision and sensitivity analysis techniques can be helpful. Jordan and Reichman (27) compared the clinical benefits of once- and twice-daily dosing regimens with theophylline over a wide range of compliance and assumed two alternative definitions of adequate therapeutic blood levels. They demonstrated that if compliance on a twice-daily-dose regimen was more than 13% worse than compliance on a once-daily regimen, clinical outcome was better with a once-daily-dose regimen, regardless of which definition of therapeutic blood levels was used. On an individual patient basis, the twice-daily regimen was hypothesized to result in an improved clinical outcome only if compliance with once- and twice-daily regimens was similar or if there was a high risk of adverse reactions on a once-daily regimen (e.g., the patient had previously demonstrated gastrointestinal distress at theophylline levels in the upper therapeutic range).

FUTURE RESEARCH DIRECTIONS

Future research should be directed toward comparing medication-taking information provided by the new electronic compliance monitoring devices with data derived concurrently from more traditional methods of compliance assessment. Using decision and sensitivity analysis concepts and supplementing compliance information with pharmacokinetic and clinical outcome data, more precise and appropriate compliance definitions can be developed. Clinically meaningful estimates of compliance, based on the extent to which a patient population's medication-taking behavior (measured with the least expensive yet effective technique) corresponds to the minimally constrained medication-taking pattern that provides satisfactory control of the disease being treated, can then be made.

ACKNOWLEDGMENTS

Some of the research reported in this paper was supported by grants from the Health Services Research and Development Service, Department of Veterans Affairs (HSR&D grant 618), the Department of Veterans Affairs Health Services Research and Development Doctoral Fellowship program, and the Department of Veterans Affairs Great Lakes Health Services Research and Development Field Program, Ann Arbor, Michigan. The author wishes to thank the Department of Veterans Affairs Hypertension Screening and Treatment Program, and Kathleen Wenzel, R.N., and Judy Martin, R.N., of the St. Louis Hypertension Screening and Treatment Program for their willing participation in compliance research, and Patricia Giles for her consistently excellent secretarial support.

REFERENCES

1. Haynes RB. Introduction. In: Haynes RB, Taylor DW, Sackett DL, eds. *Compliance in health care*. Baltimore, Maryland: Johns Hopkins University Press, 1979;1–7.
2. Pullar T, Kumar S, Feely M. Compliance in clinical trials. *Ann Rheum Dis* 1989;48:871–875.
3. Cloyd J. Compliance in epilepsy. Pharmacokinetics and medication compliance. *Epilepsy Res Suppl* 1988;1:101–107.
4. Cohn JN. Drugs used to control vascular resistance and capacitance. In: Hurst JW, Schlant RC, Rackley CE, Sonnenblick EH, Wenger NK, eds. *Arteries and veins*. New York: McGraw-Hill Information Services Company, 1990;1673–1682.
5. Weinblatt ME. Methotrexate. In: Kelley WN, Harris ED Jr, Ruddy S, Sledge CB, eds. *Textbook of rheumatology*. Philadelphia, Pennsylvania: WB Saunders Company, 1989;833–844.
6. Mäenpää H, Javela K, Pikkarainen J, Mälkönen M, Heinonen OP, Manninen V. Minimal doses of digoxin: a new marker for compliance to medication. *Eur Heart J* 1987;8(Suppl I):31–37.
7. Mäenpää H, Manninen V, Heinonen OP. Comparison of the digoxin marker with capsule counting and compliance questionnaire methods for measuring compliance to medication in a clinical trial. *Eur Heart J* 1987;8(Suppl I):39–43.
8. Black DM, Brand RJ, Greenlick M, Hughes G, Smith J. Compliance to treatment for hypertension in elderly patients: the SHEP pilot study. *J Gerontol* 1987;42:552–557.
9. Amdisen A, Nielsen-Kudsk F. Relationship between standardized twelve-hour serum lithium, mean serum lithium of the 24-hour day, dose regimen, and therapeutic interval: an evaluation based on pharmacokinetic simulations. *Pharmacopsychiatry* 1986;19:416–419.
10. Sackett DL, Haynes RB, Gibson ES, et al. Randomised clinical trial of strategies for improving medication compliance in primary hypertension. *Lancet* 1975;1:1205–1207.
11. Maronde RF, Chan LS, Larsen FJ, Strandberg LR, Laventurier MF, Sullivan SR. Underutilization of antihypertensive drugs and associated hospitalization. *Med Care* 1989;27:1159–1166.
12. Bond CA, Monson R. Sustained improvement in drug documentation, compliance, and disease control: a four-year analysis of an ambulatory care model. *Arch Intern Med* 1984;144:1159–1162.
13. Peterson GM, McLean S, Millingen KS. A randomised trial of strategies to improve patient compliance with anticonvulsant therapy. *Epilepsia* 1984;25:412–417.
14. Traub YM, McDonald RH Jr, Shapiro AP. Patient characteristics and their influence on therapy and its outcome in hypertension of the elderly. *Cardiology* 1988;75:45–55.
15. Spector SL, Kinsman R, Mawhinney H, et al. Compliance of patients with asthma with an experimental aerosolized medication: implications for controlled clinical trials. *J Allergy Clin Immunol* 1986;77:65–70.
16. Norell S. Medication behavior. A study of outpatients treated with pilocarpine eye drops for primary open-angle glaucoma. *Acta Ophthalmol* 1980;58(Suppl 143):1–28.

17. Kass MA, Meltzer DW, Gordon M. A miniature compliance monitor for eyedrop medication. *Arch Ophthalmol* 1984;102:1550–1554.
18. Yee RD, Hahan PM, Christensen RE. Medication monitor for ophthalmology. *Am J Ophthalmol* 1974;78:774–778.
19. Cramer JA, Mattson RH, Prevey ML, Scheyer RD, Ouellette VL. How often is medication taken as prescribed? A novel assessment technique. *JAMA* 1989;261:3273–3277.
20. Eisen SA, Hanpeter JA, Kreuger LW, Gard M. Monitoring medication compliance: description of a new device. *J Compliance Health Care* 1987;2:131–142.
21. Eisen SA, Miller DK, Woodward RS, Spitznagel E, Przybeck TR. The effect of prescribed daily dose frequency on patient medication compliance. *Arch Intern Med* 1990;150:1881–1884.
22. Elixhauser A, Eisen SA, Romeis JC, Homan SM. The effects of monitoring and feedback on compliance. *Med Care* (*in press*).
23. Kass MA, Gordon M, Meltzer DW. Can ophthalmologists correctly identify patients defaulting from pilocarpine therapy? *Am J Ophthalmol* 1986;101:524–530.
24. Norell SE. Accuracy of patient interviews and estimates by clinical staff in determining medication compliance. *Soc Sci Med* 1981;15E:57–61.
25. Eisen SA, Woodward RS, Miller D, Spitznagel E, Windham CA. The effect of medication compliance on the control of hypertension. *J Gen Intern Med* 1987;2:298–305.
26. Morgan TO, Adam WR, Hodgson N, Meyers J. Duration of effect of different diuretics. *Med J Aust* 1979;2:315–406.
27. Jordan TJ, Reichman LB. Once-daily versus twice-daily dosing of theophylline: a decision analysis approach to evaluating theophylline blood levels and compliance. *Am Rev Respir Dis* 1989;140:1573–1577.

*Patient Compliance in Medical
Practice and Clinical Trials*
edited by J.A. Cramer and B. Spilker
Raven Press, Ltd., New York © 1991

19

Patient Computers to Enhance Compliance with Completing Questionnaires

A Challenge for the 1990s

Bengt Dahlström and Sven-Åke Eckernäs

Professional Medical Consultants AB, Glunten, S-751 83 Uppsala, Sweden

DIFFERENTIATING BETWEEN MEDICAL COMPLIANCE AND QUESTIONNAIRE COMPLIANCE

Poor patient compliance with taking medicines is one of the most commonly overlooked problems in clinical research. Recent technical development has, however, provided tools such as the "electronic pill box" (Medication Event Monitoring System) (1) to address this problem. But compliance is not solely restricted to drug compliance.

In areas like psychiatry and pain research, in which self-ratings are of crucial importance, it is equally desirable to monitor "questionnaire" compliance (i.e., when and how patients record events on self-assessment scales). In some instances, these data are collected daily through the use of patient diaries, in which the patients are to note, for example, efficacy and adverse reaction parameters. Sometimes these data are collected when the patients return to their physician. The first approach is hampered by the lack of control of the exact time when the patient fills in his or her diary. The drawback of the second approach is that many of the emotionally influenced parameters (e.g., pain or mood) are difficult to remember at a later moment about intensity and duration. To give a true picture of the events, the patient should record them immediately when they occur. With the new portable patient computer, the MiniDoc, it is now possible to overcome the problems associated with delays by having the patients themselves enter ratings directly into the patient computer. The patient simply brings the computer along and can easily record the ratings and also the exact times of the ratings. Additionally, the use of the patient computers can solve some of the inherent problems with the traditional data acquisition method of paper and a pencil (i.e., incompletely filled in patient diaries) and the tedious work of measuring and transcribing Visual Analog Scales recordings to computer media.

A COMPUTER-BASED APPROACH TO QUALITY ASSURANCE OF SELF-ASSESSMENT DATA

The recent development of small, portable, special purpose computers and electronic devices for the monitoring of both drug and questionnaire compliance provides opportunities to record exactly when patients are taking their medicine out of the package and to record how the patient is responding to the treatment at a certain time. The key to the quality assurance is the recording of the exact time of the event. In the MiniDoc this is done by the addition of a "time tag" to every recording, thus providing valuable information on the time pattern of therapeutic effects in relation to drug intake.

THE CONCEPT OF THE MINIDOC

Previous experience of working with stationary personal computers used by investigators and/or patients for remote data entry showed that the demands to be met by the MiniDoc were the following:

- simple for the patient to use
- portable and rugged
- able to operate without recharging the batteries for extended periods of time
- flexible
- simple to program
- able to download data in ASCII format
- able to maintain a high degree of data integrity

FEATURES OF THE PORTABLE PATIENT COMPUTER MINIDOC

General

The MiniDoc is a small, lightweight (800 g), portable computer with a 256-Kb internal memory (expandable to 1 Mb). It is equipped with a graphical screen (240 × 128 pixels with 8K graphic RAM). The most prominent external feature is that the traditional keyboard has been replaced by only four buttons (see Fig. 19–1) whose functions show in clear reading just above each button. The MiniDoc can be fully operated by using only the four buttons. The function of the buttons can thus easily be changed throughout the questionnaire programs. External equipment (i.e., personal computer, printer, modem, keyboard, bar code reader) can easily be attached to the communication ports of the MiniDoc. Through another port (optically isolated), the MiniDoc can collect data from external measuring devices that provide a digital input signal (e.g., sensors for heart rate, blood pressure, or muscle tone). The MiniDoc is also equipped with an alarm, which can be used to alert the patient when it is time to take the medication or to answer the questionnaire.

Simple to Use For the Patient

The four buttons and the big graphical screen make it easy for the patient to use the MiniDoc, and only a short training session is necessary before handing over the

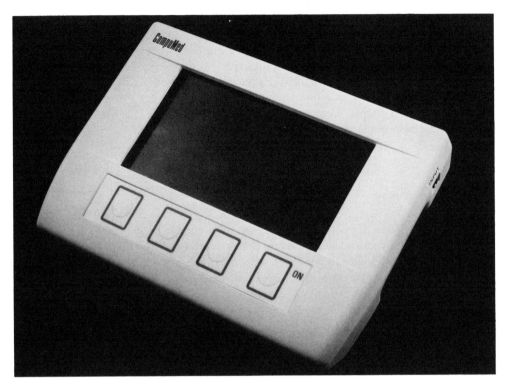

FIG. 19–1. Front view of MiniDoc.

computer to the patient. The screen size (40 characters × 16 rows) allows multiple choice questions to be presented with all choices shown on the screen simultaneously. The character size can also be increased to facilitate reading for visually impaired patients. The patient's understanding of the information presented on the screen can sometimes be enhanced by the inclusion of pictures and graphical scales. For instance, the location of pain can be entered using a picture of the human body and the degree of pain entered by using a visual analog scale. To facilitate both drug and "questionnaire" compliance, the MiniDoc can be programmed to act not only as an alarm clock but also to allow more sophisticated designs such as allowing data entry only during one or several specified time frames.

The rechargable batteries allow continuous operation of the MiniDoc for 15 hr. Thanks to the energy-efficient CMOS circuits and an automatic power shutdown when the MiniDoc is not used, it can, in the practical setting, operate for several weeks without recharging the batteries. This makes it easy for the patients to have the MiniDoc always available.

Data Integrity

The data once entered into the MiniDoc must remain unaltered until they have been transferred to a computer program in which authorized changes are permitted. Thus, the MiniDoc is designed to withstand rough treatment. It has three separate internal battery power supplies: one for the internal clock, a second rechargable battery for the computer, and a third battery supply for each individual memory chip. Should the MiniDoc be totally destroyed but the memory chips remain intact, it will still be possible to retrieve the data from that particular MiniDoc. To prevent unauthorized access to the MiniDoc, it can easily be programmed with unique access codes for different users. A patient-specific code can prevent the entry of data by, for example, other family members, and a physician-specific password can prevent unauthorized personnel from accessing the data.

Data Quality

The quality of the data obtained from a patient depends on when and how the data were collected. To address these issues, the following strategies were adopted for the questionnaire programs. First, when the patient responded to a question, he or she was immediately asked to verify whether his or her answer was correct by pressing a yes or no button. By pressing the yes button, the data were stored, inaccessible for changes by the patient or the investigator. Second, every data item was labeled with the exact time when it was entered (year, month, date, hours, minutes), thus providing vital information on the relevance of the data. Furthermore, it is not possible for the patients to leave any questions unanswered, because the program will not allow them to continue until an answer has been given.

Simple to Program and to Transfer Data

Rather than providing preprogrammed MiniDocs, they were made programmable in BASIC. The data retrieved from the MiniDoc are exported in ASCII format and can thus be directly imported into most clinical database programs. Simple communication routines have also been developed for a database program (4:th Dimension, Acius) on the Macintosh. This allows the user to incorporate MiniDoc data, clinical chemistry data from the laboratory, and other data directly entered by the investigator in the same relational database (4:th Dimension).

INTEGRATION OF THE MINIDOC IN A FULLY COMPUTERIZED DATA ACQUISITION SYSTEM FOR CLINICAL STUDIES

A fully computerized system for data acquisition from a study in rheumatology patients is now evaluated by Professional Medical Consultants AB, a Swedish clinical research organization. Data from patient self-ratings are collected from MiniDocs and are integrated with the data, which the investigator enters on electronic case record forms on his or her Macintosh computer. The complete data set for each patient is then transferred to the clinical database either via modem or on flexible disks. To this data set is also added all clinical laboratory data, which are transferred via modem from the laboratory. In this way, the time-consuming and error-generating procedure of manual data transcription has been avoided.

CLINICAL TRIALS WITH THE MINIDOC

The current experience of the MiniDoc originates from two ongoing clinical trials in rheumatology and psychiatry involving more than 400 patients. One of the studies concerns an evaluation of a new medicine for the treatment of benzodiazepine withdrawal. The objective for using the MiniDoc was to enable a rapid and reliable collection of the patients' self-ratings of anxiety. The physician's choice of dosage regimen was then based on this information until the next visit. It was also desirable to collect the self-ratings at the same time of the day (i.e., in the evening when the patients should have taken their total daily dose of the medication). The software developed for this study consisted of three main parts:

- the questionnaire (31 questions)
- patient information about the study
- general information to the patient about the use of the MiniDoc

The patient had access to the information about the study and about the MiniDoc at anytime during the day, but the questionnaire was only opened for access between 8:00 to 10:00 PM. To remind the patients to answer the questionnaire, the MiniDoc was programmed to beep every 10th min between 8:00 to 10:00 PM until the patient had made his or her self-ratings. The questionnaire contained a number of main- and subquestions, and it was decided to use a logic structure as depicted in Fig. 19–2 to

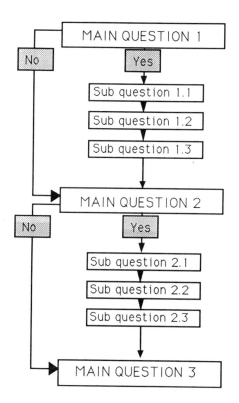

FIG. 19–2. Logic structure of questionnaire program for MiniDoc.

save the patient from answering no to each subquestion if he or she had answered no to the main question. The questionnaire also contained questions regarding the number of tablets that the patient had taken during the day. The MiniDocs were then handed over to the patients with instructions to use it every day until the next visit. At the next visit to the physician, the data in the MiniDoc were transferred to the clinical database (4:th Dimension) on the investigator's Macintosh computer.

The reliability of retrospective ratings of pain and adverse drug events in comparison with daily ratings is being addressed in an ongoing study of a new nonsteroidal anti-inflammatory medicine in patients with rheumatoid arthritis. The objective of this study is to use the MiniDoc for the collection of daily information on pain, drug intake, adverse events, and other effects during two periods of 2 weeks and to compare these results with the retrospective assessments (covering two periods of 2 weeks) of the same items, which are made when the patient comes back to see his or her physician.

Also in this study, the patients only had access to the questionnaire at a time when they should have taken their total daily dose (i.e., between 8:00 and 10:00 PM). In the software for this study, full advantage was taken of the graphic screen by presenting the visual analog scale (see Fig. 19–3). The position of the cursor, which the patient could move along the scale with the two buttons, was stored as the fraction of the total length of the scale in the MiniDoc, thus avoiding the need for additional processing of this value. Compared with the traditional way of using paper and a pencil, the MiniDoc approach will save all the effort of measurement with a ruler, calculations, and keyboard entry of the data. Another function added to this program was the alert screen (see Fig. 19–4). This was intended to urge the patient to contact his or her physician should he or she experience certain types of adverse reactions or intense drug events.

After a brief training session, the MiniDoc was handed over to the patient, who was requested to use it daily for 4 weeks. During this period, he or she visited the physician twice (every second week).

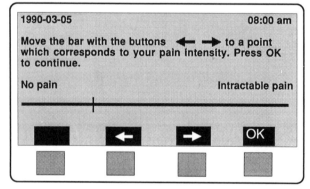

FIG. 19–3. Example of a visual analog scale for pain, which can be shown on the graphical screen of MiniDoc. The cursor, corresponding to patient's degree of pain, can be moved along the line using two buttons with arrows.

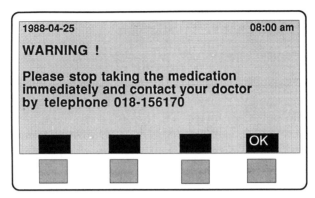

FIG. 19–4. Example of an alert screen shown on MiniDoc when certain types of adverse drug reactions were reported.

USER EXPERIENCES OF THE MINIDOC

Because the studies have not been completed yet, only interim data can be presented at the present stage. Interim results from the benzodiazepine withdrawal study show that the majority of the patients think of the MiniDoc as a helpful tool to remind them when to take their medication and to fill in the questionnaire (see Table 19–1). A few negative comments were made, revealing a hostile attitude toward computers in general and also regarding the "dementing" nature of computers.

The majority of the patients using the MiniDoc have so far been elderly patients (older than 60 years), and despite their lack of computer experience, they thought the MiniDoc was simple to use, once its function was explained to them by the physician.

The opinion of the 25 investigators has been highly positive, with a strong emphasis on the improvement in data quality that the system can bring. They also feel that this tool helps their patients to comply more strictly with the instructions for both dosage regimen and questionnaire procedures.

COST-BENEFIT OF THE USE OF THE MINIDOC IN CLINICAL TRIALS

The use of the MiniDoc for the collection of data directly from the patient saves both time and money, because no data have to be manually entered from the case report forms. Several pharmaceutical companies have estimated that the reduction of the manpower needed to handle the data may be as high as 40 to 50%. An addi-

TABLE 19–1. *Summary of comments about the MiniDoc from a group of patients (n = 21) undergoing benzodiazepine withdrawal therapy*

Positive:	19 positive statements about the MiniDoc. The reminding function (beeper) was considered as very helpful.
Negative:	1 reaction on size and noise. Does not like to take the MiniDoc on social visits. 1 reaction about the dementing nature of computers.

tional advantage is that there will be no incomplete patient records and, consequently, no need to go back to the investigator to fill in missing data afterward.

NEW POSSIBILITIES

In studies in which a close follow-up of the patients is necessary also between the visits to the physician, the MiniDoc can be connected to a central computer via a modem using the patient's own telephone line. The central computer can then automatically call the various MiniDocs in a study and retrieve the data collected during the day.

With the MiniDoc as a feedback link to the patient, it will be possible to design studies with individual dose titration schemes based on the therapeutic responses recorded by the patient. The individual dose titration concept has been successfully tested in the management of severe pain (2). To ascertain that patients who experience certain types of adverse drug reactions contact their physician, the MiniDoc can be programmed to show an alert screen, asking the patient to get in contact with his or her physician (see Fig. 19–4).

It is often difficult for the patient to remember all information given to him or her about the medication. In such cases, it can be helpful to have information about the medication and the study incorporated as a part of the program on the MiniDoc. The patient can then get this information any time by just pressing a button of the MiniDoc.

ACKNOWLEDGMENT

The development of the MiniDoc has been supported by the Swedish National Board for Technical Development. The pioneer work to use the MiniDoc in clinical studies together with Roche Produkter AB and Duphar BV is greatly appreciated.

REFERENCES

1. Editorial. *Medication Event Monitoring Overview* 1989;1:1–3.
2. Dahlström B, Tamsen A, Paalzow L, Hartvig P. Patient-controlled analgesic therapy. IV: Pharmacokinetics and analgesic plasma concentrations of morphine. *Clin Pharmacokinet* 1982;7:266–279.

PART **IV**

Analytical Issues and Approaches

Patient Compliance in Medical
Practice and Clinical Trials
edited by J.A. Cramer and B. Spilker
Raven Press, Ltd., New York © 1991

20

Statistical Approach to Subgroup Analyses

Patient Compliance Data and Clinical Outcomes

Frank L. Hurley

Biometric Research Institute, Inc., Arlington, Virginia 22209

COMPLIANCE AND CLINICAL END POINTS

Patient compliance is always a correlate of clinical outcome. Like few other correlates, however, compliance can be linked to outcome as either cause *or* effect. The approach to using compliance data is determined by the nature of its relation to outcome (i.e., cause or effect). Therefore, like any other correlate used to define subgroups for analysis, the hypothesized relation between compliance and the safety and effectiveness end points must be specified before a clinical trial begins. Thus, the usefulness of compliance data in an analysis depends on pretrial postulation of the relation of compliance to outcomes.

The effects of compliance on clinical outcomes are mediated through pharmacokinetics and pharmacodynamics, and the key to determining the effect of various compliance patterns is understanding the nature of this relation. Pharmacokinetics and pharmacodynamics are complex issues as they relate to clinical outcomes, and understanding how such data relates to compliance data generally requires consultation with a pharmacokineticist.

For example, occasionally or even consistently missed doses may have little therapeutic impact if the medicine's half-life is substantially longer than the recommended interdose interval. In other cases, full compliance with the number of recommended doses may leave significant gaps in therapeutic coverage depending on the timing of the doses—as John Urquhart says, "BID is not equivalent to Q 12 hours" (1). Thus, a rational approach to the evaluation of the effects of various compliance profiles requires careful consideration of the complexities of the disease or condition treated as well as the properties of the medicine.

At the same time, there is wisdom in the age-old aphorism that "drugs don't work for people who don't take them." A simplistic hypothetical example can illustrate most clearly how the underlying compliance profile in a clinical trial can overwhelm even strong drug effects. Table 20–1 presents the results of intent-to-treat analyses for three hypothetical studies. The results range from those in Study 1, slightly favoring placebo, to those in Study 3, which show a highly significant effect favoring the active treatment.

TABLE 20–1. *Mean response to treatment (change from baseline) intent-to-treat analysis*

	Active	Placebo	p Value
Study 1	3.2	3.25	0.50
Study 2	6.0	3.25	0.05
Study 3	7.1	3.25	0.001

In the first hypothetical study, the changes from baseline values were 3.2 for the active group and 3.25 for the placebo group. In Study 2, changes from baseline were 6.0 and 3.25 for the active and placebo groups, respectively, and in Study 3, active and placebo group changes were 7.1 and 3.25. Thus, in all three trials, the placebo group showed a change of 3.25, whereas the active groups' changes ranged from 3.2 to 7.1. Resulting p values were 0.50, 0.05, and 0.001, ranging from nonsignificant in Study 1 to highly significant in Study 3.

How can these results be reconciled? Could they possibly represent the same active medicine for the same indication? Reference to Table 20–2 shows the compliance-specific effect rates underlying all three studies. That is, if subjects are stratified according to compliance profile, Table 20–2 shows the expected therapeutic response for high, medium, and low compliance. Although real-life research requires that compliance be defined in relation to the complexities of pharmacokinetics and pharmacodynamics, for these hypothetical studies the categories of high, medium, and low compliance have been assigned.

These compliance-specific effect rates reflect a truly active product, demonstrating that compliance with the regimen dramatically increases response to treatment: The medicine works for people who take it! A similar although far less pronounced pattern, however, is apparent in the placebo group. The most obvious reason for this pattern lies in the rarity of treatment of a disease or condition with a single-dimensional therapy. Most often, therapy involves multiple medications and/or some modification of life-style. Better compliance with a prescribed drug regimen is likely to be accompanied by better compliance with other facets of treatment, making predictable the observed compliance-correlated response in the placebo group as well as in the active group. Likewise, no difference between effects of active and placebo treatment would be expected in the low-compliance group.

How can these same compliance-specific effect rates underly all three studies with such different intent-to-treat results? Differential compliance profiles provide the explanation (Table 20–3).

Study 2 shows the same compliance profiles for active and placebo groups, with 25% falling into low and medium compliance categories, whereas high compliance is reported for 50% of each group. Recent publication of compliance results in a variety of clinical settings demonstrate this type of pattern (2–4).

TABLE 20–2. *Relation of compliance to clinical end points: mean response to treatment by subject compliance category*

Compliance category	Active	Placebo
Low	2.0	2.0
Medium	6.0	3.0
High	8.0	4.0

TABLE 20–3. *Compliance profiles*

| | Percent of group | | | | | |
| | Study 1 | | Study 2 | | Study 3 | |
Compliance	A	P	A	P	A	P
Low	75	25	25	25	10	25
Medium	15	25	25	25	15	25
High	10	50	50	50	75	25

In Study 1, the active group shows a high percentage in the low compliance category and markedly lower percentages in the medium and high compliance categories. Thus, in comparison with the typical pattern of Study 2, Study 1 shows an abnormally high percentage of subjects in the active group in the low compliance category, whereas the reverse is true for Study 3.

Although in practice one should have serious questions about the reasons for such differential compliance patterns between the active and placebo groups, these patterns are presented here to illustrate an important point. Looking only at compliance-specific response to treatment as presented in Table 20–2 and applying the compliance profiles for active and placebo populations to unadjusted mean response reveals a highly significant difference in Study 3 (p value of 0.001), borderline significance in Study 2 (p value 0.05), and no significance in Study 1 (p value 0.50).

Using compliance-adjusted mean response, however, produces exactly the same mean response for all three studies (Table 20–4). Although the results of these three studies appear different in Table 20–1, applying any of several compliance adjustment techniques produces an identical adjusted mean response in all cases.

It can be concluded that the underlying compliance profiles of the treatment groups can have a significant effect on the intent-to-treat analysis and can even overwhelm drug effect. This conclusion raises several questions. Should equivalent compliance be expected in active and placebo groups? Is such equivalence an earmark of a "good study"? Finally, should simple *post hoc* stratification or equivalent covariate analysis be performed to adjust for compliance?

To address these questions, a somewhat less arbitrary hypothetical study is suggested, specifically a weight loss program. This study entails a multifaceted therapeutic approach, including medicine as well as patient-specific diet and exercise programs. Although compliance with the drug regimen is not influenced by drug effects, compliance with the overall program is highly correlated with results. Results in our

TABLE 20–4. *Effect of compliance profiles on unadjusted mean response to treatment percent of group*

| | Study 1 | | Study 2 | | Study 3 | |
Compliance	A	P	A	P	A	P
Low	75	25	25	25	10	25
Moderate	15	25	25	25	15	25
High	10	50	50	50	75	25
Mean response	3.2	3.25	6.0	3.25	7.1	3.25
Compliance adjusted mean response	6.0	3.25	6.0	3.25	6.0	3.25

INTENT-TO-TREAT RESULTS   CORRELATION OF COMPLIANCE
MEAN WEIGHT LOSS   WITH WEIGHT LOSS

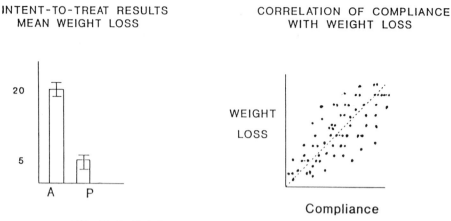

FIG. 20–1. Relationship of compliance to clinical endpoints.

hypothetical weight loss program indicate that the medicine is extremely effective in 50% of patients, moderately effective in 25%, and ineffective in the remaining 25%.

Figures 20–1 and 20–2 summarize the results. Based on the intent-to-treat analysis, the medicine is effective, producing an average weight loss of 20 pounds versus an average loss of 5 pounds in the placebo group. When correlation of drug regimen compliance with the pounds-lost end point is analyzed, however, weight loss is clearly dependent on compliance. This finding is not surprising because one of the assumptions was that overall program compliance was clearly related to achieving the desired weight loss effect.

If compliance-adjusted analysis is conducted using any of various techniques, the active–placebo results are identical. This study shows that in some instances, compliance can be a surrogate measure of the end point. Thus, in this case the simple-minded *post hoc* stratification, analysis ignores the relation between lack of placebo effect and low compliance. That results in attributing the observed difference to differential compliance among the groups rather than to the response feedback effects on compliance. To a large extent, given what is known about weight loss pro-

COMPLIANCE PROFILE   COMPLIANCE ADJUSTED RESULT

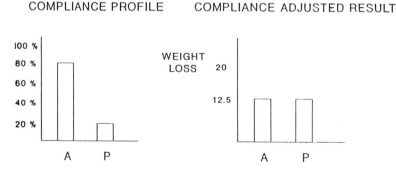

FIG. 20–2. Relationship of compliance to clinical endpoints.

grams, results reflect not necessarily drug effects but compliance with the entire therapeutic program.

The statistical conclusion to this example is that blinded use of statistical techniques to achieve compliance-adjusted analysis is inappropriate. The proper analytic approach must be based on a *study-specific assessment of the determinants of compliance*.

DETERMINANTS OF COMPLIANCE

Determinants of compliance include patient and behavioral parameters, regimen parameters, and response feedback parameters. Patient and behavioral parameters involve issues such as personality and life-style. Compliance with a therapeutic regimen is a different matter for a patient who works an 80-hr week and travels a great deal than for another person with similar personality characteristics who receives constant care in a nursing home.

Route of administration and dose interval are obvious regimen parameters; compliance with an intravenous regimen involving frequent office visits requires much greater personal commitment than compliance with a once-daily oral regimen.

Response feedback parameters can be critical factors in determination of compliance with various treatment regimens. These response feedback parameters can reflect either positive or negative drug effects or what happens as a result of an entire therapeutic regimen, as exemplified by the hypothetical weight loss example.

The potential impact of compliance determinants must be taken into account when deciding on what analytical approach best applies to a study. Patient parameters, like other baseline patient characteristics, should be equivalently distributed by randomization into active and placebo groups. Regimen parameters are usually equivalent by study design, except when those parameters are themselves under study, as in trials comparing two different dosing regimens of the same medicine.

Response feedback parameters merit particular attention in determining the appropriate use of compliance data. Response feedback may be rapid-positive (e.g., insulin or heroin), rapid-negative (e.g., scopolamine-induced nausea), slow-positive (e.g., Protropin) or slow-negative (e.g., quinidine, flecainide). Some agents have both components; tricyclic antidepressants, for instance, often have rapid-negative feedback parameters (dry mouth, blurred vision) followed by slow-positive parameters (relief of depression). An analgesic producing quick pain relief and subsequent gastrointestinal distress has the opposite combination of response feedback (i.e., rapid-positive and slow-negative).

The classic problem of pediatric antibiotic treatment presents a response feedback pattern that demonstrates that obvious therapeutic effect does not always result in good compliance: In this case, therapeutic effect is often accompanied by premature discontinuation of therapy.

APPROACH TO ANALYSIS

Consideration of appropriate approaches to analysis should be separated into comparison of treatment groups and estimation of effect rates. Response feedback effects of the therapeutic regimen on compliance are not controlled by study design or randomization and, if present, will produce differential response profiles in the active and placebo groups. *Thus, response feedback is the key to analysis and interpretation of compliance results.* If there is no response feedback, noncompliance from other sources increases variability in outcomes and therefore diminishes the efficiency of the study. Statistical analysis techniques can restore some of but not all the statistical power of the study. If response feedback effects are present, their nature and magnitude must be explained to define appropriate analytical approaches.

COMPARISON OF TREATMENT GROUPS

If response feedback effects are negligible, the active and placebo compliance profiles should be equivalent. Standard statistical approaches can be used to reduce variance when essential baseline factors are equivalent by study design or by randomization into treatment groups. Variable patient compliance profiles introduce variance into results just as variable demographics introduce variance in results (e.g., response variation in a hypertension study with a wide patient age span). Just as baseline variables can be used as covariates to reduce unexplained variance in response, standard statistical approaches using compliance results to stratify patients or as a covariate will greatly increase the efficiency of analysis.

If, however, response feedback effects are potentially significant, different compliance profiles are likely for active and placebo groups and the cause–effect relation between drug effect and compliance must be carefully examined. This requires examination of both the nature of the relation (i.e., the types of effects operating) and the time course of events. Pilot studies to define the nature of response feedback effects and other compliance factors should be considered before clinical trial design is finalized. Obviously, causal events must precede effect events.

In studies in which compliance is affected by response feedback, a change in a patient's compliance profile during the course of the study will naturally occur. Detailed dose-by-dose compliance information should be used to identify the time of the change, and correlation to clinical records will provide insight into the nature of the relation. For example, decreased compliance after reported adverse reactions signals a different relation than increased compliance after reduction in symptoms or, conversely, decreased compliance after elimination of symptoms.

Parenthetically, it should be noted that analysis of these patterns can provide compelling explanations for both isolated adverse reactions and dramatic therapeutic failures in individual patients. The hypothesized nature of the response feedback relation and the resultant predicted compliance profiles can then be specified based on pharmacokinetics and pharmacodynamics. This will allow proper definition of compliance subgroups before pivotal studies, so these predefined relations can be used to improve the efficiency of analysis.

ESTIMATION OF EFFECT RATES

In addition to comparing results among two or more treatment groups, results of phase III trials are used to estimate rates for adverse events as well as effectiveness. A recent trend in reporting results for a proposed therapeutic regimen is meta-analysis, in which results from a number of studies are combined to produce an overall rate (5–9). This technique often requires use of actuarial analysis based on length of exposure to the medicine to distinguish acute and chronic effects, thus providing more useful labeling to the prescribing physician. That is, rather than using the total number of patients exposed to the medicine (regardless of the length of exposure) as the denominator to determine chronic use adverse reaction rates, the effective denominator would be adjusted to account for differing lengths of exposure.

For example, consider two studies of an antihypertensive: a short-term 1,000 patient study, and a long-term follow-up of 100 patients. If 20% of the patients in long-term follow-up experienced serious angina, a simple safety summary might report overall incidence of angina of 1.8% (20/1,100). This would significantly obscure the risk associated with use of the product by including in the denominator the 1,000 patients not at risk of the long-term effect.

Differential exposure caused by variable compliance can similarly obscure true adverse reaction rates. This could be particularly true for patient subgroups that, because of other circumstances, have unusually high compliance profiles relative to the clinical trial group. For example, if 25% of the patients in an antihypertensive trial had a low compliance profile (essentially, did not take the medication), the adverse reaction rates from this study would underestimate full compliance adverse reaction rate by at least 33%. One would therefore be likely to see higher than expected adverse reaction rates in nursing homes in which medication compliance is presumably improved by staff attention. The prescribing physician should have access to this information in choosing between alternate medications.

CONCLUSIONS

Compliance data are critically important to realistic interpretation of the results of clinical trials. This is true both when comparing differential results between treatment groups and particularly for proper estimation of event rates.

In comparisons between treatment groups, use of compliance information can significantly increase the efficiency of the analysis. Careful analysis of differential compliance patterns can also provide valuable insights into drug effects in individual patients. Adverse reaction rates that include noncompliant patients in the denominator sharply underestimate the actual rate of those events in a fully compliant population. Similarly, anticipated effects or prediction of full-dose efficacy needs to be presented in relation to compliance. The prescribing physician should know the effects of compliance on these rates to tailor treatment to a particular patient population. If patients are going to be treated in a setting that compels greater compliance (e.g., a nursing home) than is the norm in the usual patient population, the impact of that enforced compliance on treatment effects should be available.

Finally, proper consideration of compliance data can provide a significant increase in the efficiency of the analysis. Compliance should be treated like any other correlate of clinical outcome used to define subgroups for analysis, and the hypothesized relation for the subgroup must be specified before the clinical trials begin.

REFERENCES

1. Urquhart J. Therapeutic implications of real-time compliance data. ASCPT Annual Meeting, 1990.
2. Kass MA, Gordon M, Morley RE, et al. Compliance with topical timolol treatment. *Am J Ophthalmol* 1987;103:188–193.
3. Cramer JA, Mattson RH, Prevey ML, et al. How often is medication taken as prescribed? A novel assessment technique. *JAMA* 1989;261:3273–3277.

4. Coats AJS, Adamopoulos S, et al. Effects of physical training in chronic heart failure. *Lancet* 1990;335:63–66.
5. Jenicek M. Meta-analysis in medicine: where we are and where we want to go. *J Clin Epidemiol* 1989;42:35–44.
6. Ellenberg SS. Meta-analysis: the quantitative approach to research review. *Semin Oncol* 1988;15:472–481.
7. Naylor DC. Meta-analysis of controlled clinical trials. *J Rheumatol* 1989;164:424–426.
8. L'abbé KA, Detsky AS, et al. Meta-analysis in clinical research. *Ann Intern Med* 1987;107:224–233.
9. Hedges LV, Olkin I. *Statistical methods for meta-analysis.* Academic Press, 1985.

Patient Compliance in Medical
Practice and Clinical Trials
edited by J.A. Cramer and B. Spilker
Raven Press, Ltd., New York © 1991

21

Regulatory View

Use of Subgroup Data for Determination of Efficacy

Russell Katz

Division of Neuropharmacological Drug Products, Office of Drug Evaluation I, Food and Drug Administration, Rockville, Maryland 20857

This chapter describes the position the United States Food and Drug Administration adopts with regard to the appropriate use of subgroup data in determining the efficacy of a drug product. Further, it presents the results of an informal survey undertaken to document how well commercial sponsors appear to comply with current Food and Drug Administration guidelines in this area. In this chapter, particular attention will be paid to the issue of compliance and how it relates to subgroup analyses. The views expressed in this chapter are those of the author and do not represent an official statement of the Food and Drug Administration.

PUBLIC POSITION OF THE FOOD AND DRUG ADMINISTRATION

The Food and Drug Administration has no official policy regarding the use of specific subgroup data for the determination of efficacy of a drug product. Having said this, however, it should be clear that certain principles are generally applied to the analysis of any data set. That is, there is a general approach the Food and Drug Administration would like to see used in all cases, but based on data to be presented later, it appears that this approach is largely misunderstood or, unfortunately, ignored.

The approach that the Food and Drug Administration endorses can be found in the *Guideline for the Format and Content of the Clinical and Statistical Sections of New Drug Applications,* published by the Food and Drug Administration in July 1988 (1). This document provides detailed guidance to sponsors of new drug applications regarding the type of data and statistical analyses that should be included in a new drug application. It is intended, among other things, to encourage uniformity in applications submitted to the Food and Drug Administration.

In the guidelines, the following statement concerning the appropriate statistical analyses a sponsor should submit appears:

> As a general rule, even if the applicant's preferred analysis is based on a reduced subset of the patients with data, there should be an additional "intent-to-treat" analysis using all randomized patients (p. 61).

(The definition most often used for an intent-to-treat analysis is an analysis that includes patients who have received at least one dose of medicine and have had at least one efficacy assessment.)

Further, the guidelines state the following on the subject of dropouts and their appropriate analysis:

> If the data sets in the intent-to-treat analysis and the applicant's preferred analysis are substantially different, comparability of treatment groups in both sets should be examined and any other reasons for such differences should be discussed.

Later, the guidelines specifically refer to patients who drop out of a study because of poor compliance but who have available data. Data from these patients should be included in an intent-to-treat analysis.

It is worthwhile to elaborate somewhat on these positions.

One important point that emerges from the guidelines is that the intent-to-treat analysis is clearly not always the only analysis that will be accepted as valid by the Food and Drug Administration. The guideline is intentionally vague about when certain subgroup analyses might be considered acceptable (because a general guideline could not possibly predict when such a procedure would be valid), but it is explicit about the fact that the Food and Drug Administration is willing to consider an alternative analysis as primary. To be sure, a sponsor must be able to defend such an alternative analysis, but the Food and Drug Administration is on record as agreeing to judge the merits of each case.

Another important point incorporated into the guidelines is that the Food and Drug Administration does have great interest in seeing the results of an intent-to-treat analysis. The Food and Drug Administration view is that such an analysis has the great advantage of not introducing the kind of bias that postrandomization exclusions can produce. Such biases can lead to erroneous conclusions, as shall be seen. Intent-to-treat analyses are not without problems, but they do provide critical information. Clearly, the Food and Drug Administration feels that the intent-to-treat analysis is the standard against which other analyses must be compared; after all, it is the only analysis that the Food and Drug Administration specifically requires be included in all new drug applications. But, again, it bears repeating that it is not necessarily the *only* analysis that may be judged to be acceptable.

VALUE OF THE INTENT-TO-TREAT ANALYSIS

The Food, Drug, and Cosmetic Act requires that before the Food and Drug Administration may approve a new drug application, that application must contain (among other things)

> substantial evidence that the drug will have the effect it purports or is represented to have under the conditions of use prescribed, recommended, or suggested in the proposed labeling thereof. . . .

The law defines "substantial evidence" as

> evidence consisting of adequate and well-controlled investigations, including clinical investigations, . . . on the basis of which it could fairly and responsibly be concluded . . . that the drug will have the effect it purports to . . . have. . . .

Although the definition of an adequate and well-controlled clinical investigation depends on the medicine and disease under question (e.g., the design of a study to determine the efficacy of a general anesthetic is not appropriate for the study of a hypnotic medicine), the "gold standard" is undoubtedly the randomized controlled trial. The randomized controlled trial is generally accepted by the scientific community as the primary method by which the efficacy of any new drug product should be determined. In those circumstances in which such a trial can ethically be conducted, it is widely regarded as the only acceptable experimental design capable of yielding valid conclusions about drug efficacy.

In such a trial, patients are randomly allocated to one of several treatment groups, and the purpose (usually) is to detect a difference in outcomes between the control group and the new treatment. Such a trial is best able to

> distinguish the effect of a drug from other influences, such as spontaneous change in the course of the disease, placebo effect, or biased observation. [21 Code of Federal Regulations 314.126(a)]

Randomized controlled trials should not, ordinarily, be considered to recreate or mirror clinical practice. They are highly idealized, "artificial" scientific experiments that have as their goal to determine if the medicine under study is safe and effective. Because randomized controlled trials are rigorous scientific endeavors and not clinical practice, their interpretation is dependent on the application of scientific principles that may or may not be applied in the clinical setting. For example, if a physician prescribes a medicine to a patient, the patient takes the medicine, and the patient's condition improves, all concerned conclude that the medicine was effective. Conversely, if the patient does not take the medicine and does not improve, their noncompliance is considered to be (part of) the explanation of their lack of improvement. This sort of *post hoc, ergo propter hoc* reasoning, however, cannot be relied on to determine adequately if the medicine in question was actually responsible for the effect seen. To determine efficacy validly, a randomized controlled trial is usually necessary.

WHY CONDUCT A RANDOMIZED CONTROLLED TRIAL?

A controlled clinical trial is generally necessary to determine if a medicine is effective. The choice of one or more adequate control groups will permit the conclusion that the medicine is or is not effective. Randomization of patients to treatment or control is a fundamental aspect of an adequate trial design. Randomization is critical for at least two reasons:

1. Random allocation of patients to treatments will tend to create groups that are comparable in those factors, both known and unknown, that may have an effect on their response to treatment (i.e., prognostic criteria).
2. The statistical tests usually employed to analyze data are dependent on randomized assignment to treatment for their validity (2).

Once it is accepted that the randomized controlled trial is the appropriate paradigm for the assessment of drug effect, the experiment must be carried out "according to the rules," and according to the rules, an adequate analysis of the data relies on the comparison of randomized treatment groups, for the reasons just elucidated.

The major problem with comparing subgroups of patients, therefore, is that randomization may not have been preserved. Because the basic assumption that the groups to be compared have been created randomly (the fulfillment of which is necessary to give validity to significance tests) may have been violated, it can be difficult (or impossible) to interpret meaningfully any results obtained.

DATA FROM NONCOMPLIERS

The Food and Drug Administration considers patients who withdraw from studies because of noncompliance as a subgroup that should be included in any intent-to-treat analysis. Advocates of excluding data from noncompliers in the definitive analysis of a clinical trial usually use an argument based on "common sense" grounds. They state that if a medicine is not taken (or not taken in sufficient dosage), it cannot possibly be expected to work. Therefore, to include data from such patients is illogical and, in some sense, unfair, because the medicine itself, in these cases, is not being tested. This argument has great intuitive appeal. However, excluding these patients after randomization results in the comparison of nonrandomized groups and can lead to misleading conclusions.

A widely publicized example of such reasoning demonstrates one of the serious objections to such analyses.

The Coronary Drug Project was a randomized controlled trial that was designed to compare the effects of five lipid-lowering medicines and placebo with respect to prevention of coronary heart disease (3). The primary outcome measure was total mortality, and each patient was followed for a minimum of 5 years or until death. Concern will be directed to two treatment groups: the clofibrate and placebo groups. The 5-year total mortality of the 1,103 patients receiving clofibrate was 20.0%; for the 2,789 patients receiving placebo, the total mortality was nearly identical, 20.9%. The effects of compliance on the results were also determined. Patients were allocated to one of two groups: good compliers, defined as those patients who took greater than or equal to 80% of the prescribed dose (as determined by pill count), and poor compliers, those patients who took less than 80% of the prescribed dose. In the clofibrate groups, good compliers had a significantly decreased mortality when compared with poor compliers (15.0% versus 24.6%, respectively; p value of 0.00011). At first blush, this "subgroup" analysis seems to support the view that clofibrate is beneficial (because patients who actually took the medicine seemed to benefit). However, a similar analysis of patients in the placebo group revealed a similar statistically significant decrease in mortality in the good compliers as compared with the poor compliers (15.1% versus 28.2%, respectively; p value of 4.7×10^{-16}). Because the difference in outcome in the placebo subgroups cannot be due to "drug effect," it must be due to some fundamental difference between the subgroups of compliers.

The authors of the study attempted to determine if the differences in the two placebo subgroups could be established through the use of multivariate statistical methods. A multiple linear regression analysis of 5-year mortality and compliance was carried out on 40 baseline characteristics used as adjusting variables. This analysis yielded an adjusted mortality for good compliers of 16.4% and 25.8% for poor compliers. The minimal differences between the unadjusted and adjusted mortality rates demonstrate that differences in these baseline variables account for little of the differences in outcome between the subgroups defined by compliance. Clearly, then, other fundamental differences between the patients in the subgroups have not been detected by this detailed analytic procedure. What this implies is that compliers are, in some unknown and perhaps unknowable way, different from noncompliers.

The authors also attempted to determine if patients who complied with the prescribed clofibrate regimen were benefited, despite the absence of any overall effect on mortality. They concluded that there was no clearly valid way to arrive at this conclusion, primarily because it was impossible to identify the appropriate placebo comparison group. For example, the 5-year mortality for poor clofibrate compliers was 24.6% but was only 19.4% for all placebo patients. Alternatively, mortality in the good clofibrate compliers was only 15.0%, as compared with 19.4% for the placebo patients. However, the argument can be made that the use of all placebo patients as the control group is inappropriate, because it is known that the two compliance subgroups have dissimilar outcomes.

One then could compare the between-treatment responses within compliance strata (i.e., clofibrate good compliers compared with placebo good compliers, and the corresponding poor compliers), which would give still different results. The authors suggest that any conclusion could be justified, depending on which groups are compared, but that any of the results of these subgroup comparisons are unreliable, because there is absolutely no assurance that the compliers in the placebo group are the same as the compliers (or noncompliers to noncompliers) on both known and unknown factors that might affect outcome. It is possible, for example, that the reasons for compliance (or noncompliance) are different between treatment groups and that those differences might have an effect on the outcome. It has been seen that at least in this case, detailed statistical manipulation was unable to detect any systematic reason for the differences between the two subgroups of compliers, yet clearly differences must exist. The only way to be assured that groups are comparable in all relevant respects (i.e., on those factors that may affect outcome), both known and unknown, is through the randomization process. Excluding patients after randomization, however "logical" the maneuver appears to be, can result in groups unbalanced on (unknown) critical factors, thereby introducing bias into the trial. Analyzing all patients randomized to treatment allows the assumptions on which the successful interpretation of the data rely to be fulfilled and hence gives meaning to significance testing.

Other examples of the introduction of bias into studies in which noncompliant patients are excluded from the analysis exist. In a study comparing propanolol, atenolol, and placebo given to patients at the time of myocardial infarction, overall mortality at 6 weeks was comparable between the three treatment groups (4). However, more patients in the beta-blocker groups discontinued secondary to adverse reactions (bradycardia, hypotension) than in the placebo group, although the number of discontinuations was the same in all three groups (placebo patients discontinued more often because of nonspecific reasons). Mortality in those patients in the propanolol and atenolol groups who discontinued was 15.9% and 17.6%, respectively, whereas in the compliers the mortality was 3.4% and 2.6%, respectively. There was no difference in mortality between subgroups of placebo patients. Because it is unlikely that the increased mortality in the noncomplier groups receiving beta-blockers was drug-related, the occurrence of adverse reactions in this subgroup appeared to have identified those patients already at increased risk for death. This example illustrates that the comparison of good compliers in each treatment group, although "logical," introduces substantial bias, because omitting the noncompliant patients from the analysis biases the results in favor of the active medicines by removing patients who are at high risk.

Including the data from patients who are not fully compliant with a drug treatment in the analysis of a trial designed to determine if that drug treatment is effective appears, on face, to be paradoxical. How can the efficacy of a treatment be fairly judged if patients do not receive the treatment? The answer lies in the principle, stated earlier, that the analysis of clinical trial data is dependent on certain rules and that primary among those rules is that randomized groups need to be compared. Excluding patients after they have been randomized and received treatment results in the comparison of nonrandomized groups and allows for the introduction of bias. Often, this bias is undetected and undetectable, and therefore it is difficult to interpret the significance testing performed.

The intent-to-treat analysis is predicated on the (albeit "conservative") assumption that if a mistake in judgment is made, it is better to reject a claim of efficacy than inappropriately overestimate a particular therapy's effectiveness. This principle is reflected in the generally accepted method of hypothesis testing employed in most clinical trials. That is, the maximum allowable type I error (the probability of falsely concluding that a treatment is effective when the null hypothesis is true) is prospectively fixed, whereas the probability of incorrectly concluding that the treatment is ineffective when the null hypothesis is false (type II error) is not (2). The comparison of nonrandomized groups allows for the introduction of serious bias. Because the extent and effect of that bias may be unknowable, the basic principle of the analysis of randomized controlled trials can be placed in serious jeopardy.

Intent-to-treat analyses are imperfect. Indeed, Feinstein (6) gives an (albeit hypothetical) example of a situation in which the intent-to-treat analysis supports the incorrect conclusion of a drug effect, while the compliers only analysis yields the correct answer of no treatment effect. For these reasons, the Food and Drug Administration solicits and reviews alternative analyses and evaluates, on a case-by-case basis, any discrepancies between the intent-to-treat analysis and any other analysis of the sponsor's choosing. However, the Agency places great emphasis on the results of the intent-to-treat analysis, because it generally prevents the introduction of the sorts of bias potentially introduced into the analysis of subsets of the fully randomized treatment groups.

It is often stated that the *prospective* designation of subgroups (defined by some definition of compliance or other factor) makes an analysis of the resulting groups acceptable. As has been seen, however, serious bias can be introduced into a study if compliance and outcome are confounded, and the prospective designation of these categories offers no protection against the introduction of bias. Therefore, in most cases, even the prospective designation of a "compliance" analysis runs the risk of producing an unreliable result.

A number of attempts are currently being made to determine more accurately the degree of patient compliance in clinical trials. Traditionally, compliance in clinical trials has been assessed by counting the number of pills a patient has left at a given visit to the clinic. However, estimates of the degree of compliance based on pill counts or patient reports can be severely inaccurate. In an attempt to quantify compliance, a number of products are being evaluated that can measure compliance more accurately. Most of these products are similar and consist of a pill bottle that has a mechanism to electronically record each time the bottle is opened by the patient. In this way, an investigator can accurately determine how often and when, during a clinical trial, a patient has opened the bottle. Although this does not prove that the medication was actually taken by the patient, it does provide considerably more objective evidence than patient reports and pill counts. Armed with this data, proponents of using compliance data argue that this information can be used to analyze clinical trial results in several ways that give more reliable results than the intent-to-treat analysis. First, because compliance data are now more accurate, the exclusion of patients who are truly noncompliant can be done more appropriately. More interesting, however, are the current attempts to obtain valid dose-response information from such data (5). Specifically, because it is felt now that the actual doses that patients received can be known accurately, it should be possible to regress response on dose and derive a valid dose–response curve from the results of the clinical trial.

Such attempts are interesting and exciting. However, it should be emphasized that the new technology and the resultant novel statistical approaches cannot solve the problem created by analyzing groups created in a nonrandom way. To reiterate, as long as the possibility exists that compliance and outcome can be confounded (and it has been seen that they can be, and the nature of the relation is often unknowable), the potential is real for the introduction of potentially serious bias.

CURRENT PRACTICES IN THE HANDLING OF COMPLIANCE DATA

Although the Food and Drug Administration requires that a sponsor perform an intent-to-treat analysis for each clinical trial performed, as stated earlier, any other analysis may also be performed. Analyses that exclude noncompliers are often performed, and attempts are made by sponsors to justify their exclusion. Such analyses are evaluated on a case-by-case basis by the review divisions. Further, it is undoubtedly true that the inclusion of partial or noncompliers in an analysis has certain consequences. It is true that the inclusion of these data makes a true drug effect (should one exist) more difficult to detect and increases the number of patients needed to detect it. Further, the inclusion of noncompliers often raises the question of how to handle missing data, because such patients routinely have incomplete outcome (and safety) data. Therefore, the collection of compliance data can be important, and by extension, it seems reasonable to assume that the entire issue of compliance (e.g., definitions, data collection, analytic plans) should be addressed in protocols for definitive efficacy trials.

In an attempt to determine the current state of this issue, the author undertook an informal survey of protocols for such trials. To be included in the survey, a protocol had to fulfill four criteria:

1. submitted by a commercial sponsor
2. recently submitted (within the past year)
3. randomized controlled trial
4. definitive phase II/III trial (one intended to fulfill the requirements of an adequate and well-controlled trial)

Thirty-five protocols were found that met the above criteria. All but one were multicenter trials, and all were for studies of investigational medicines intended to treat psychiatric or neurologic illness. The sample was not a random sample and was not necessarily perfectly representative of the practice of the entire industry, because some sponsors were represented more frequently than others. However, no sponsors were intentionally excluded; any protocol found in an approximately 1-month search that met the criteria above was included in the survey.

The first question asked was: How many protocols mention compliance? To be included in the count of protocols that referred to compliance, a liberal interpretation was used. Any protocol that included the word or any reasonable variant of the word *compliance* was counted, regardless of how often or in what part of the protocol it appeared.

Applying this definition, 24 of 35 (69%) of the protocols addressed the issue. Almost one-third of protocols for definitive efficacy trials apparently ignored the issue. It should be noted that all protocols mentioned dropouts or noncompleters and how they would be accounted for, and all protocols stated that medication would be counted at each study visit, but only 69% explicitly mentioned compliance.

Definitions of compliance fall into three general categories. The first category can be defined as *the percentage of prescribed medication,* in which compliance is defined by the percentage of pills prescribed that were actually taken. This is the definition of compliance most commonly referred to in the literature. Of the 24 protocols that mentioned compliance, six, or 25%, defined compliance according to the percentage of prescribed pills taken. Five of the six defined a patient as compliant if he or she took 80% or more of the prescribed medication; one of the six defined a complier as one who took 75% or more of the prescribed medication.

The second category can be defined as the *number of pills taken (or not taken) over a specified time period.* Seven of the 24, or 29%, fell into this category. The chart below details how sponsors defined compliance in this category:

2—Twenty days total off medication or 6 consecutive days off medication.
2—No medication for 24 hr
1—Three consecutive days off medication
1—Misses more than four capsules in 1 week
1—Medication for at least 8 days and reaching a certain blood level

These protocols were of varying lengths, so it is impossible to determine from these definitions how they relate to total study duration. Also, with regard to the last definition, it is interesting to note that a patient who may have been 100% compliant by the routine definition of the word might not have reached the designated blood level and hence would have been considered noncompliant by the protocol.

The third category can be defined as the *name calling* category, an appellation that conveys the subjective and almost judgmental approach taken by these sponsors in defining compliers. In these protocols, compliance was never defined, it was simply named. Ten of the 24 (42%) protocols "defined" compliance in the following ways:

4—"significant noncompliance"
2—"noncompliance"
2—"poor compliance"
1—"do not comply with protocol"
1—"number of pills taken is substantially different from the number prescribed"

What is striking about all these definitions of compliance is their arbitrariness. Even the first two categories, which appear to be somehow quantitative, have no particular rationale. The importance or potential danger of these arbitrary definitions will become evident later.

The next important question was: What will happen to compliers (or more accurately, to noncompliers) during the course of the study, and how will they be accounted for in the analysis?

All 24 protocols that mention compliance state that patients found to be noncompliant will be discontinued from the study. This is of great interest for a number of reasons, not the least of which is that it is the only facet of compliance on which all protocols agree.

The next question is to determine how sponsors plan to make use of the data generated by these patients.

To answer this question, it is necessary to divide the 24 protocols into two groups, based on their definitions of compliers. Protocols that fall into the first two groups described earlier (percentage, and number of pills) are examined separately from those in the name calling group. This is necessary because of the latter group, one cannot tell who the sponsor intends to include in the primary analysis. For example, the protocol may say that patients who complete at least 8 of 12 weeks will be included in the primary analysis, but that "noncompliers" will be withdrawn. It is possible, in such a case, that noncompliers may be withdrawn after 9 weeks of the study and thus be included in the analysis.

Looking at the first group (which consists of 14 protocols) 12 of 14, or 86%, do not include data from noncompliers in the primary analysis. In one of 14, compliers were not mentioned in the statistical section, and in only one of 14 cases (7%) were these patients to be included in the primary analysis. Turning to the name calling category, there is somewhat greater scatter in the data. The following list describes which patients were to be included in the primary analysis:

4—only evaluable patients (evaluable patients defined in the protocol)
2—only evaluable patients (evaluable patients not defined)
2—cannot tell
2—included in the primary analysis

With regard to the first category, as mentioned earlier, it is impossible to determine if the evaluable patients category included noncompliers, although it is likely that it did not. It is likely also that the two protocols that did not define evaluable patients did not intend to include noncompliers as evaluable.

From these data, it is clear that few protocols that mention compliance actually intend to include these patients in a primary efficacy analysis. That percentage is probably three of 24, or 12.5%, but to be charitable, if the four from the first category above are included (an extremely liberal interpretation), the total is seven of 24, or 29%, which is still a low percentage.

It is useful to determine how many of the protocols state the sponsors' intentions to perform an intent-to-treat analysis. It should be recalled that the Food and Drug Administration guidelines currently require that all sponsors perform an intent-to-treat analysis.

Of the 35 protocols reviewed, only 16, or 46%, even mention an intent-to-treat analysis. The following list describes how the sponsor intends to use the intent-to-treat analysis:

10—as primary analysis
 3—as secondary analysis
 2—initial analysis
 1—unclear if primary or secondary

The protocols that stated that the intent-to-treat analysis was to be the initial analysis were vague about the meaning of "initial"; apparently, an intent-to-treat analysis was to be performed before other analyses, but the protocols were silent on the question of which would be "primary."

The most obvious conclusion to be drawn from this survey is that more than half the protocols simply did not state any intention on the part of the sponsor to perform an intent-to-treat analysis, despite the guideline's explicit instruction to do so. As has been noted, the intent-to-treat analysis is certainly not the only analysis that the Food and Drug Administration will find acceptable under all circumstances, but is clearly an analysis that should be included in all applications. That mention of it is not made in most of the protocols surveyed is somewhat unsettling. What is perhaps mildly encouraging is the fact that of the protocols that do mention an intent-to-treat analysis, the majority explicitly state that it is to be the primary analysis.

Finally, it would be useful to see how those protocols that do list the intent-to-treat analysis as primary define and handle (non)compliers.

Seven of the ten (70%) make no mention of compliance at all. Of the remaining three, two fall into the name calling category, and one falls into the "compliance defined" category. This is interesting, although perhaps not surprising. That is, because the primary efficacy analysis will include data from all patients, it can be seen as unnecessary to define, at least for purposes of the analysis, what a complier is. However, in such protocols it is not certain that compliance (however defined) will not be a factor in deciding whether to withdraw a patient (after all, all these protocols have rules for dropping patients early). Therefore, it would be useful in these protocols to try to define compliance, but only if noncompliance will result in early withdrawal. Of course, it is possible that in these protocols, no degree of noncompliance would result in patient withdrawal.

Eleven of the 35 protocols made no mention of compliance at all. Seven of these 11 are protocols in which the intent-to-treat analysis is primary. This is somewhat reassuring, because as noted above, a prospective definition of compliance is less critical if all patients are to be included in the final analysis. Of course, it is still important, because if patients are to be withdrawn because of noncompliance, they will have incomplete data, which may effect the outcome.

In six of 16 protocols that mention an intent-to-treat analysis, that analysis is not clearly the primary analysis. Also, 19 of the 35 protocols do not mention an intent-to-treat analysis at all, although some of these 19 mention a primary (not sole) analysis. Therefore, in 25 of 35 (71%) of the protocols, the intent-to-treat analysis can be considered not to be the primary analysis. The question can then be asked: Does the sponsor state the course of action they will take if in any of these 25 protocols there is a discrepancy between the outcome of the primary analyses and any other analyses (specifically the intent-to-treat analysis) they perform? The answer is that in *no* protocol does a sponsor prospectively address this contingency. Although it may be impossible to detail specifically how such discrepancies will be handled before inspection of the data, the fact that the issue is not addressed at all in these protocols is of some concern in light of the great emphasis that the guidelines place on addressing any such discrepancies.

One protocol, which describes both an intent-to-treat and completers analysis, contains the following statement:

> If there are a large number of patients not completing the study, then the "intent-to-treat" population is considered to be the more important of the two populations.

This was the only protocol that even addressed the question of potential discrepancies in outcomes. (Note that, in fact, it does not actually discuss discrepancies in the *outcomes* of the two different analyses; it discusses which analysis will be primary depending on the number of patients left in the study. Theoretically, if few patients did not complete, the completers analysis might be primary, even if it differed from the intent-to-treat results.)

COMPLIANCE BASED ON PLASMA LEVELS

Before summarizing the important results of this survey, a particular problem recently seen in several protocols is mentioned. These protocols define compliance in terms of achieving certain predefined plasma levels of medicine. This is of particular interest in the anticonvulsant area, in which blood level monitoring is routinely performed and in which well-defined therapeutic ranges are believed to exist. However, certain problems with these protocols need to be addressed.

First, blood levels are, at best, an indirect measure of compliance. Intersubject variability can be great, and prospectively designating a certain plasma level as a marker of compliance is problematic. Further, and more importantly, a more objective "measure" of compliance, like plasma levels, still does not address the fundamental problem that arises when analyzing a subgroup of the data, discussed in detail earlier.

A protocol recently submitted to the Food and Drug Administration described a randomized, parallel group, placebo-controlled trial of an anticonvulsant medicine. The protocol called for the removal of patients who did not achieve a certain prespecified plasma level of drug by a certain time after initiation of treatment. The use of this rule had the potential to introduce serious bias into the study, because it would have resulted in patients from only one treatment group being removed (for this reason) after randomization (because placebo patients were not at risk, by definition, for being dropped for this reason). Also, as mentioned earlier, some patients might actually have been completely compliant as that word is ordinarily understood (i.e., they took all their medication) but still might not have achieved the appropriate levels for other reasons. Such patients would have been inappropriately withdrawn under this rule.

Another problem with this paradigm is a sort of variant of the first problem. As mentioned, this protocol allowed some period of time after initiation of therapy before the plasma level rule took effect. This reflects the thinking noted earlier, that the medicine needs to have a chance to work; that is, it is only fair to judge the efficacy of the medicine when it reaches a therapeutic level. This sort of thinking is especially common in the anticonvulsant area, in which well-defined therapeutic ranges are believed to exist for many anticonvulsants.

Another trial was recently submitted in which the outcome measure was a 6-month seizure-free interval. If a patient had a seizure before the "therapeutic level" was reached, it was not counted. This was found to be unacceptable. The discarding of this event as somehow unfair to the medicine was predicated on the unstated assumption that if the level had been therapeutic, the seizure would not have happened. This is a clear example of positing the efficacy of the medicine before it is demonstrated. In other words, the sponsor is assuming that the medicine would have been effective at the therapeutic level, when that is exactly what the trial was supposed to determine!

SURVEY CONCLUSIONS

The main findings of the survey of definitive efficacy protocols are summarized.

First, a number of caveats are in order. This was not a random sample and may not be representative of current practice throughout the industry. In addition, this was not a survey of new drug application submissions. That is, it is possible that when a sponsor submits a new drug application, some of the deficiencies noted in the protocols may be corrected (e.g., intent-to-treat analyses may be performed). However, some of the deficiencies noted cannot be corrected after the fact, and beyond that, to the extent that a protocol should be a detailed, prospective statement describing the sponsor's intended conduct and analysis of the trial, it should be as complete a statement as possible. Such a protocol will serve to prevent the arguments that often accompany what might appear to be data-conditioned analyses.

To the extent that gathering compliance data is important, it is disturbing that approximately one-third of the protocols reviewed make no mention of compliance. The definitions of compliance used in most (or all) of these protocols are nonstandardized, idiosyncratic, arbitrary, and often uninterpretable in a prospective way. Further, to the extent that an accurate accounting of compliance is important, it is difficult to believe that many of the rules that define compliance can actually be applied (e.g., how reliably can an investigator tell if a patient took no medicine for 3 consecutive days?).

Next, the only point of agreement in the protocols that describe compliance is that when noncompliance is determined, those patients are withdrawn from the study. It may be useful to raise the question of the propriety of this procedure. For example, in those trials in which the intent-to-treat analysis is to be primary, why should these patients be dropped? Further, there are little data on patterns of patient compliance during the course of a study. If a patient is found to be noncompliant at some point in the study, does that predict future noncompliance in the study if allowed to remain in the trial? If levels of compliance change, perhaps these patients should remain in the study. Allowing such patients to continue should yield more usable data. One objection to the intent-to-treat analysis that carries forward a patient's last score is that such a maneuver may be misleading. Allowing patients who have been noncompliant to remain in the study longer would be helpful in this regard.

The vast majority (87.5%) of protocols that mention compliance apparently do not intend to include these patients in an intent-to-treat analysis, and the overall percentage of protocols in which the intent-to-treat analysis is clearly primary is only 29%. Although the guidelines do allow for alternative analyses, these numbers raise serious questions because the guidelines (and good statistical practice) call for an intent-to-treat analysis in all cases, as well as a detailed explanation for any discrepancies seen between the two analyses. In this regard, it is sobering to recall that only 46% of the protocols even mention an intent-to-treat analysis and that none of the protocols describe how any discrepancies might be explained.

REFERENCES

1. Food and Drug Administration. *Guideline for the format and content of the clinical and statistical sections of new drug applications.* U.S. Department of Health and Human Services, July 1988.
2. Pledger GW. Compliance in clinical trials: impact on design, analysis and interpretation. In: Schmidt D, Leppik IE, eds. *Compliance in epilepsy (Epilepsy Res. suppl 1).* Elsevier Science Publishers B.V., 1988;125–133.

3. The Coronary Drug Project Research Group. Influence of adherence to treatment and response of cholesterol on mortality in the coronary drug project. *N Engl J Med* 1980;303:1038–1041.
4. May GS, DeMets DL, Friedman LM, Furberg C, Passamani E. The randomized clinical trial: bias in analysis. *Circulation* 1981;64(4):669–673.
5. Efron B, Feldman D. *Compliance as an explanatory variable in clinical trials. Technical Report No. 129.* Public Health Service Grant 5 R01 GM 21215-13, March 1989.
6. Feinstein AR. "Compliance bias" and the interpretation of therapeutic trials. In: Haynes RB, Taylor DW, Sackett DL, eds. *Compliance in health care.* Baltimore, Maryland: Johns Hopkins University Press, 1979;309–322.

Patient Compliance in Medical Practice and Clinical Trials
edited by J.A. Cramer and B. Spilker
Raven Press, Ltd., New York © 1991

22

Biometric Issues in Measuring and Analyzing Partial Compliance in Clinical Trials

Joerg Hasford

Biometric Center for Therapeutic Studies, D-8000 München 2, West Germany

The history of compliance is as old as the traditional handing down of medical treatments. Even Hippocrates was aware that "patients are often lying when they say they have regularly taken the prescribed medicine" (1). The results of poor compliance might have been negligible or even beneficial for centuries, as long as almost no pharmacologically effective therapies were available. Since the early days of antibiotics such as streptomycin, isoniazid, and penicillin, compliance has become an important issue of effective patient care.

DEFINITION

Compliance is defined in the context of this chapter following Haynes, as a patient's behavior in terms of taking medication, following prescribed diets, or executing medically recommended life-style changes (1). In addition, compliance measures the extent to which a person's behavior coincides with medical or health advice. Thus *compliance* is both a term for a behavior and a measure of it.

There is little evidence that regular attendance at follow-up examinations and the like does provide a valid index for the proper administration of the prescribed medicine. Roth et al. (2) have analyzed the correlation between the percentage of missed appointments and the percentage of prescribed medicine taken in 105 patients. The correlation coefficient of $r = 0.12$ is low and strongly indicates that follow-up rates should not be used even as a surrogate measure of compliance in the context of the analysis of clinical trials.

Correct prescribing specifies the medicine, type of preparation, dosage, time, regularity, and method of application. Even more specific details may be important to add (e.g., take before or after meals, avoid intake with dairy products). The physician might also ask the patient to not take certain other medicines. In clinical trials, such a prohibition is standard with regard to the respective control therapies. Thus, compliance is a complex and heterogeneous construct.

Compliance assessments may be highly diverse. Patients can administer more, less, or exactly as much medicine as prescribed. Patients may take medicines erratically (i.e., sometimes taking more and sometimes less than prescribed). Finally, patients may neglect the recommended method of administration of the medicine or may take unauthorized medicines. Disregarding these complexities, the measure of compliance is most often expressed by a simple ratio, relating the actual medication use (i.e., what is taken) to the amount specified in the protocol or the physician's prescription (i.e., what should be taken).

ROLE AND SIZE OF COMPLIANCE IN CLINICAL TRIALS

The effect of therapy is expressed based on the assumption that the medicine has been taken. If no therapy has been administered, there can be no therapy-related effects. This holds true not only in routine medical care, but also for participants of clinical trials. Risks of partial compliance in clinical trials have to be taken even more seriously, however, as not only the therapy of individual patients might become complicated, but it is also likely that incorrect judgments about efficacy and safety of the particular medicine will occur, and this may affect many future patients.

The rationale of all efforts to keep compliance as high as possible and to correct the trial's results for partial compliance can be explained by a simple model: Assuming the medicine under investigation has an effect at all, patients with poor compliance will show no or only small effects in comparison to highly compliant patients, who consequently will show great effects (Fig. 22–1). Thus, varying compliance within treatment groups leads to a larger variance of the end point values and can cause a distortion in the observed difference Δ between treatment groups. Both these effects can falsify the results of statistical tests. The following example might be simpler than the reality of data obtained in most clinical trials but nevertheless demonstrates the issue (Fig. 22–2).

When

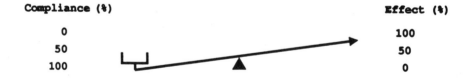

Compliance (%)		Effect (%)
0		100
50		50
100		0

then

varying compliance

- increases variability of the outcome
- may bias size of outcome

FIG. 22–1. Implications of varying compliance on treatment effects.

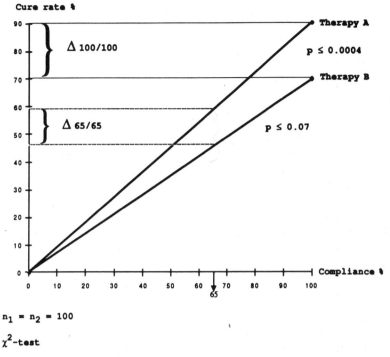

FIG. 22–2. Cure rate and effect size difference Δ in dependence on compliance.

Assuming that treatment A has a compliance rate of 100% and a response rate of 90% and treatment B correspondingly has a response rate of 70%, the difference Δ then amounts to 20%. This difference shows with $n_1 = n_2 = 100$ patients using the chi²-test, a $p \leq 0.0004$. If compliance falls identically in both groups, lower response rates and proportionally smaller deltas are observed. Poor compliance leads to a distortion of Δ (13% versus 20%), and the difference between A and B becomes statistically insignificant when compliance has reached 65% in both groups. Distortions in the other direction are also possible.

The problems encountered with partial compliance in clinical trials have been well perceived and described by Dixon et al. (3), who stated in 1957:

Many chemotherapy trials based on unsupervised oral medication have probably been built on very unsure foundations. However carefully they were controlled statistically and scientifically, the results may have been vitiated by inadequate consumption of prescribed drugs.

Partial compliance presents a considerable problem in medical care. In an extensive overview, Sackett and Snow (4) reported a mean compliance between 33% and 94% for drug therapies and between 8% and 70% for recommended dietary interventions. The problem of partial compliance can also be of considerable size in clinical trials. Taking the Helsinki Heart Study (5) as a recent example among many possible others, compliance proved to be good in less than two-thirds (63.8%) in a subsample of 1,739 patients examined. Seventeen and one-half percent of the participants were classified as intermediate and 18.5% as poor compliers (5).

BIOMETRIC TASKS AND PROBLEMS

The major objectives of formally including compliance data into the statistical analysis of the outcome criteria of clinical trials are

1. to adjust statistical analysis results for the impact of partial compliance
2. to estimate treatment effects and the difference between the treatment groups under the assumption of 100% compliance.

Biometricians and textbooks of clinical trials methodology almost always oppose the formal integration of compliance data into the statistical analysis of outcome criteria (6–8). Their prime example, which has been repeatedly cited as proof for this position, is a publication of the Coronary Drug Project, analyzing the data of the clofibrate and of the placebo group in compliance-stratified subgroups (9). There is a clear positive compliance–effect relation in the clofibrate group, with an almost identical placebo compliance–effect relation (Table 22–1). In a long-term trial, such a positive placebo compliance–effect relation does not make sense. Subsequently, this result was considered to be an artifact generated by a misuse of subgroup analysis. The concluding statements of the authors (9) represent the opinion expressed in major textbooks:

> It is doubtful if any valid conclusions can be drawn from such analyses because there is no way of ascertaining precisely how or why the patients in the clofibrate and placebo groups have selected themselves or have become selected into the subgroups of good and poor adherers. . . . In conclusion, analyses of data from the Coronary Drug Project have demonstrated the great difficulty, if not impossibility, of drawing any valid conclusions from findings about mortality or morbidity in subgroups defined by patients' responses—such as adherence or biochemical response—to a treatment.

The scepticism expressed in these statements is understandable from a biometrician's point of view. The uneasiness of physicians who are confronted with statements about results of trial treatments that include noncompliers in the statistical analyses of outcomes is also understandable. There is also an asymmetry present, as nobody would seriously attribute an adverse reaction to a treatment that had never been administered. In addition, it seems that up to now, the inherent methodological problems have hardly been analyzed in sufficient detail and that there should be a more differentiated point of view. Therefore, a set of criteria in the format of a decision tree is presented (Fig. 22–3). This tool may be used to decide whether the inclusion of compliance into the statistical analysis of the outcome criteria is or is not appropriate.

TABLE 22–1. *Compliance–response relation: Coronary Drug Project, 5-year mortality, clofibrate versus placebo, stratified for compliance[a]*

	Clofibrate		Placebo	
Compliance	n	Mortality (%)	n	Mortality (%)
Less than 80%	357	24.6 ± 2.3	882	28.2 ± 1.5
Greater than or equal to 80%	708	15.0 ± 1.3	1,813	15.1 ± 0.8
Total	1,065	18.2 ± 1.2	2,695	19.4 ± 0.8

[a]From ref. 9, with permission.

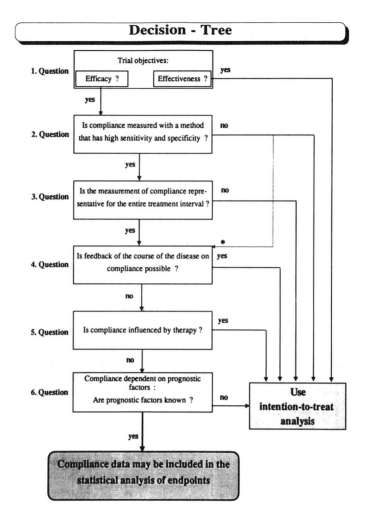

FIG. 22–3. Decision tree.

DECISION TREE

Objective of the Trial: Efficacy or Effectiveness?

The first question of the decision tree asks for a specification of the trial's objectives: efficacy or effectiveness.

According to Cochrane (10), efficacy is defined as "the effect of a particular medical action in altering the natural history of a particular disease for the better under ideal conditions of use." In the context of clinical trials, this means usually phase II or III trials or applying the *explanatory approach* (11), when one wants to know whether and how a medicine works. Administration of the treatment as prescribed is a substantial part of "ideal conditions of use." Thus the inclusion of compliance data in the statistical analysis of the outcome criteria of such a trial is indicated by its objectives.

"Effectiveness" in contrast is defined as "the effect of a particular medical action in altering the natural history of a particular disease for the better in routine clinical practice." This concerns mainly late phase III and phase IV trials and can also be called a *pragmatic approach* (11). As partial compliance is an indispensable part of all therapeutic efforts in routine medical practice, it does not make sense to correct the treatment effects observed for the impact of partial compliance. The aim of such trials is, among others, to find out whether a therapy will work sufficiently despite partial compliance. This aim corresponds to the principle of the intention-to-treat analysis.

Most often it will not be difficult to answer this first question in the decision tree. When there are difficulties, however, as with secondary prevention trials, it is wise not to waste too much time with attempts to find the right answer but to proceed to the next question. Although the use of compliance data as an explanatory variable in effectiveness trials is inappropriate, there may be sound reasons for measuring and analyzing compliance as a dependent variable (e.g., to find out whether a treatment is accepted by the patients).

Measurement of Compliance: Sensitivity and Specificity

The second question in the decision tree concerns the sensitivity and specificity of the measurement of compliance. Only when the measurements of individual patients' compliance are correct can a more precise estimation of the treatment effects be achieved. Several studies demonstrated that all indirect methods of measurement such as the common pill count, patient interview, impression of physician, and the presence or absence of a clinical response provide only low to moderate sensitivity in the detection of noncompliance (Table 22-2). Only one study has reported greater than 65% sensitivity of an indirect method of detecting noncompliance. For specificity, the situation is not much better.

The occurrence of specified clinical responses like the decrease of blood pressure as an indicator of compliance with diuretic therapy proved to be disappointing. In addition, there is a risk of circular reasoning in a clinical trials setting: The blood pressure decreased, therefore the patient had really administered the medicine beforehand. This conclusion requires the statement that the medicine always affects blood pressure. The impression of the physician or the nurse has a sensitivity of about 50 to 65% and usually overestimates the true compliance (12,13). The information provided by the patient either by interview or by a medication diary again considerably overestimates compliance when compared with measurement by pill count or by direct methods and provides a sensitivity in the range between 20 and 55% (14-20). It seems, however, that when a patient admits noncompliance, this information can be trusted (14,21).

The pill count shows a sensitivity between 44 and 80% when compared with direct methods. The results of pill counts and of direct measurements correlate with an $r = 0.41$ to 0.80 (22,23). There are evident problems in assessing the sensitivity and specificity of direct methods such as drug or marker level monitoring. Definition of

TABLE 22–2. *Sensitivity and specificity of methods measuring compliance*

Author (ref.)	Method	Standard	n	Sensitivity (%) (noncompliance)	Specificity (%) (compliance)
Craig (14)	Clinical response	Drug level	40	40	80
	Pill count	Drug level	40	60	70
	Patient interview	Drug level	40	40	100
Mäenpää et al. (15)	Pill count	Marker level	1,739	44	89
	Patient interview	Marker level	1,739	20	98
Paulson et al. (16)	Patient interview	Drug level	49	52	100
Finney et al. (22)	Pill count	Drug level	33	80	75
Wing et al. (17)	Documentation by patients	Marked items	25	54	92
Inui et al. (18)	Patient interview	Pill count	241	55	88
Park and Lipman (19)	Patient interview	Pill count	117	50	96
Rickels and Briscoe (20)	Patient interview	Pill count	301	36	94
Mushlin and Appel (12)	Impression of physician	Pill count	89	65	45
Moulding (13)	Impression of physician or nurse	Medication monitor	116	51	78

a standard with which to compare other than direct observation of the patients under investigation is difficult.

Direct methods like plasma drug level monitoring are specific and prove that the medicine has been administered beforehand.

The evaluation of medication monitors faces similar problems. A medication monitor is a pill box, with an electronic device in its cover, recording any opening of the box by day, hour, and minute for a time period up to several months. However, the medication monitor cannot prove that a medicine has really been administered. When the pill box has been opened at regular intervals during a longer time period, it seems reasonable to conclude that the patient has actually administered the medicine. Partial compliance can safely be assumed, when there are longer intervals recorded that do not fit into the prescribed regimen and when the pill box contains more pills than it should. There will always be some patients who try to cheat the medication monitor, but one can doubt that there will be many. At present, the available medication monitors cannot record the amount of the medicine taken at each opening. Medication monitors have also been developed to allow the monitoring of the compliance with externally administered medicines like eyedrops, lotions, and creams.

When discussing methods for measuring compliance, the different components of compliance (Table 22–3) have to be considered, too, as the compliance status cannot validly be classified dichotomously in a simple yes or no. In the context of clinical trials, it can be extremely important to assess compliance in the placebo group,

TABLE 22–3. Capacity of direct and indirect methods to measure compliance and its various components

Components of compliance	Direct methods					Indirect methods			
	Proof of medicine	Proof of marker	Direct observation	Pill count	Medication monitor[a]	Impression of physician	Patient interview[b]	Clinical response	Filling of prescription
Drug	yes	yes	yes	no	yes	no	no	no	no
Dosage	yes[c]	yes[c]	yes	no	no	no	no	no	no
Time of application	yes[d]	yes[d]	yes	no	yes	no	no	no	no
Regularity of application	yes[e]	yes[e]	yes	no	yes	no	no	no	no
Method of application	no	no	yes	no	no	no	no	no	no
Use of placebo	no	yes	yes	no	yes	no	no	no	no
Use of unauthorized medicines	yes[f]	no	no[g]	no	no	no	no	no	no

[a]Assessed under the assumption that openings reflect actual use.
[b]Patients admitting noncompliance can usually be trusted.
[c]When there is an invariant dose–response curve.
[d]When there is an invariant dose–response curve over time.
[e]Infeasible when treatment has to be administered repeatedly over time.
[f]Only if test is available.
[g]Unless inpatients are observed continuously.

which is impossible with direct methods unless a marker is used, and to be able to exclude the administration of medicines that are not permitted in the trial or in the particular treatment group.

There is at present not a single method that can cover all these components at the same time (Table 22–3). Direct observation is an unrealistic approach, and direct measures, whether drug or marker monitoring, again are usually not feasible for more than a couple of time points. Medication monitors seem to represent important progress, as they allow measurement of compliance over time and also in a routine setting. Medication monitors are not useful for detecting the administration of medicines that should not be taken. Thus, one has to think about the major aims and pitfalls of compliance monitoring in a particular trial first and then decide on the most appropriate methods that can be combined (e.g., medication monitors and plasma level monitoring of prohibited medicines).

The criteria at this step in the decision tree—sensitivity and specificity—are extremely important. It should be standard practice not to use data that are invalid or unreliable. *When compliance has not been measured with satisfactory sensitivity and specificity, compliance cannot be integrated into the statistical analysis.* The intention-to-treat analysis is then the only possible choice of method.

Representativeness of the Compliance Data

The third criterion of representativeness is one that has been largely neglected. Most treatments have to be administered repeatedly over time. A measurement of compliance at a single or a few time points will then not provide data that allow a correct assessment of the patient's compliance at the different "should be" time points of treatment administration. Thus, to get a correct assessment of the compliance patterns of individual patients over time, compliance has to be measured either at all "should be" time points of treatment administration or at a probability sample of them. The latter will allow valid inferences regarding the population of "should be" time points of treatment administration. Even direct methods of measurement at regular scheduled follow-up examinations will not generate the true pattern of compliance over time. Gordis et al. (24) compared physician visit compliance with compliance measured with direct methods at a random sample of treatment days (Table 22–4). Taking the random sample measurements as standard, the sensitivity

TABLE 22–4. *Sensitivity and specificity of compliance measurements using a nonrepresentative sample (physician visit compliance), random sample compliance being the standard[a][b]*

Physician visit compliance	Random sample compliance				
	0–25%	26–50%	51–74%	75–100%	Total
0–25%	24	4	3	5	36
26–50%	7	11	3	8	29
51–74%	1	—	1	2	4
75–100%	1	4	7	22	34
Total	33	19	14	37	103

[a]From ref. 24, with permission.
[b]Sensitivity (0–25%): 24/33 = 73%; specificity (75–100%): 22/37 = 60%; overall agreement: 58/103 = 56%.

of detecting noncompliance was only 73%, and overall agreement existed for a mere 56% of the 103 patients. This study shows empiric evidence that compliance measurements using nonprobability samples do not contribute to a more precise statistical analysis, as this requires correct compliance data. Including such invalid compliance data into the statistical analysis could even be harmful, as bias will be introduced in the analyses, and wrong conclusions will be almost inevitable then.

Therefore, when compliance has not been assessed at probability samples or with the population of "should be" time points of treatment administration, the analyses should be restricted to the intention to treat approach. From a biometric point of view, this last criterion is extremely important, as the validity of statistical analyses cannot be better than the quality of the data itself.

At present, only medication monitors can provide the data that fulfill the requirements of this criterion. It seems to be practically unfeasible to assess compliance by drug or marker level monitoring for all "should be" time points of a treatment prescribed to be repeatedly administered over time.

Feedback on Compliance

A major aim of therapeutic research is to hypothesize and test causal links between treatments and the course of disease. Planning, executing, and the analysis of clinical studies have to be done in such a way that cause-and-effect relations can be derived. The eminent advantage of the randomized trial related to its experimental character is that it provides a framework for reliable causal interpretation. One prerequisite is that the alleged cause precedes the effect. By introducing a variable into the statistical analysis of the outcome criteria as a stratifying factor or as a covariable that has been measured *after* the therapy has been administered, this prerequisite will no longer be fulfilled. Compliance has to be considered as a dependent variable unless there is convincing evidence that it is not. Therefore, one has to check carefully whether feedback of the course of disease on compliance was possible.

The empirical knowledge about feedback effects on compliance is limited and contradictory in the sense that both positive and negative feedback mechanisms have been reported. Joyce (25) has analyzed the effects of phenylbutazone, an experimental medicine called C, and placebo in patients with rheumatoid arthritis in compliance stratified subgroups (Table 22–5). He reported statistically significantly ($p \leq 0.05$) more toxic reactions and adverse symptoms in the patients with poor compliance compared with the patients with good compliance. A subsequent conclusion that "poor compliance leads to increased toxic reactions and adverse reactions" would be pure nonsense. A feedback mechanism of the toxic symptoms and the adverse reactions on these patients' compliance may more plausibly explain these observations.

Another well-known phenomenon is that an improving course of disease can have a negative feedback on compliance. In antibiotic trials, it has been observed that patients with disappearing infections showed poor compliance (26). Patients, thinking that antibiotics were harmful medicines, stopped administering them as soon as they felt better. Analyzing the relation between compliance and course of disease in a clinical trial when negative feedback is present produces the concept that the less medicine taken, the more efficacious it is. The nonsense of this type of analysis can be easily recognized with the examples mentioned. But there are more possible ef-

TABLE 22–5. *Feedback as possible explanation: compliance versus number of toxic reactions and adverse symptoms in a trial on rheumatoid arthritis*[a]

	Number of toxic reactions ($\bar{x}$)					Number of adverse symptoms ($\bar{x}$)				
	PBZ[b]	C[c]	P[d]	$\bar{X}$		PBZ[b]	C[c]	P[d]	$\bar{X}$	
Patients with good compliance ($n = 33$)	0.9	1.8	0.8	1.2		7.4	8.4	8.3	8.0	
		$p < 0.001$			$p < 0.05$		$p = 0.2$			$p < 0.05$
poor compliance ($n = 27$)	1.3	1.7	1.6	1.5		8.7	10.9	10.6	10.1	
		$p > 0.2$					$p < 0.001$			

[a]From ref. 25, with permission.
[b]Phenylbutazone.
[c]Experimental drug C.
[d]Placebo.

fects of feedback mechanisms that are often impossible to detect as long as results are in accord with present medical reasoning. When feedback mechanisms are possible, causal compliance–effect relations can no longer be safely derived. The intention-to-treat analysis is then indicated.

There are many diagnoses including gallstones and asymptomatic risk factors such as hyperuricemia or hyperlipidemia in which patients are ignorant of the course of disease as long as the physician does not provide them with the relevant information. At present, it seems difficult to solve the feedback problem as neither the course of disease nor compliance is continuously measured over time.

Compliance—Independent from Therapy

This criterion again concerns causal interpretation. Compliance must enter the statistical analysis as a prognostic factor and not as an end point itself. This requires that compliance is an *independent* variable. One way to check this assumption is to compare the compliance distributions in the different treatment arms by using a statistical test. If a statistically significant result is obtained and the sample sizes are large, it is important to determine whether the difference in the compliance distributions has real relevance. The disadvantage of the statistical test is that when there is a nonsignificant result, one must not conclude that there is no difference, as it is not then possible to specify the error probability. An alternative approach might be to apply the procedures common in examining bioequivalence [e.g., Westlake's (27)]. An example for compliance probably being a dependent variable is provided by the Lipid Research Clinics Coronary Primary Prevention Trial (Table 22–6) (28). Compliance was indirectly measured by package count. The data show that in the cholestyramine group, there is a trend toward an increasing proportion of patients with lower compliance in comparison with the placebo group, in which a reverse trend can be observed. In the case in which the analyses indicate different compliance distributions, the intention-to-treat analysis is appropriate.

Reasons for compliance being therapy-dependent may be a complex scheme of drug administration, safety devices of the drug package (e.g., childproof closures), or the perceptibility of the placebo, to name just a few.

TABLE 22–6. *Compliance probably being a treatment-dependent variable:
compliance distributions in the cholestyramine resin group and the placebo group of the
Lipid Research Clinics Coronary Primary Prevention Trial[a][b]*

Mean daily package count	Cholestyramine resin (n = 1,900) (50.1%)	Placebo (n = 1,893) (49.9%)
0–1	68.9%	31.1%
1–2	64.7%	35.3%
2–3	60.5%	39.5%
3–4	59.8%	40.2%
4–5	48.9%	51.1%
≥ 5	43.1%	56.9%

[a]From ref. 28, with permission.
[b]χ^2-test: test statistic = 143, DF = 5, p value < 0.000001; test of linear trend: test statistic = 139, DF = 1, p value < 0.000001.

Compliance Dependent on Prognostic Factors

Attempts to integrate compliance data into the statistical analyses of outcome criteria aim to extract the true pharmacodynamic effect as precisely and as unbiased by partial compliance as possible. Thus, a necessary condition is that compliance is not determined by prognostic factors (29). Otherwise the observed change of the difference Δ with better compliance cannot safely be explained only by the treatment but also by a different prognostic factor mix in the patients with better compliance. A prognostic factor is a variable measured *before* the start of treatment, which determines the course of disease. There are unspecific prognostic factors such as the International Federation of Gynecology and Obstetrics (30) stages of cancer and the New York Heart Association (31) functional class, but treatment-specific prognostic factors such as the estrogen receptor status exist, too. When no differences are found in the compliance distributions between treatment groups, it is usually reasonable to assume that the different compliance levels have not selected themselves based on different prognostic factor mixes between the treatment groups. It is important, however, to examine whether the different compliance levels represent heterogeneous prognostic factor mixes within a treatment group. The evidence gained by these analyses is as strong as the knowledge about prognostic factors. There are even diseases such as vitamin or endocrine deficiencies in which the main prognostic factor seems to be compliance with supplementary therapy itself.

As long as the relevant prognostic factors are known, possible interactions between compliance and prognostic factors can be allowed for by statistical means. In the case in which the prognostic factors of the course of disease are unknown, statistical analyses should be conducted according to the intention-to-treat strategy.

Directions for Using the Decision Tree

The decision tree should not be used as an aid in deciding whether it is appropriate to integrate compliance data into the statistical analysis of the outcome criteria only after a trial has been completed. From the biometric point of view, such decisions should be made early in the planning phase of a trial. The results of *a priori* planned analyses are obviously more convincing than of those performed *a posteriori*. As the measurement of compliance can be cumbersome and costly, *a priori* use of the decision tree may be economically more rewarding, too. The decision tree, especially the first and the last three criteria (Fig. 22–3), does not relate to the use of compliance as a dependent or outcome variable.

The aim of the decision tree is to make rational and transparent decisions possible. Its use guarantees that the most important pitfalls will be considered. The decision tree should, however, not be misunderstood as a law to which one must strictly adhere. In clinical trials, one must first define the objectives. When using the decision tree in phase II or III of drug development, the question might be whether to continue the development of a medicine. Thereafter, the issue is how much risk is acceptable (i.e., how large a deviation from the decision tree criteria is necessary to find a satisfactory treatment effect by integrating compliance data). Lack of sensitivity, specificity, and representativeness of the measurements should be absolute criteria for not integrating compliance data. The other criteria have to be judged cautiously and without bias. The more valid the results of an analysis are to be and the less one is ready to accept the risks of wrong conclusions, the more strictly the last three criteria should be adhered to. In addition, avoidance of some of the obstacles mentioned is aided by appropriate specification of the study design.

Assessment of the much-cited clofibrate versus placebo trial publication (9) with the decision tree shows that compliance should definitely not have been included into the statistical analysis. The major reason is the lack of sensitivity, specificity, and representativeness (the second and third questions of the decision tree) of the methods used to measure compliance in this study. In the Coronary Drug Project trial, patients' compliance was assessed by the attending physicians at the regularly scheduled follow-up visits. The physician interviewed the patient, counted or estimated the number of capsules returned, and estimated then the mean number of capsules taken per day for the 4-month follow-up periods. These estimates were averaged over the 5-year period (9). When the paper (9) was published, there was already sufficient evidence available to show that such a procedure would not provide valid data.

INDEXING PATTERNS OF COMPLIANCE

When a treatment is prescribed to be administered only once, compliance need only be assessed once, and its result can easily be integrated in further statistical analyses. If the treatment has to be administered repeatedly over time, compliance data should be the result of repeated measurements (see the third criterion), which have to be aggregated before they can be integrated into the statistical analysis. The calculation of compliance depends on the method of measurement. When direct methods are used, compliance is calculated by the number of positive tests divided by the number of all tests performed times 100. This procedure ensures that by definition, compliance can never exceed 100%, which is a serious drawback of this formula.

An alternative would be to use the information gained with drug, metabolite, or marker level monitoring in a qualitative manner (i.e., to classify each measurement with respect to the size of compliance necessary to achieve the actually measured value). However, intraindividual and interindividual variations of the levels measured present a serious obstacle in routinely following this alternative. When indirect methods such as medication monitors are used, compliance is calculated as the ratio of the amount of actually missing medicine to the amount of medicine that is expected to be missing under the assumption that the study protocol had been strictly adhered to or correspondingly by relating the pattern of drug package openings. Although the latter procedure has the advantage of allowing for compliance greater than 100%, both have severe drawbacks. There is the neglect of the pattern of compliance and of the possibly different impact of compliance on the course of disease over time. From a medical point of view, it can be highly relevant whether a patient is compliant during the first phase of therapy and noncompliant in the second or vice versa, or whether the patient omits every second dose. The resulting course of disease measured as therapeutic efficacy may be different, although the compliance index may be the same for all different compliance patterns. It should also be remembered that the time window of the maximum possible treatment efficacy must not stretch over the whole treatment period (e.g., the risk of myocardial reinfarction is higher during the first 6 months after myocardial infarction than afterward, thus compliance with β-blocker therapy during the first 6 months is more important than later on). The common practice of averaging compliance results over the whole treatment period often leads to considerable bias.

A solution to the problems mentioned might be a hierarchical ranking of the different compliance patterns with respect to the *a priori* knowledge about the pharmacodynamics and pharmacokinetics of the particular medicines and about the impact of treatment, which may vary according to the time administered in relation to the course of the disease.

STATISTICAL ANALYSIS

The main objectives of using compliance data in statistical analyses are:

- to estimate the treatment effects unbiased by compliance
- to estimate the treatment effects under the assumption of excellent compliance
- to reduce the possible impact of partial compliance—increased variance of the outcome criterion—on the result of the statistical test
- to find the degree of compliance necessary for the achievement of the clinically relevant therapeutic effects.

The first steps of analysis should be directed toward identifying a relation between compliance and treatment effects. The size of the treatment effect and its difference between treatment groups should be descriptively displayed for different compliance levels.

The different compliance levels should be chosen either with regard to known pharmacologic properties of drug action or with regard to traditional biometric procedures (e.g., percentiles or quartiles of compliance). A dichotomous classification such as compliant: yes/no or compliance greater than 80% or less than or equal to 80% is not recommended, as it is too crude to identify a compliance–effect relation.

When no relation can be seen, further statistical analyses are fruitless. A couple of possible reasons for this should be considered:

- the therapies may not be efficacious
- compliance itself may not vary as much as is necessary to detect a compliance–effect relation

- the dosages are such that efficacy is, to a large extent, independent of compliance
- the therapy works in such a way that it is, to a large extent, independent of compliance

If a positive relation between compliance and therapeutic effects exists, one should check the treatment effect size in strata with near zero compliance. There should be no evident differences between groups, otherwise the assumption of comparability of the treatment strata has to be rejected. The size of treatment effects and their difference between treatment groups in the excellent compliance strata (~100%) indicates the effect size for administered-as-prescribed therapy. When a plateau of the effect sizes has been reached, considering compliance levels below 100%, too, neither increased efficacy with increased dosage nor decreased efficacy with slightly decreased dosage can be expected. When there is a steep slope between compliance and effect size, even minor differences in the compliance in the treatment groups can bias the estimate of the effect difference considerably. In addition, the variance of the outcome criteria will be unduly increased. Appropriate statistical adjustment will then be rewarding. In the case of a shallow slope, further statistical efforts will show only minor gains. Descriptive analyses of the relation between compliance and effect size thus provide highly relevant insights.

Few papers discuss the integration of compliance into the inferential statistical analysis of clinical trials (32). The author suggests using transparent and well-known procedures such as unifying test statistics (e.g., the Mantel-Haenszel procedure) (33) over compliance homogeneous strata.

CONCLUDING REMARKS

The consideration of compliance as a major condition of treatment efficacy has been long neglected. In the past centuries, this reflected that the history of therapy was primarily a history of placebo. During this century, this reflected that there were no proper means to measure compliance. This latter situation has dramatically changed in recent years with new methods of measuring and monitoring compliance continuously by medication monitors. The heavy financial burden of drug development makes it essential to minimize the risks of wrong judgments about the efficacy of new medicines in phases I to III. Compliance monitoring and the integration of compliance data into the statistical analysis can help to avoid wrong decisions, which until now has been the case because of partial and unknown compliance. To achieve this goal it is absolutely indispensable that compliance is measured with highly sensitive and specific methods at all time points of treatment administration as prescribed or a representative sample of all them.

Only reliable compliance data can contribute to a more accurate assessment of treatment effects. There are further possible pitfalls, as compliance might be a dependent variable. The decision tree presented here should be of considerable help in determining whether the integration of compliance data is appropriate and in assessing the strength of evidence gained. The decision tree can be used either in the planning or in the analytic phase of a trial. The tree must be used by experienced researchers in close cooperation with a biostatistician.

The decison-tree-aided review of the much-cited publication of the Coronary Drug Project (9) shows that it is a poor example attempting to argue against the use of compliance data (34).

Monitoring compliance as a dependent variable, either in the pre- or postmarketing phase, will also provide useful data and insights. Little empirical knowledge is available about compliance dependence on sex, age, disease, medicine, formulation, or treatment duration, just to mention a few factors. Strategies aimed at improving compliance can now be properly evaluated. It is surely no exaggeration that compliance monitoring in clinical practice, in which compliance will be regarded as a dependent variable, can considerably help improve patient therapy.

ACKNOWLEDGMENTS

This chapter is dedicated to Professor Karl Überla.

The author wishes to thank Ms. D. Dickson, MSc, for patiently assisting in preparation of the English version of the manuscript, Ms. M. Baedeker for typing it, and both editors for their critical review of the first draft.

REFERENCES

1. Haynes RB. Introduction. In: Haynes RB, Taylor DW, Sackett DL, eds. *Compliance in health care*. Baltimore, Maryland: The Johns Hopkins University Press, 1979;1–7.
2. Roth HP, Caron HS, Hsi BP. Estimating a patient's cooperation with his regimen. *Am J Med Sci* 1971;262:269–273.
3. Dixon WM, Stradling P, Wootton IDP. Outpatient P.A.S. therapy. *Lancet* 1957;II:871–872.
4. Sackett DL, Snow JC. The magnitude of compliance and noncompliance. In: Haynes RB, Taylor DW, Sackett DL, eds. *Compliance in health care*. Baltimore, Maryland: The Johns Hopkins University Press, 1979;11–22.
5. Mäenpää H, Manninen V, Heinonen OP. Comparison of the digoxin marker with capsule counting and compliance questionnaire methods for measuring compliance to medication in a clinical trial. *Eur Heart J* 1987;8(suppl I):39–43.
6. Bulpitt CJ. *Randomised controlled clinical trials*. London: Martinus Nijhoff Publishers, 1983.
7. Friedman LM, Furberg CD, DeMets DL. *Fundamentals of clinical trials*, 2nd ed. Littleton, Massachusetts: PSG Publishing Co., 1985.
8. Weiss NS. *Clinical epidemiology—The study of the outcome of illness*. New York: Oxford University Press, 1986.
9. Coronary Drug Project Research Group. Influence of adherence to treatment and response of cholesterol on mortality in the Coronary Drug Project. *N Engl J Med* 1980;303:1038–1041.
10. Cochrane AL. *Effectiveness and efficiency—Random reflections on health services*. The Nuffield Provincial Hospitals Trust, 1972.
11. Schwartz D, Flamant R, Lellouch J. *Clinical trials*. London, New York: Academic Press, 1980.
12. Mushlin AI, Appel FA. Diagnosing potential noncompliance. *Arch Intern Med* 1977;137:318–321.
13. Moulding TS. The unrealized potential of the medication monitor. *Clin Pharmacol Ther* 1979;25:131–136.
14. Craig HM. Accuracy of indirect measures of medication compliance in hypertension. *Res Nurs Health* 1985;8:61–66.
15. Mäenpää H, Javela K, Pikkarainen J, Mälkönen M, Heinonen OP, Manninen V. Minimal doses of digoxin: a new marker for compliance to medication. *Eur Heart J* 1987;8(suppl I):31–37.
16. Paulson SM, Krause S, Iber FL. Development and evaluation of a compliance test for patients taking disulfiram. *Johns Hopk Med J* 1977;141:119–125.
17. Wing RR, Epstein LH, Norwalk MP, Scott N, Koeske R. Compliance to self-monitoring of blood glucose: a marked-item technique compared with self-report. *Diabetes Care* 1985;8:456–460.
18. Inui TS, Carter WB, Pecoraro RE. Screening for noncompliance among patients with hypertension: is self-report the best available measure? *Med Care* 1981;19:1061–1064.
19. Park LC, Lipman RS. A comparison of patient dosage deviation reports with pill counts. *Psychopharmacologia* 1964;6:299–302.
20. Rickels K, Briscoe E. Assessment of dosage deviation in outpatient drug research. *J Clin Pharmacol* 1970;10:153–160.

21. Gordis L. Conceptual and methodological problems in measuring patient compliance. In: Haynes RB, Taylor DW, Sackett DL, eds. *Compliance in health care*. Baltimore, Maryland: The Johns Hopkins University Press, 1979;23–45.
22. Finney JW, Friman PC, Rapoff MA, Christophersen ER. Improving compliance with antibiotic regimens for otitis media. *Am J Dis Child* 1985;139:89–95.
23. Roth HP, Caron HS, Bartholomew PH. Measuring intake of a prescribed medication—a bottle count and a tracer technique compared. *Clin Pharmacol Ther* 1969;11:228–237.
24. Gordis L, Markowitz M, Lilienfeld AM. Studies in the epidemiology and preventability of rheumatic fever. IV. A quantitative determination of compliance in children on oral penicillin prophylaxis. *Pediatrics* 1969;43:173–182.
25. Joyce CRB. Patient co-operation and the sensitivity of clinical trials. *J Chronic Dis* 1962;15:1025–1036.
26. Daschner F, Marget W. Treatment of recurrent urinary tract infection in children. II. Compliance of parents and children with antibiotic therapy regimen. *Acta Paediatr Scand* 1975;64:105–108.
27. Westlake WJ. Use of confidence intervals in analysis of comparative bioavailability trials. *J Pharm Sci* 1972;61:1340–1341.
28. Lipid Research Clinics Program. The Lipid Research Clinics coronary primary prevention trial results II. The relationship of reduction in incidence of coronary heart disease to cholesterol lowering. *JAMA* 1984;251:365–374.
29. Feinstein AR. Biostatistical problems in "compliance bias." *Clin Pharmacol Ther* 1974;16:846–857.
30. International Federation of Gynecology and Obstetrics, ed. *Annual report on the results of treatment in gynecological cancer*. Stockholm, 1979.
31. Criteria Committee, New York Heart Association. *Diseases of the heart and blood vessels. Nomenclature and criteria for diagnosis*, 6th ed. Boston: Little Brown and Co., 1964;114.
32. Efron B, Feldman D. *Compliance as an explanatory variable in clinical trials*, (Technical Report No. 129). Stanford: Division of Biostatistics Stanford University, 1989.
33. Mantel N, Haenszel W. Statistical aspects of the analysis of data from retrospective studies of disease. *JNCI* 1959;22:719–748.
34. Hasford J. *Compliance und Wirksamkeitsaussagen in randomisierten Studien* (Habilitationsschrift). München: Ludwig-Maximilians-Universität, 1989.

*Patient Compliance in Medical
Practice and Clinical Trials*
edited by J.A. Cramer and B. Spilker
Raven Press, Ltd., New York © 1991

23

Antihypertensive Drug Trials

Contributions from Medication Monitors

Peter Rudd, Shaheda Ahmed, Valerie Zachary, Carol Barton, and
Delphine Bonduelle

*Department of Medicine, Stanford University Medical Center,
Stanford, California 94305–5475*

This chapter explores what might be learned from adding electronic medication monitors to antihypertensive drug trials. It describes the paradigm of the clinical drug trial and the application of the new technology to a particular study among ambulatory hypertensives.

The Drug Trial Paradigm

At first glance, the paradigm of the antihypertensive drug trial appears simple and unambiguous. First, the investigator identifies a group of stable and generally uncomplicated ambulatory hypertensive patients, confirming their baseline status by clinical and laboratory evaluation. Second, the group undergoes a placebo washout phase to establish baseline blood pressures and randomization to receive one or another medication. Third, periodic monitoring occurs to determine comparative efficacy and safety. The clinician–investigator evaluates each patient's progress toward the therapeutic goal and adjusts the regimen in accord with the study protocol. If a patient fails to reduce blood pressure below a specified level, the investigator may escalate the prescribed dose or add other antihypertensive agents. Fourth, at each return visit, the investigator queries the patients about interval symptoms and possible adverse reactions. Finally, most protocols include some measure of compliance, such as patient self-report and/or pill counts of remaining medication. These traditional measures primarily serve as a quality control maneuver for trial execution rather than as an outcome variable of the study itself.

Ambiguities in the Paradigm

This simple paradigm for the antihypertensive drug trial contains a number of potential ambiguities, especially in assessing compliance and in interpreting the study's results. For example, some investigators have long suspected that some patients do not adhere closely to the clinical prescription. It has been impolite to remark on discarded study pills in the parking lots outside study centers or to notice that patients' blood pressure readings are often lower at scheduled rather than at unscheduled clinical assessments. These and other observations have cast doubt on the validity of existing compliance measures, but few feasible alternatives existed. Most observers acknowledge that drug ingestion may produce prompt hypotensive responses and that a patient may successfully avoid taking all pills until a few hours before a clinic visit and still exhibit satisfactory blood pressure control. The nagging suspicion has remained: What would be discovered if a more precise and dynamic measure of medication-taking behavior were applied to a clinical drug trial, especially if proper compliance were essential for judging full efficacy.

OVERVIEW OF THE TRIAL ITSELF

The study consisted of a randomized, double-blind, parallel comparison of two oral antihypertensive agents: isradipine (a dihydropyridine calcium channel blocker) (1–4) and enalapril (a nonsulfhydryl angiotensin converting enzyme inhibitor) (5–9). After a 3-week, single-blind placebo washout phase, the study patients randomly received either isradipine (1.25–5.0 mg twice daily) or enalapril (2.5–20.0 mg twice daily). Each medication was titrated upward over the first 6 of 10 weeks of active treatment.

Standards of Compliance

The study protocol specified that patients should take their study medicines before breakfast and before dinner approximately 12 hr apart during all study phases, including taking their morning dose on the day of each clinic evaluation. Explicit standards of medication compliance were given: Patients would be considered noncompliant and would be discontinued and replaced if they missed an average of six or more doses for any 2-week interval during the first 6 weeks of the double-blind treatment phase. This criterion corresponded to a tolerated threshold of 21% noncompliance: six omitted doses of 28 possible doses twice daily during 2 weeks. The protocol further specified that patients had to display at least 80% compliance by pill count during the placebo phase to proceed to randomization. Similarly, the analysis would exclude any patient exhibiting more than 20% omitted doses during the entire study. No mention was made about medication-taking patterns that exceeded 100% of the prescription, although all subjects received 150% of the tablets necessary to cover any scheduled intervisit interval. Thus, the entry and maintenance criteria were selected for a highly compliant population, at least as measured by pill count.

Electronic Medication Monitoring

Patients received the study medications in a special vial (Medication Event Monitoring System-1, Aprex Corporation, Fremont, California), which contained a microprocessor capable of recording the precise times of opening and closing the vial and retaining information for as many as 350 consecutive events. Patients were told that the dispensing vials allowed follow-up on how medication was taken but no other mention was made of monitoring their compliance nor of the possibility of excluding them from the study for suboptimal levels of compliance.

At each return visit, the remaining pills were counted surreptitiously and the same medication monitor was reissued to the patient with a new supply of tablets. When the study ended, a microcomputer was used to download the information from the monitor and carry out formal data analysis.

The monitor recorded vial openings and closings rather than tablet consumption *per se*. Patients were explicitly urged to (a) keep all study medications in the special vials, (b) remove only one pill at a time, and (c) avoid removing multiple doses at a time for delayed administration. It was assumed that the absence of any recorded openings during an interval indicated nonconsumption of medicine. Further, it was believed to be improbable that anyone would systematically open and close the vial over weeks without actually taking the tablet. The pill counts served to validate the vial-generated data.

Compliance End Points

At each return visit, patients were asked, "When did you take your last pill of the study medication," the specific self-reported time being noted to (a) establish the probability of full drug effect from the morning's dose and (b) assess the accuracy of self-report compared with the monitor. Compliance was calculated by four measures: (a) pill count, [number of missing pills/number of pills prescribed for the interval] $\times$ 100; (b) total openings, [total openings per intervisit interval/total number of pills prescribed for the interval] $\times$ 100; (c) two-dose days, [number of days in which two dosings occurred by the monitor/number of days in the interval] $\times$ 100; and (d) optimal intervals, [number of interdose intervals corresponding to the near-optimal 10 to 14 hr/total number of vial openings for the interval] $\times$ 100.

Descriptive statistics, chi-square analysis with Yates' correction for continuity for categorical data and the t-test statistic, correlation, and linear regression for continuous variables were employed. The upper limit of statistical significance was $p = 0.05$.

TRADITIONAL TRIAL RESULTS

The study's outcomes may best be described by contrasting those results available by traditional analyses from those available only with the electronic monitor.

Patients

Of 24 patients entering the trial, three failed to meet blood pressure entry criteria or developed intolerable symptoms on placebo treatment. The remaining 21 patients were predominantly middle-aged (mean age, 57; range 33–71) with chronic, mild, stable hypertension; 76% were white and 67% were male. Their duration of known hypertension was 8 years (range, 0.5–21 years). The two subgroups from randomization were similar in sociodemographic features; none of the differences was statistically significant.

TABLE 23–1. *Change in blood pressure with treatment*

	Enalapril (mm Hg; mean ± SEM) (n = 11)	Isradipine (mm Hg; mean ± SEM) (n = 10)
Systolic		
pretreatment	147.2 ± 3.6	152.5 ± 3.4
posttreatment	138.4 ± 3.6[a]	133.1 ± 2.7[a]
Diastolic		
pretreatment	98.1 ± 1.0	99.4 ± 0.8
posttreatment	86.9 ± 2.0[a]	84.7 ± 2.1[a]

[a]$p < 0.01$.

Antihypertensive Response

If one used only traditional measures, the trial successfully demonstrated that each of the medicines significantly lowered mean sitting diastolic blood pressure from the end of the placebo washout phase to the last two visits on stable effective therapy. Table 23–1 summarizes the mean (± SEM) values for pre/post blood pressures. The two drugs achieved statistically equivalent reductions in pressures, with an overall 8% decrease in sitting systolic and 13% decrease in sitting diastolic pressures.

Adverse Reactions

Similarly, by traditional measures, both medicines produced an array of mild adverse reactions, which were both clinically and statistically insignificant, within groups and between groups. Three of 11 patients received enalapril and two of ten patients on isradipine remained asymptomatic throughout the active treatment phase. The other patients reported one or more adverse reactions not previously cited during the placebo washout interval, including headache, dizziness, fatigue, constipation, tinnitus, and urinary frequency. None of the symptoms was severe or persistent enough to prompt withdrawal from the trial. By history alone, none of the symptoms could be unambiguously ascribed to the study medication. No significant changes were detected in laboratory findings nor any directly attributable to either study medication.

Pill Count Compliance

The traditional measures of compliance indicated outstanding performance and no perceived obstacles to following the prescription by patient self-report. Overall, the two medication regimens produced similar compliance rates by pill count (mean ± SEM): enalapril 91.5±1.6% and isradipine 98.7±2.3% (NS). For most patients, compliance rates by pill count for each 1- to 2-week interval clustered at 100±20%, but the range extended from 0 to 135%.

MONITOR-DERIVED DATA

Monitor Concordance with Pill Count

Functional monitor-generated data were available for 18 patients. Figure 23–1 illustrates the concordance between tablet count for each intervisit interval and the respective data from monitor vial openings. Although the majority of points cluster along the line of identity ($r = 0.243$, $p < 0.02$), the scatterplot confirms that most outliers corresponded to low compliance by monitor despite near-perfect compliance by pill count. The distribution indicates that only ten of 105 intervals showed less than 80% compliance by pill count, whereas 27 (26%) were suboptimal by electronic monitor (chi-square $= 8.40$, df $= 1$, $p < 0.001$). The most deviant patient exhibited a mean compliance rate of 93% by pill count for eight return visits during 98 days. In contrast, this monitor confirmed only 21% appropriate opening for the interval. Without the monitor's data, such major deviation in medication-taking behavior would have remained either unsuspected or unconfirmed.

Levels of Compliance

The distribution of medication-taking compliance depends largely on the criteria selected for assessment. Table 23–2 demonstrates that mean values fall progressively below 100% compliance as the criteria become more stringent; the distribution by medication also become more dissimilar. None of the intergroup differences reach statistical significance, in part because of small sample size.

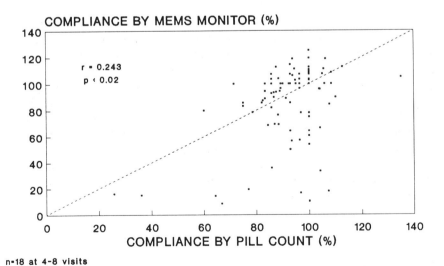

n=18 at 4-8 visits
for each subject

FIG. 23–1. Concordance in compliance measures; pill count versus electronic monitor at 1–2 week intervals. Distribution of values for simultaneous measurement of medication-taking behavior among 18 hypertensive patients followed for 13 weeks, comparing pill counts with electronic medication monitors, which recorded each pill vial opening.

TABLE 23–2. *Comparison of compliance measures by increasingly stringent criteria[a]*

Compliance measure	Enalapril (percent; mean ± SEM) ($n = 11$)	Isradipine (percent; mean ± SEM) ($n = 10$)
Pill count (all visits)	91.5 ± 1.6	98.7 ± 2.3
Total openings (all visits)	84.0 ± 5.1	95.4 ± 3.3
Two-dose days (exactly two openings/ day)	57.4 ± 6.8	69.1 ± 5.2
Optimal intervals (openings at 10–14-hr intervals)	34.5 ± 4.7	43.1 ± 4.8

[a]Intergroup differences: none significant at 0.05 level.

Less than half of all the vial openings occurred at the prescribed interval of 12 ± 2 hr. The distribution was unimodal, centered over the desirable interval. Even if one extends the acceptable limit to 12 ± 6 hr, about 25% of the vial opening took place outside this generous range.

Impact of Scheduled Visits

Such disheartening results might be easily obscured by improved medication-taking behavior immediately before scheduled visits. The approach of the visit might prompt well-intentioned but nonrepresentative behavior, much as many people brush their teeth especially well before going to see the dentist. Traditional pill counts would generally miss such discrepancies, because overdispensing or even massive pill-dumping at the end could compensate for previous underdispensing.

Figure 23–2 compares the distribution of days versus doses. If concordance were perfect, one would expect the number of days between scheduled visits to be proportional to the number of vial openings during the interval. Three days before each scheduled return visit were arbitrarily selected as the period of special interest, because it approximated five half-lives of the shorter-acting preparation and potentially steady-state conditions. The percentage formed by the 3 days before the scheduled visit compared with the entire interval in days versus the percentage of openings for the same ratio of times was plotted. Most points lie close to the line of identity, consistent with a steady-state distribution ($r = 0.731$, $p < 0.001$). Six points lie substantially above the line of identity ($>20\%$ deviation), suggesting overdispensing before the scheduled visit. Five additional points indicate that no doses were taken in the 3 days immediately preceding the scheduled assessment. Overall, seven of these 11 deviant points were attributable to two of the 18 patients, whereas the remaining four points corresponded to unusual deviation for four patients.

Monitor Concordance with Self-Report

Much in the same way, major deviations were observed only in a subset of medication-taking intervals by self-report. Because oral antihypertensive agents may have a prompt impact on blood pressure level, knowing the last dosing interval is essential for interpreting the medication's effect on hypertension. The patients claimed that the last dose of medicine was taken 0.2 to 14 hr before the scheduled visit (mean ± SEM = 3.67 ± 0.24 hr). In contrast, the monitor indicated a range of

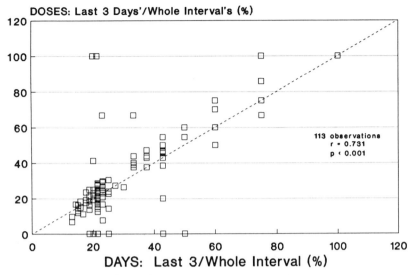

Monitor data, n=18, 4-8 visits each

FIG. 23-2. Homogeneity of drug-taking: impact of scheduled visits. Correlation between doses taken (vial openings) and days passed; if scheduled visits stimulate atypical medication-taking behavior, one would expect that the percentage formed by the last 3 days compared with the entire interval between visits would not correlate with percentage of doses taken in the last 3 days compared with those taken during entire intervisit interval.

openings from 0.5 to 208 hr for the same intervals (mean $\pm$ SEM = 14.43 $\pm$ 2.94 hr; $r = 0.023$, NS). Thus, self-reported compliance, even by short-term recall, correlated imperfectly with openings by the monitor. Not surprisingly, such discrepancies may distort proper interpretation of clinical observations like blood pressure at a scheduled visit.

LESS TRADITIONAL ANALYSES

Dose–Response Relations

The heterogeneous compliance rates undermine any search for traditional dose–response relations between prescribed dosage of the antihypertensive agents and the blood pressure response. Correlation coefficients for prescribed dose and change in sitting diastolic blood pressure response were low and statistically insignificant for both enalapril ($r = -0.037$) and isradipine ($r = -0.286$) by this analysis.

Prescribed versus Administered Dosage

In contrast, administered rather than prescribed dosage was focused on, as measured by the medication monitor. Twenty-four hours was selected as the critical interval before each scheduled return visit because the antihypertensive effect might last as long as 24 hr with chronic administration. The distribution of blood pressure changes by dose administered in the preceding 24 hr was wide. None of the correlations achieved statistical significance, in part because of small subsample sizes. It was observed, however, that five of 18 subjects (28%) had an unambiguously positive dose–response relation: Three patients on enalapril and two on isradipine had progressive declines in diastolic pressures as the administered dose in the 24 hr increased. One patient on isradipine had an inverse response with less blood pressure reduction on higher doses. The remaining 12 patients exhibited equivocal responses. There was no temporal trend for blood pressure change during the 10 weeks of active drug treatment.

Natural Experiments of Dosing

Because patients' medication-taking behavior frequently varied from day to day, the monitor could be used to define the apparently administered dose and to examine the effect of the patient's own titration. The monitor was able to indicate both "under-" and "overdosing" beyond the prescribed range. In the case of both study medicines tested, relatively flat dose–response relations emerged, consistent with relative independence of the blood pressure lowering effect from the particular dose used. This interpretation necessarily assumes that each monitor opening corresponds to drug consumption. Unfortunately, finding modest overdispensing in the few days before scheduled visits muddles confidence in this interpretation. One would need an independent and dynamic measure of blood pressure variability between scheduled visits to reduce the ambiguity.

Probes for Reported Adverse Reactions

With the goal of further reducing ambiguity, it was found that the monitor provided a method to probe both adverse reactions and secondary resistance to treatment. To illustrate the first capability, Fig. 23–3 depicts the medication-taking pattern of a patient who reported approximately 1 week of vertigo on the follow-up visit. The figure plots every monitor opening for each day in a vertical stack on the ordinate. On the day preceding the onset of the presumptive drug-induced symptom, the monitor recorded seven openings rather than the customary one to three openings per day. Although the timing of possible overdispensing may be coincidental, it serves as a useful probe for possible causal associations. Unfortunately, no further information nor rechallenge with high doses was possible.

Evaluating Secondary Resistance to Treatment

In similar ways, loss of responsiveness to treatment may be clarified by using the medication monitor. Such secondary resistance may reflect individually or collectively the biology of the disease, the pharmacology of the medication, or the behavior of medication-taking. One patient was observed who achieved good blood pressure control (sitting diastolic pressure <80 mm Hg) when the prescribed dose of isradipine was raised from 2.5 to 7.5 mg/day. At the last visit, however, his pressure unexpectedly rose back to baseline levels. The monitor's data allowed contemporaneous assessment of prescribed versus administered dose, mean interval for the prior four openings, and the interval from the last dose's vial opening to the clinical

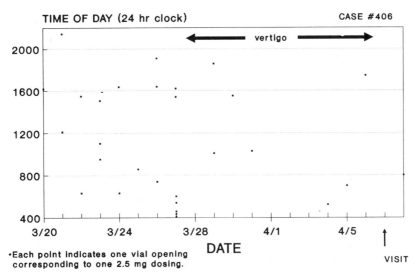

FIG. 23–3. Patient-reported vertigo after "hypercompliance" with enalapril, using monitor-generated data. Data from medication-taking of patient #406, who reported 1 week of vertigo on the return visit on 4/7/88. Each *dot* represents one medication vial opening. On the day preceding onset of symptoms, monitor showed 7 openings rather than the usual 1–3 per day. The symptom, in turn, prompted less medication-taking.

assessment. Only one of these measures changed in parallel to the relapse in blood pressure. The monitor confirmed that the interval from the last dose to the visit rose from 3 to 5 hr to more than 20 hr at the last visit. In this case, the secondary resistance most plausibly becomes a matter of suboptimal medication-taking rather than biological or pharmacological resistance (see Fig. 23–6).

Interpreting the Clinical Experiment

The test of the monitor's ultimate value lies in whether or not it helps interpret the clinical experiment. When a patient fails to achieve the desired therapeutic response, can the monitor better distinguish suboptimal medication-taking or partial compliance compared with traditional pill counts?

Near Optimal Compliance and Blood Pressure Response

Of 168 possible return visits, usable pill count and simultaneous blood pressure data were available for 165 (98%). Overall, the compliance rate by pill count exceeded 80% in 93% of the return visits. Focusing on the 90 data pairs representing active treatment rather than placebo administration, it was observed that 58 (72%) reflected both achievement of goal blood pressure (sitting diastolic pressure <90 mm Hg) and near-optimal compliance (89–119%). In contrast, 23% of the visits were associated with failure to achieve goal blood pressure despite near-optimal compliance by pill count. Only four of 81 visits (5%) were associated with suboptimal compliance by pill count, often with achievement of goal blood pressure.

The distribution of near-optimal compliance was moderately shifted by adding the electronic monitor's data. In this context, we defined optimal compliance as (a) mean interopening interval for the four prior openings to be less than 16 hr and (b) the interval from the last opening to the clinical assessment to be less than 24 hr. With this definition, the desirable combination of achieved goal blood pressure and near-optimal compliance was more difficult to attain. The rate fell to 61% ($n = 49$) of all visits for which both monitor and blood pressure data were available. The overall proportion of visits judged to have near-optimal compliance thus declined by 15%. Eight patients at 15 visits gave evidence of inferior medication-taking by monitor than by pill counts, whereas pill counts indicated inferior compliance compared with the monitor for three patients at three visits. If one accepts the monitor as reliable, it can be concluded that pill count misclassified patients' responses in 18 of 81 occasions (22%).

If the focus is on only the visits at which patients were receiving active treatment and for which both monitor and pill count data were available, there was one occasion when the monitor confirmed that poor blood pressure control was associated with markedly prolonged intervals between dosings just before the visit. On two other occasions, despite less than 80% compliance by pill count, the monitor confirmed sufficiently improved medication-taking just before the visit to achieve goal blood pressure. On these three occasions, the pill count would have offered potentially misleading clues about why the hypotensive effect was different than expected. Pill counts exceeded 120% of the prescribed regimen in four patients (range, 123–350%).

Timing versus Taking

The relatively high rate of imperfect medication-taking becomes most striking when contrasting the overall taking of medications with their precise timing. Using data from the electronic medication monitor, each patient's compliance rate (number of vial openings as a percent of the prescribed dosings for the entire monitored interval) was plotted against the same patient's timing of dosing (percent of prescribed doses taken in the optimal window of 12 ± 3 hr).

Figure 23–4 displays these data, each patient ($n = 18$) represented by one point superimposed on two coordinates to establish standards of "taking the pills" regardless of when taken versus "timing the pills" as prescribed. The vertical coordinate is placed at 80%. It represents a standard widely cited in the literature as the minimum level of taking medication for acceptable compliance. In the original work by Sackett (10), it was observed that ambulatory hypertensives had to consume at least 80% of their prescribed regimen by pill count to achieve goal blood pressure at a surprise home visit. Thus, all points to the right of the vertical coordinate reflect taking at least 80% of the prescribed dose. In contrast, the horizontal coordinate represents the reasonable but arbitrary expectation that 67% of the dosings will occur in the timing window of 12 ± 3 hr. All points above this line indicate taking at least two-thirds of the prescribed doses with the proper timing. Finally, the line of identity has been drawn to indicate the relation between taking and timing, if the two were perfectly linked.

Figure 23–4 confirms that all the data points lie well below the line of identity.

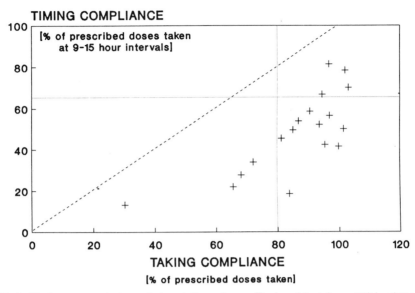

FIG. 23–4. Timing errors during a twice-daily regimen. Each subject (*n* = 18) is plotted with one point, reflecting percentage of total number of prescribed doses taken (regardless of precise time) versus percentage of total number of prescribed doses taken as prescribed (every 12 hr). A narrow margin of 3 hr is permitted on either side of precisely 12 hr. Vertical coordinate represents threshold of 80% compliance (cf. ref. 10), and horizontal coordinate reflects arbitrary expectation of taking at least two-thirds of the doses with the prescribed timing.

They suggest that more patients succeed at taking medication at some time or another than at precisely timing the medication-taking to correspond to the prescription. Fully 14 of 18 (78%) exceeded the 80% compliance threshold, whereas only four of 18 (22%) fulfilled the generous window of having at least two-thirds of vial openings occur in the range of 12 ± 3 hr. These data support the view that most patients, even among a cohort preselected for high levels of compliance by pill count, may be unsuccessful in attaining moderate compliance for the correct timing of doses.

Shifting the Distribution of Timing Errors

This form of analysis points to another strategy for improving clinical outcome despite suboptimal timing of doses. A longer-acting preparation, still prescribed at 12-hr intervals, could increase the proportion of time that patients would receive therapeutic benefit, even with the same timing errors. The distribution itself would improve, just by having the medicine last longer. In essence, some pharmacokinetic redundancy would compensate for poor timing of doses. Figure 23–5 replots the data, using the more generous window of 12 ± 6 hr. By this maneuver, the same 14 of 18 subjects meeting the greater than or equal to 80% pill-taking criterion are retained but triple the proportion achieving satisfactory timing of doses to 12 of 18 (67%). The entire distribution, moreover, is shifted more closely to the line of identity, compared with Fig. 23–4.

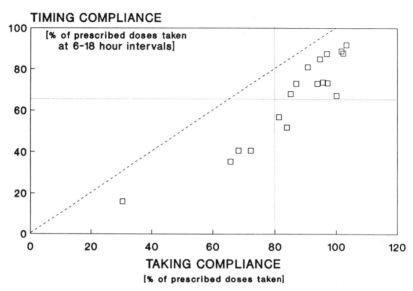

FIG. 23–5. Timing errors during a twice-daily regimen. Format of the figure is identical to that of Fig. 23–4 except the margin of acceptable dosing times has been extended (12 ± 6 hr). With this single change, the points more closely approximate the line of identify and the proportion of subjects meeting both taking and time compliance criteria triples from 22 to 67%.

IMPLICATIONS FOR CLINICAL TRIALS AND PRACTICE

The present report summarizes experience with applying a new technology to the monitoring of medication-taking behavior within an antihypertensive drug trial.

Trade-offs with the Electronic Monitor

The technology's special attraction lies in three characteristics. First, the device measures medication-taking in a dynamic mode, hour by hour and day by day. This is in contrast to lumping the data together into static averages (e.g., pill counts), which reflect the entire interval from the last visit. Second, the measure records close to the actual tablet-dispensing event, rather than hours or days afterward (e.g., a blood level drawn later) when the medication has reached steady state in the sampled body fluid. Third, the monitor closely approximates a standard vial in size, shape, weight, and operation, minimizing the likelihood that the measurement process itself will change patients' behavior in uncharacteristic ways.

The existing technology, despite its promise, is still imperfect. The vial circuitry can record each opening but cannot ensure actual drug consumption. To confirm concordance between the numbers of vial openings and missing pills, the investigator must still perform pill counts. The most hard-core skeptic may still require a biologic assay, even on a random sampling basis, to confirm that medication consumption actually occurred. A proportion of patients could manipulate the data by opening the vial and deliberately or inadvertently fail to consume the medication. Systematic vial opening over weeks to months is improbable without actual pill dispensing and ingestion.

Relevance to Clinical Drug Trials

Application of such electronic monitors to a drug trial is hardly coincidental. Many clinical investigators succeed in controlling for most features that might influence outcome variables except whether ambulatory patients return to visits as scheduled and whether they take their medications as prescribed. By reducing ambiguity about medication compliance, the ability to interpret variability in the biology of disease and the pharmacology of the medicine may be improved.

Partial Compliance and Therapeutic Sufficiency

A remarkable discrepancy has been found between the precise timing of medication-taking and the simplistic notion of whether medication is taken at all. Traditional pill counts reflect the crude concept that each missing pill represents a tablet consumed. The electronic monitor adds timing, the extra layer of sophistication that allows new questions: (a) What is the minimal amount of medication required for a particular therapeutic effect? (b) What is the distribution of interopening intervals and does it reflect therapeutic sufficiency? or (c) Are there large gaps in dosing times during which the medicine's effect will likely wear off and the patient will lose the benefit of treatment or run the risks of withdrawal?

The monitor encourages the investigator to focus on whether the medication-taking behavior is sufficient rather than whether it corresponds exactly to a particular prescription. Our own data suggest that patients have more trouble attaining the proper timing, even if they excel in removing the proper number of pills from the container. The discrepancy is all the more notable because it emerged among a cohort of patients with chronic, stable, uncomplicated hypertension, carefully chosen for near-optimal compliance by pill count.

The data support previous reports that partial compliance is both highly prevalent and apparently random rather than systematic in its occurrence (11,12). Most patients appear to take most of their prescribed tablets most of the time. When they deviate from the prescription, they are more likely to undertreat rather than overtreat.

Insufficiency of Pill Counts

Such deviations must be detected to produce a response. Imperfect measures (e.g., pill counts), which prompt patients to "dump" pills to appear fully compliant, confound many reports in the compliance literature, if they are the only measure. The confounding occurs especially when medications are supplied by the study without charge or when near-perfect compliance is required for study continuation. Although less than half of the vial openings in our study occurred at the prescribed interval of 12 ± 2 hr, the traditional measure of pill count was insensitive to this gross deviation. Even patients' accuracy in reporting the interval since the last dosing appeared suspect.

A patient may invalidate the entire pill count process by discarding many unused doses sometime before the scheduled visit. Moreover, pill counts offer no capability to evaluate secondary resistance to treatment nor a way of correlating drug-taking

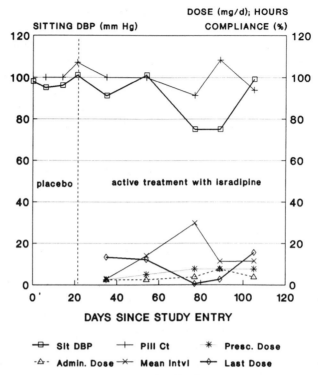

FIG. 23–6. Interpreting secondary resistance. Pill counts versus monitor (Case #452).

patterns with reported adverse drug reactions, two capabilities illustrated in the present report.

Search for the Optimal Dose Range

Somewhat surprisingly, we noted an apparently flat dose–response curve for antihypertensive efficacy, after correcting for administered rather than prescribed dose. Miller et al. (13) cautioned that one explanation for observing an early plateau in the dose–response relation is that initial dose selection might be too high, either in dose amount or in dosing frequency. They claim that failure to demonstrate a plateau indicates that only a portion of the effective dose range was sampled during therapeutic testing. The monitor allowed examination of the antihypertensive effect of under- and overdosing beyond the range of prescribed dosages.

Primacy of Good Measures

The entire field of medication compliance has suffered in the absence of good measures. Because all science is measurement, no clinical situation can be well-defined, diagnosed, or treated without practical and unambiguous measures. The infrastructure of our understanding about suboptimal medication compliance is suspect: its prevalence, determinants, impact, detection, and amelioration. Much of this uncertainty reflects building our previous dogma on a foundation of questionable measures: self-report, pill counts, biological assays, and therapists' opinion (14). Improved measures may correct the situation.

Impact of Partial Compliance on Trial Interpretation

Our data confirm others' work that medication-taking behavior is imperfect among ambulatory patients, even when preselected for high levels of compliance by pill count. Such levels of partial compliance, especially in trials of small sample size, may dilute intergroup differences among the treatment arms. For example, after partial compliance, one might predict a lower than maximal therapeutic effect from active treatment. More subtly, such partial compliance may obscure the frequency and impact of adverse drug reactions. As patients try to minimize toxicity, they may take less than the prescribed amount, especially if the toxicity occurs promptly and induces lower levels of medication-taking.

Natural Experiments in Nature

Electronic monitoring of medication-taking should permit several new kinds of studies, which exploit experiments in nature. Patients dose themselves in several ways, easily detectible for the first time with devices like the Medication Event Monitoring System. Cramer et al. (15) recently described application of the electronic monitor to ambulatory patients with seizure disorders. They observed that only 76% of 7,413 antiseizure doses were taken as prescribed and that only 13% of patients with suboptimally low compliance were detected by pill count. In their experience, the compliance rate was linearly related to the prescribed dosing frequency (1–4 times/day; $p<0.01$, ANOVA). Most impressively, 12 of 16 seizures were associated with missed doses as documented by the electronic monitor among patients with chronic antiepileptic regimens. Optimal management, then, should focus on improving medication compliance rather than on escalating the regimen, in contrast to common clinical practice.

Implications for Drug Development

The present study also underscores several implications for drug development, which often relies heavily on clinical trials to establish efficacy against placebo, identify the therapeutic range of doses, and monitor for untoward reactions. First, partial compliance appears to be ubiquitous, variable, and elusive. It is both difficult to measure and resistant to simplistic, unifactorial, and nonreinforced approaches. These characteristics make it a worthy opponent for further investigation rather than an unsavory or disreputable embarrassment.

Second, one should explore simple strategies before trying expensive tactics to reduce the consequences of partial compliance. The industry has largely accepted the desirability of once-daily dosing whenever possible. Yet once-daily dosing alone may be insufficient. As long as patients omit doses on a frequent basis, the proper focus should be on the sufficiency of the regimen for a particular clinical purpose. Such sufficiency is enhanced by a built-in redundancy for timing. A medicine that lasts 36 to 48 hr may still be prescribed every 24 hr, assuming no accumulation to toxicity. Such prescribing would cover for the important subset of patients who err on the side of taking less than the full prescription. This approach does not pretend to "fix" partial compliance but merely to compensate better for it. Many technical problems still prevent finding long-acting preparations for all circumstances.

Summary

The electronic monitor allows more assessment in depth of smaller numbers of patients with more information generated per patient. This stands in contrast to blind insistence on larger trials with focus limited to the average effect, and classification of patients by "intention-to-treat". Using medication compliance as a covariable, stratification of the outcome data may reveal new and important drug effects for both efficacy and safety. Subtle toxicities resulting from or resolving with drug "holidays" may emerge for the first time. The increasing number of "n-of-1" trials may employ such electronic monitoring to confirm the use of the intervention variable (16). The electronic monitor transforms many regimens into patient-initiated experiments in variable dosing. Clinical practice may then shift away from the common pattern of frequent medication-switching in favor of "fine tuning" once compliance has been confirmed.

Overall, the field of medication monitoring is shifting from rigid counts of pills prescribed and returned. It seeks to identify a regimen that is sufficient for a clinical purpose despite imperfect compliance. Such sufficiency is more important than insisting on perfect concordance between prescription and behavior. The technology also moves clinical pharmacology beyond the traditional focus on peak and trough levels and identifies the holes between the periods of compliance. Better measures should facilitate more thoughtful and successful tactics for partial compliance and imperfect clinical response.

ACKNOWLEDGMENTS

The authors acknowledge (a) the understanding of Dr. Leonard Gonasun and the financial support of Sandoz Research Institute for underwriting the clinical drug trial, (b) the helpful suggestions of Dr. John Urquhart and John Bell of Aprex Corporation, and (c) the technical assistance of Yvonne Nakahigashi in preparing the manuscript.

REFERENCES

1. Tse FL, Jaffe JM. Pharmacokinetics of PN 200-110 (isradipine), a new calcium antagonist, after oral administration in man. *Eur J Clin Pharmacol* 1987;32:361–365.
2. Clifton GD, Blouin RA, Dilea C, et al. The pharmacokinetics of oral isradipine in normal volunteers. *J Clin Pharmacol* 1988;28:36–42.
3. Chellingsworth MC, Willis JV, Jack DB, Kendall MJ. Pharmacokinetics and pharmacodynamics of isradipine (PN 200-110) in young and elderly patients. *Am J Med* 1988;84(suppl 3B):72–79.
4. Schran HF, Jaffe JM, Gonasun LM. Clinical pharmacokinetics of isradipine. *Am J Med* 1988;84(suppl 3B):80–89.
5. Schwartz JB, Taylor A, Abernethy D, et al. Pharmacokinetics and pharmacodynamics of enalapril in patients with congestive heart failure and patients with hypertension. *J Cardiovasc Pharmacol* 1985;7:767–776.

6. Reams GP, Lal SM, Whalen JJ, Bauer JH. Enalaprilat: an intravenous substitute for oral enalapril therapy; humoral and pharmacokinetic effects. *J Clin Hypertension* 1986;3:245–253.
7. Lees KR, Reid JL. Age and the pharmacokinetics and pharmacodynamics of chronic enalapril treatment. *Clin Pharmacol Ther* 1987;41:597–602.
8. Kubo SH, Cody RJ. Clinical pharmacokinetics of the angiotensin converting enzyme inhibitors; a review. *Clin Pharmacokinet* 1985;10:377–391.
9. Hockings N, Ajayi AA, Reid JL. Age and the pharmacokinetics of angiotensin converting enzyme inhibitors enalapril and enalaprilat. *Br J Clin Pharmacol* 1986;21:341–348.
10. Sackett DL. Hypertension in the real world: public reaction, physician response, and patient compliance. In: Genest J, Koiw E, Kuchel O, eds. *Hypertension: physiopathology and treatment.* New York: McGraw-Hill, 1977;1142–1149.
11. Rudd P, Byyny RL, Zachary V, et al. Pill count measures of compliance in a drug trial: variability and suitability. *Am J Hypertension* 1988;1:309–312.
12. Rudd P, Byyny RL, Zachary V, et al. The natural history of medication compliance in a drug trial: limitations of pill counts. *Clin Pharmacol Ther* 1989;46:169–176.
13. Miller L, Dalton M, Vestal R, Perkins JG, Lyon G. Delays in the drug approval process: recent trends. *J Clin Res Drug Devt* 1988;2:31–45.
14. Rudd P, Marshall G. Resolving problems of measuring compliance with medication monitors. *J Compliance Health Care* 1987;2:23–35.
15. Cramer JA, Mattson RH, Prevey ML, Scheyer RD, Ouellette VL. How often is medication taken as prescribed? A novel assessment technique. *JAMA* 1989;261:3273–3277.
16. Guyatt GH, Keller JL, Jaeschke R, Rosenbloom D, Adachi JD, Newhouse MT. The *n*-of-1 randomized controlled trial: clinical usefulness; our three-year experience. *Ann Intern Med* 1990;112:293–299.

Patient Compliance in Medical
Practice and Clinical Trials
edited by J.A. Cramer and B. Spilker
Raven Press, Ltd., New York © 1991

24

Patient Compliance as an Explanatory Variable in Four Selected Cardiovascular Studies

John Urquhart

Aprex Corporation, Fremont, California 94539; and University of Limburg Department of Pharmaco-Epidemiology, 6200 Maastricht, The Netherlands

This chapter reviews four clinical trials in the cardiovascular field in which data on patients' compliance with the prescribed intervention has played an important role in analysis and interpretation of the results. One of the aims in doing so is to examine how compliance data have been used or misused in an effort to increase the amount of scientifically valid, clinically useful information obtained from clinical investigations.

WHY LOOK AT COMPLIANCE?

A measure of compliance is an estimate of the dose that the patient actually took, which often differs from the dose that was prescribed or assigned. Variation in dose of any agent with pharmacological activity means variation in drug response. From the pharmacological perspective, dose–response relations are a fundamental property of any medicine, but it is a property often difficult to measure. For this reason alone, it is a lost opportunity if not a scientific lapse to study a medicine's effects in circumstances in which dose is both highly variable and undefined. To ignore variable compliance is to consign dose-dependent variation in drug response to the category of unallocated variance in drug response, discarding useful information about the human effects of the medicine. Dose–response relations are usually nonlinear, so variable dosing changes the mix of drug effects and thus the margin between therapeutic and toxic effects. Furthermore, learning why the dose taken differed from the dose prescribed is another basic aspect of understanding the human response to the medicine.

Yet there is a school of thought in clinical trials analysis that holds that any attempt to analyze trial results in relation to doses actually taken by trial participants is so tainted by bias (1) as to preclude any useful information being derived therefore. Thus there is a conflict between purely statistical and purely pharmacological perspectives. It is naive to ignore potential biases, but it is also naive to let fear of bias stymie properly controlled analyses of the most basic attribute of any medicine— the dose dependency of its effects.

Thus, a second aim of this chapter is to try to reconcile this conflict in views, by showing

1. contributions that well-controlled analyses by compliance can make to trials interpretation
2. peculiarities of the trial whose results have provided the main support to the argument against using compliance data to interpret trials results (1)

HOW VARIABLE IS COMPLIANCE IN CLINICAL TRIALS AND PRACTICE?

As many chapters in this book describe, studies with a variety of methods for measuring compliance show that compliance varies among patients between 0 and somewhat more than 100% of prescribed doses taken, in both outpatient drug trials and clinical practice. It is unrealistic to dichotomize compliance of individual patients into "good" and "poor," for the distribution of compliance in the patient population is a continuum. An approximate summary of compliance (as percent of prescribed doses taken) with chronic-use drug regimens that do not afford symptomatic relief is as follows:

> Half to two-thirds of patients manage to take more than four-fifths of prescribed doses. Another 30 to 40% of patients are aptly described as "partial compliers" in that they take between two- and four-fifths of prescribed doses, with many delays and omissions of scheduled doses. The balance is divided between small minorities who take (a) very few doses or (b) more doses than prescribed.

However, compliance improves in the few days before and after a scheduled visit to the physician (2–5), so short trials with frequently scheduled visits may show a higher overall compliance than the foregoing figures.

Even when more or less correct numbers of doses are taken, however, dose timing is often markedly at odds with the assumptions of drug developers. Thus the percentage of prescribed doses taken within pharmacodynamically appropriate intervals is lower than the percentage of prescribed doses taken (without classification in regard to timing). The impact of vagaries in dose timing is a problem in trials interpretation beyond the scope of this chapter, because the studies reviewed here used preelectronic methods for measuring compliance that could not show dose timing. There is, however, abundant evidence in experimental pharmacology to show that too-short intervals between doses can lead to toxicity and that too-long intervals between doses allow drug action to cease. There is also a toxicity problem in relation to too-long intervals between doses of medicines that have hazardous rebound phenomena, as illustrated by the recent finding of a four- to fivefold relative risk of incident coronary artery disease in partially compliant hypertensives prescribed beta-blockers (6). These are issues for the future.

The four trials reviewed in this chapter are

1. A trial of the effects of exercise in heart failure performed at the John Radcliffe Hospital in Oxford (7)
2. The Lipid Research Coronary Primary Prevention Trial of cholestyramine (8,9)
3. The Helsinki Gemfibrozil Trial (10,11)
4. The Coronary Drug Project trial of clofibrate (1,12)

For convenience, these trials are referred to, respectively, as the Oxford study, the Lipid Research trial, the Helsinki trial, and the Coronary Drug Project trial.

OXFORD STUDY

In this study, exercise was compared with rest for the treatment of chronic heart failure. In a random-order, cross-over design, the comparisons were an 8-week program of periodic exercise on a stationary bicycle and an 8-week program of rest. Compliance with the prescribed exercise regimen was measured by the cumulative change in the bicycle's odometer reading, expressed as a percentage of the value expected from full compliance with the prescribed regimen. Compliance with the comparison regimen of rest was thought to have been secured by making the stationary bicycles unavailable to the patients. There was no evidence of significant carryover effects to complicate the interpretation of results. Eleven of 12 patients completed the trial. One patient died during the rest program, his first randomized treatment.

An intent-to-treat analysis revealed that the exercise group had a statistically significant increase in exercise time and peak oxygen consumption, together with significant improvements in tiredness, breathlessness, daily activity, and general well-being, but without change in chest pain. Heart rates at rest and at submaximal exercise were lower after the exercise program than after the rest program, and peak heart rate occurred at a higher workload after the exercise program. The product of heart rate and blood pressure at submaximal exercise was lower at the end of the exercise program than at the end of the rest program, indicating that the exercise program resulted in a more efficient performance.

Compliance with the exercise regimen spanned a wide range—26 to 110% of the prescribed amount, with a mean of 74%. These values for range and mean are strikingly similar to the range and mean of compliance with drug regimens in chronic, prophylactic therapy, when drug regimen compliance is similarly defined as percent of prescribed amount taken (2–4,13–17).

With the efficacy of exercise proved in the primary analysis, the wide variation in compliance created the opportunity to explore a wide range of exercise-dependent change in cardiac function and oxygen consumption. According to the authors (7),

> compliance with the exercise regimen seemed to be the one factor necessary to achieve benefit. Even though exercise had significant effects in an intention-to-treat analysis, there was a clear correlation between the compliance with exercise and the improvement achieved, indicating the specificity of the improvements seen to the training programme itself. It was not the patients with the most severe heart failure who had low compliance, but paradoxically, those least severely affected, which may indicate a lesser incentive to exercise in these subjects.

These findings extend and amplify the results of the trial, giving physicians useful information to use in reviewing a program of exercise with patients.

In effect, the patients' variable adherence to the prescribed regimen converted a "fixed-dose" trial of exercise into a "variable-dose" trial. The wide range in levels of exercise led to a wide range of exercise-dependent cardiorespiratory responses. Because the patients chose the exercise level after randomization, however, a bias might arise if those with the best prognosis also happened to be the ones who best complied. Fortunately, the investigators sought to learn the reasons for good, partial, or poor compliance. The results led to the surprising paradox that the best compliers had the most severe heart failure. The investigators believed that the severity dependence of compliance arose from patients' incentives to help their relatively poor condition. It would have been useful to know if patients with more severe failure might have had quicker perception of benefit. A continuous measure of compliance showing its time dependence might have added useful information.

Thus, the trial illustrates the value of learning as much as possible about the determinants of compliance, not only to discover possible biases linked to variable compliance, but also for its heuristic value for future trials and its clinical value in routine care.

LIPID RESEARCH TRIAL

This large, long, multicenter trial, costing $150 million (18), was the first to demonstrate that intervention to lower cholesterol levels reduces the risk of coronary heart disease (8,9). Sponsored by the United States National Institutes of Health, the trial involved 3,806 men with cholesterol levels greater than 265 mg/dL but without clinical evidence of overt coronary heart disease, selected from more than 480,000 men screened. Participants were randomized to two groups: one treated with cholestyramine, and the other with placebo. Each group received the same dietary recommendation aimed at effecting a moderate reduction in cholesterol levels.

Cholestyramine is an awkward pharmaceutical, for its cholesterol-lowering effect not only requires a large dose, but its physical properties require its formulation with a large quantity of excipient. The recommended full dose of cholestyramine was (and is) 24 g of active agent per day, accompanied by 30 g of excipient—54 g of powder that the patient must reconstitute daily as a slurry in several divided doses. This large dose is at the uppermost fringe of daily doses in all pharmacotherapy. The trial planners (19) recognized that a substantial fraction of patients would find compliance difficult and so included procedures for a regular measure of compliance, based on counts of returned unused packets of medicine. The packets contained 4 g of medicine plus 5 g of excipient in the "active" limb of the trial, and 5 g of excipient plus 4 g of a biologically inert silica mixture in the "passive" limb (19). Patients were examined bimonthly for an average of 7.4 years, and the bimonthly compliance data were averaged over that period. Trial methods included a special procedure to compute compliance during longer than bimonthly periods when appointments were missed (9).

Several of the exclusion criteria for the trial were related to the likelihood of good compliance: missing or failing to fast before more than one of four prerandomization appointments; significant gastrointestinal symptoms or disease that would preclude taking cholestyramine; another household member participating in the Lipid Research trial or taking cholestyramine. A prescient aspect of the design was a prerandomization exclusion of patients who showed a large drop in cholesterol level in response to the diet program, which was initiated in the prerandomization period (19). Excluding such patients minimized the likelihood that an association between compliance behavior and cholesterol reduction would arise if compliance with the placebo regimen was linked to compliance with the dietary regimen.

Appendix D in the pretrial report (19) suggests that the trial planners thought of compliance more in terms of total cessation of dosing than as a spectrum of variable dosing. They projected a "noncompliance rate" of 5% per year, leading to a cumulative 35% of patients being noncompliant by the trial's end after 7 years. The results showed that 294 (15.5%) of the active recipients and 133 (7.0%) of placebo recipients (on average) had returned packet counts indicating almost total noncompliance with the regimen (Table 24–1).

TABLE 24–1. *Compliance in active and placebo limbs of Lipid Research trial*

Mean daily dosage taken (packets)	Number of patients	Percentage of patients
Cholestyramine recipients		
0–1	294	15.5
1–2	145	7.6
2–3	135	7.1
3–4	156	8.2
4–5	205	10.8
5–6	965	50.8
total	1,900	100.0
Placebo recipients		
0–1	133	7.0
1–2	79	4.2
2–3	88	4.6
3–4	105	5.6
4–5	214	11.3
5–6	1,274	67.3
total	1,893	100.0

Measuring compliance was a formidable task in this large trial. More than 30 million packets of drug or placebo were prescribed during the 7-year trial. On average, two-thirds of the packets appeared to have been used, requiring the counting of approximately 10 million unused, returned packets, not including extra packages dispensed as reserve supplies and also returned unused.

Cholestyramine is supposed to be nonabsorbed, and its action is to sequester bile acids, thereby diverting substrates for cholesterol synthesis toward increased bile acid production, and reducing both total and low-density lipoprotein–cholesterol levels in plasma. The trial results showed that a substantial fraction of cholestyramine recipients who were fully compliant by the packet count measure were able to achieve greater than 25% reductions in plasma cholesterol levels (9). However, some patients whose packet counts indicated full compliance had little or no reduction in cholesterol levels; presumably many of these patients discarded packets to create the appearance of full compliance. Their data were nevertheless used to advantage in the secondary analyses, as noted below.

A primary outcome assessed in the trial was "risk of coronary heart disease," defined as the combined incidence of death definitely caused by coronary heart disease and/or nonfatal myocardial infarction. Plasma levels of cholesterol and its various fractions were also followed, with particular focus on low-density lipoprotein cholesterol.

The intent-to-treat analysis showed a statistically significant average reduction in risk of coronary heart disease of 19% in the active group, compared with the placebo group, associated with an 8.5% lower level of total cholesterol and a 12.6% lower level of low-density lipoprotein cholesterol (8). The 19% reduction in risk arose from comparing the cumulative 7.4-year incidence of coronary heart disease as 7% in the cholestyramine group and 8.6% in the placebo group. Other measures of occurrence of coronary heart disease—newly positive exercise tests, the development of angina, and the occurrence of coronary bypass surgery—were comparatively reduced by 20 to 25% in the active group. All-cause mortality, however, was only slightly and not significantly lower in the active group, because of their inexplicably larger number of violent deaths. A total of 68 and 71 patients died of any cause, respectively, in the active and placebo groups, representing cumulative mortality rates of 3.6% and 3.7% of the corresponding groups (8).

Thus, the primary analysis (8) led to the conclusion that cholestyramine treatment had definitive efficacy in reducing the risk of coronary heart disease:

> The LRC-CPPT findings show that reducing total cholesterol by lowering LDL-C[holesterol] levels can diminish the incidence of CHD [coronary heart disease] morbidity and mortality in men at high risk for CHD because of raised LDL-C levels. This clinical trial provides strong evidence for a causal role for these lipids in the pathogenesis of CHD.

The interpretation focused not only on the efficacy of cholestyramine *per se,* but also on the general point that intervention to reduce cholesterol levels was beneficial.

The trial created a need to relabel cholestyramine, for it greatly expanded information about the medicine's effects during long-term use. In 1985, the results of both primary and secondary analyses of the Lipid Research trial were incorporated by the Food and Drug Administration into new labeling for cholestyramine.

Figure 24–1 shows the principal results of the secondary analysis of the Lipid Research trial included in the medicine's relabeling (20). The intent-to-treat average levels of coronary risk reduction and cholesterol reduction are shown by the lower of the two horizontal dashed lines. Three levels of compliance-dependent reduction in coronary risk and of total cholesterol levels are shown by the open and closed circles. The distribution of patients among the three groups were as follows: 965 (50.8%) in the highest compliance group, 496 (26.1%) in the intermediate group, and 439 (23.1%) in the lowest group. This analysis was not included in the trial reports (8,9) but was done as part of the Food and Drug Administration's review that translated the Lipid Research trial findings into new labeling for cholestyramine. As Lasagna pointed out (21), there is some misunderstanding about the nature and origin of these dose-dependent efficacy claims for cholestyramine. The relabeling is

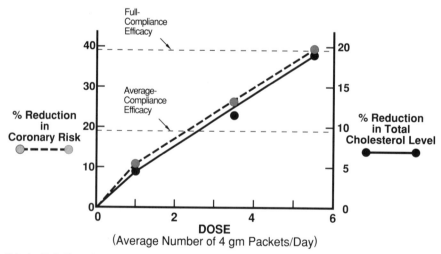

FIG. 24–1. Relations between cholestyramine dose, coronary risk reduction, and reduction in total cholesterol level. The definition of coronary risk reduction, the numbers of patients in each compliance stratum, and the basis on which the curves were derived are given in the text. (Copyright Aprex Corp., 1988, reproduced by permission.)

based on the conservative approach of comparing reductions in coronary risk and in cholesterol levels within compliance strata, between active and placebo groups. Naturally, the labeling also includes results of the intent-to-treat analysis based on all participants, irrespective of compliance (20).

The authors of the published report (9) approached the assessment of dose-dependent efficacy in a less conservative manner than the Food and Drug Administration, as follows:

> Many participants in the cholestyramine group, especially those who took five or more packets of medication daily, sustained levels of TOTAL-C[holesterol] and LDL-C[holesterol] at least 25% and 35% below their respective baseline levels, while many others who adhered less well had little or no change. This wide range of decreases in TOTAL-C and LDL-C within the cholestyramine group provided an opportunity to study the relation between the degree of cholesterol lowering and the incidence of CHD. Furthermore, analysis of the placebo group, which contained adherent and nonadherent participants who differed little from each other with respect to changes in TOTAL-C and LDL-C levels, made it possible to investigate whether self-selection influenced this relationship.

They used the Cox proportional hazards model to project a 49% coronary risk reduction expected from full-dose cholesterol reductions.

Both interpretations take advantage of a postrandomization "experiment of nature," in which patients arrayed themselves across a wide range of compliance with the prescribed regimen. The average compliance in the trial was 4.2 packets per day in the first year and 3.8 packets per day in the last year (i.e., roughly two-thirds of prescribed doses taken). Thus, the average compliance was slightly lower than the average found with the exercise regimen in the Oxford trial, but the range was about the same.

As shown in Table 24–1, compliance was substantially better in the placebo group than in the active group, presumably because of the medicine's gastrointestinal adverse reactions of flatulence, bloating, and dyspepsia. Compliance with the placebo was surprisingly good: Even though excipients are supposed to be "inert," 54 g of any kind of material is a great deal to swallow daily for more than 7 years.

This systematic difference in compliance between active and placebo groups indicates a greater disincentive for patients to comply in the active group. In that sense, the compliance differences between the two groups are interpretable as reflecting different degrees of global dissatisfaction with the regimens. The difference also reflects the fact that drug intake is not only a measure of the magnitude of the independent variable in a clinical trial, but may also be a dependent or outcome variable, in that it is sometimes influenced by patients' responses to the medicine. This is a potential source of bias.

Depending on the type and severity of adverse reaction, their negative impact of compliance can be considerable, as Kruse et al. (22) have graphically shown for the nausea induced by ethinyl estradiol. Efron and Feldman (23) describe a procedure for adjusting for the active placebo difference in compliance, to facilitate statistical analysis of compliance–response data. Although analytically useful, this statistical adjustment does not obviate the need to learn why patients comply partially or poorly and the basis for differences in compliance observed between treatment groups. Without such understanding, statistical comparisons of compliance-linked results may mislead. The presumption in the Lipid Research trial is that the observed differences in compliance relate to patients' responses to unpleasant but not serious gastrointestinal symptoms. There was no evidence found in this trial to link the severity of adverse reactions to the magnitude of the medicine's cholesterol-reducing effect.

The authors of the Lipid Research trial report were cognizant of the potential problems of bias in equating compliance-correlated outcomes with drug dose dependence. They found several lines of evidence to support the validity of linking the incidence of coronary heart disease to compliance, drug dose, and cholesterol reduction. One was the lack of significant association between compliance with placebo and incidence of coronary heart disease or changes in cholesterol levels. Another was that the observed cholesterol changes were a sufficient explanation of the incidence of coronary heart disease in the Cox proportional hazards model, with compliance behavior *per se* having almost no influence other than through its dose-dependent impact on cholesterol levels. As the authors (9) noted,

> This result implies that participants in the cholestyramine group who had high [compliance] but little change in TOTAL-C[holesterol] or LDL-C[holesterol] levels had essentially the same incidence of CHD as those who did not take the drug at all.

A third line of evidence was that all analyses were adjusted for baseline levels of the known major risk factors for coronary heart disease, making it unlikely that hidden risk factors linked to compliance behavior preexisted the study and could have explained the compliance-correlated differences in outcome. A fourth line of evidence is that the foregoing relations were quantitatively consistent with the mean differences found in the intent-to-treat analyses for incidence of coronary heart disease and cholesterol levels between treatment groups. Thus, a careful search failed to find bias lurking within the various relations between compliance and outcomes.

Note that the issue of potential bias in the compliance analysis does not bear on the proof of efficacy, which was settled by the primary analysis. The question here is whether the compliance–response relation can be interpreted as a dose–response relation, to predict the magnitudes of beneficial action in patients who take the full dose or partial doses. Undetected biases might act to give the compliance-response relation a steeper slope than the dose-response relation. However, a well-documented strong bias acts in the opposite direction when compliance is measured, as in the Lipid Research trial, by counting returned, unused medication. This bias, sometimes called the *parking lot effect* (24), refers to patients' discarding of unused medication to create the appearance of good compliance; it leads to an underestimate of partial compliance and an overestimate of full compliance (15) and dilutes the estimate of efficacy in the presumed full-dose subgroup. As a result, the slope of the compliance-response relation underestimates the slope of the dose–response relation.

One practical consequence of the "parking lot" bias is an overestimated cost of treatment needed for a given benefit (25,26). Oster and Epstein (26) noted the misreading of cholestyramine's dose–effect relations in an earlier cost-benefit analysis for the full 24-g daily dose and the average 16-g daily dose in the Lipid Research trial (27). Because of the likelihood that the medicine's dose-response relation was underestimated by the compliance-response relation, all the published studies probably overestimate the costs needed for a given level of benefit.

The overall conclusions of the Lipid Research trial analysts (9) were as follows:

> The consistency of the reductions in CHD manifestations observed with cholestyramine resin in this controlled trial . . . leaves little doubt of the benefit of cholestyramine ther-

apy. These results could be narrowly interpreted to apply only to the use of bile acid sequestrants in middle-aged men with cholesterol levels above 265 mg/dL. . . . The trial's implications, however, could and should be extended to other age groups and women and, since cholesterol levels and CHD risk are continuous variables, to others with more modest elevations of cholesterol levels. The benefits that could be expected from cholestyramine treatment are considerable. In the LRC-CPPT, treatment was associated with an average cholesterol fall of 8.5% beyond diet, and an average 19% reduction in CHD risk. Moreover, [an analysis] that looks at cholesterol reduction and CHD more closely indicates that a 49% reduction in CHD incidence would be predicted for subjects who obtained a 25% fall in plasma cholesterol levels, or a 35% fall in LDL-C[holesterol] levels, which are typical responses to 24 g of cholestyramine resin daily.

The ensuing relabeling of cholestyramine allowed its manufacturers to make a new claim that the medicine reduces the risk of coronary heart disease. With promotion of this claim, together with the increasing medical and public attention to the virtues of cholesterol reduction, United States sales of cholestyramine increased from under $5 million to more than $100 million per year within several years, indicating that many more patients were not only prescribed the medicine, but were taking it as well.

Although experts may differ on the wisdom of broad intervention to change cholesterol levels, it is both sound science and good public policy that the debate be informed about the dose-dependent effects of a medicine and the likely distributions of dosing and dose-dependent effects in populations treated under normal conditions of use. A randomized, placebo-controlled trial does not represent normal conditions of use, for many reasons, including that the patients cannot know either the extent of treatment benefits or whether they are receiving active treatment. An assessment of patients' usage of cholestyramine in routine practice, together with its attendant cholesterol-lowering effects, would complement the information from the Lipid Research trial.

HELSINKI TRIAL

This 5-year placebo-controlled trial (10,11) of the lipid-altering agent gemfibrozil involved 4,081 asymptomatic men, aged 40 to 55, who had on two consecutive occasions a total cholesterol level minus high density lipoprotein cholesterol greater than or equal to 5.2 mmol/liter. All patients were encouraged to follow a cholesterol-lowering diet, to engage in physical activity, and to reduce weight and smoking. Randomization resulted in 2,046 and 2,035 patients, respectively, in the drug and placebo groups. Follow-up examinations were done quarterly for 5 years, with a full medical examination done yearly. The cardiovascular end points were fatal and non-fatal myocardial infarction and cardiac death, composed of sudden cardiac death, unwitnessed cardiac death, and definite nonfatal myocardial infarction.

The primary analysis showed that gemfibrozil treatment led to a statistically significant reduction in serious coronary events (10). The secondary analysis focused mainly on estimating the respective influences of decreased low-density lipoprotein cholesterol and increased high-density lipoprotein cholesterol (11). (Gemfibrozil differs from cholestyramine in having distinctly opposite effects on these two lipid fractions.)

The prescribed dosages of active medicine or the identical placebo were two 300-mg capsules taken twice daily. Compliance measures included counts of returned, unused capsules and a semiannual measurement of urinary levels of gemfibrozil. In addition, in the last quarter of the third year of the trial, a special study was done to compare compliance assessment by (a) low-dose digoxin as a marker substance added to the capsules, (b) a special questionnaire, and (c) capsule count (16,28). The main analysis of the trial data did not use results of the special study, which will be commented on later.

Compliance was expressed as percentage of prescribed doses taken. In applying the capsule count method in the trial, it was the practice to dispense 400 capsules to each patient for the 3-month interval (i.e., a 100-day supply), and thus a small excess in relation to the amount prescribed. This dispensing policy precluded capsule counts indicative of either substantial overdosing or exuberant discarding, as Rudd et al. (29) have observed.

On a year-to-year basis, in the 5-year study, the average levels of capsule-count compliance were, in percentages, 85, 85, 84, 84, and 82 in the active group and 85, 86, 86, 86, and 83 in the placebo group (10). Based on the 5-year average results of the capsule counts, the patients were divided into quartiles of compliance, with the boundaries between quartiles being 69%, 85%, and 93% compliance. Thus, by the capsule count criterion, at least half the patients took less than 85% of the prescribed dose. The inverse statement, that half the patients took more than 85% of the pre-scribed doses, is not valid, for counting returned, unused dosage forms underesti-mates poor or partial compliance by at least half (15) for reasons already noted. At least a quarter of the patients took less than 69% of the prescribed doses.

The relations between the capsule count measure of compliance and lipid changes are shown in Fig. 24–2. There is no sign that any of the lipid levels varied with compliance in the placebo group, whereas a clear association with compliance is evident in the active group. Note that the reduction in triglyceride levels appeared

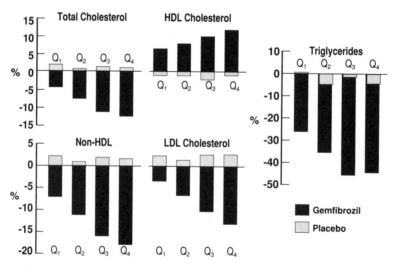

FIG. 24–2. Percentage changes in serum lipid levels in the Helsinki Heart Study by treatment and quartile of compliance. The break points between quartiles of compliance are given in the text. HDL, high-density lipoprotein; LDL, low-density lipoprotein. (Redrawn from ref. 11, with permission.)

to reach its maximum in the third quartile of 85 to 93% of prescribed capsules taken, whereas there was a progressive, compliance-related increase in drug effect on the other lipid fractions, without evidence of maximum effects having been reached.

Figure 24–2 shows that variable dosing with the active agent created a wide range of lipid responses, whose impact on coronary heart disease was subjected to multivariable analysis. This was the "experiment of nature" nested within the ostensibly fixed-dose trial. The contrasting results between active medicine and placebo in Fig. 24–2 demonstrate the specificity of the drug treatment to the lipid effects produced. Had there been substantial cross-coupling in lipid effects between compliance with the capsule regimen and compliance with dietary, exercise, weight loss, or smoking recommendations, such effects should have been evident from compliance-associated changes in lipid fractions in the placebo group, but none occurred.

Constancy of lipid-altering effects throughout the 5-year study in the highest-compliance quartile demonstrated that the medicine's action is maintained (11). This observation is helpful, for undetected gradual decline in compliance can create the illusion of tolerance to a medicine's actions.

Data on the relations between compliance and adverse reactions were not reported but would have been informative. The similar compliance levels in active and placebo groups suggest that drug adverse reactions were not strong enough to influence average compliance, but a comparison of the actual distributions of compliance in the two groups would also have been informative. The efficacy data in Fig. 24–2 suggest that a still higher dose of gemfibrozil might elicit even larger changes in the cholesterol fractions. Such information, however, has to be balanced against other evidence on the relations between dose and adverse reactions.

The trial analysts were well aware of the potential complications in interpreting the effects of compliance-dependent lipid changes on the incidence of coronary heart disease. The issue was greatly simplified, although not completely disposed of, by the absence of compliance-dependent lipid changes in the placebo group. To assess possibly hidden influences of compliance behavior *per se,* the trial analysts used the proportional hazards model to investigate whether compliance had independent effects, other than those mediated through its dose-dependent effects on lipid levels. That analysis showed no influence of compliance behavior *per se* on the incidence of coronary heart disease.

One of the main conclusions of the trial was "that the effect of gemfibrozil therapy on CHD risk is mediated through its actions on HDL and LDL cholesterol" (11). The clear dependence of the lipid levels on compliance adds the useful information that those patients who take less than the recommended dose can expect a lesser reduction in the risk of coronary heart disease.

This large trial has many other important features, including the differential effects of the medicine in the different types of dyslipidemias, that are outside the limited focus of this chapter.

As in the Lipid Research trial, however, the statistically lower mortality caused by coronary heart disease in the gemfibrozil group did not lead to a reduction of all-cause mortality. In the 5-year trial, the drug and placebo groups had cumulative death rates of 2.19% and 2.07%, respectively, for any cause—approximately the same annual mortality rate as in the Lipid Research trial.

In light of the results of the Helsinki trial, the American labeling for gemfibrozil (30) now includes a claimed 34% reduction in serious coronary events and a 37% reduction in incidence of nonfatal myocardial infarction. Unlike the cholestyramine labeling, however, the gemfibrozil labeling does not make dose-dependent efficacy claims.

Some Additional Points

The semiannual measurements of urinary gemfibrozil excretion appeared to add little but cost and trouble to the study. The trial report comments that relative to the findings shown in Fig. 24–2, the "lipid responses in relation to compliance measured by gemfibrozil in urine revealed similar but weaker trends" (11). This result is not surprising, because the medicine's 1.5-hr plasma half-life and lack of evidence for accumulation (30) indicate that a single dose of medicine taken a few hours before urine collection will produce urinary gemfibrozil levels that are scarcely different from those in patients who have dosed regularly for weeks. It is well-recognized that many partially compliant patients improve their dosing in the day or so before a scheduled visit (2–5).

Returned capsule counts undoubtedly underestimated the extent of poor or partial compliance in the trial, as already noted. Thus, as in the Lipid Research trial, it would be expected that the compliance-response relation shows a lower slope than the medicine's true dose-response relation. As noted for cholestyramine, this discrepancy would lead to an overestimate of the drug cost needed to obtain a given level of benefit.

Results of the Special Compliance Methods Study

A special study conducted in the last quarter of the third year compared three methods for measuring compliance: capsule counts, marker-digoxin excretion, and a questionnaire (16). This special study involved 1,739 participants from the drug and placebo groups in the main trial.

The authors noted that all three methods were more reliable for detecting poor rather than good compliance. The marker-digoxin measurement provided unambiguous evidence in respect to drug intake but applied only to a small fraction of the time intervals between examinations. A pretrial evaluation (28), showed (Fig. 24–3) that the method misclassified many partial or poor compliers as good compliers, and many partial compliers as poor or good compliers.

According to the digoxin marker analysis, 1,109 (64%) of the 1,739 participants were classified as good compliers. Of these, however, 117 returned more than 25% of dispensed capsules and so could not have been satisfactorily compliant throughout the 3-month interval. An additional 20 participants reported taking fewer than 75% of the prescribed doses. Using the lowest compliance detected in each patient by the three methods, the authors concluded that 57% of the treated group were good compliers (16). This percentage is similar to what was found in other chronic treatment situations in which pain relief is not involved: by Kass et al. (2–4) in asymptomatic glaucoma patients, by Cramer et al. (13) in epileptic patients, and by Kruse and Weber (14) for a variety of patients seen in general medical care.

As one might expect from the results shown in Fig. 24–3, the marker method also missed a number of poor compliers: 222 patients, or 13% of the study group, were found to be poor compliers by capsule count or by questionnaire but had digoxin excretion values indicative of good compliance. This probably reflects the previsit

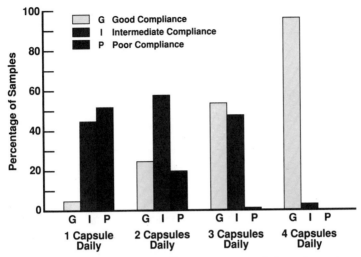

FIG. 24–3. Distribution of three-strata compliance assessments based on urinary excretion of marker digoxin, by dose taken, in the special compliance study during the Helsinki Heart Study. (Redrawn from ref. 28, with permission.)

surge in compliance, which Cramer et al. (5) found to persist as long as 5 days before a scheduled visit.

On the basis of the special study, the authors recommended against dichotomizing compliance into "good" and "poor," noted the value of using multiple methods to assess compliance, and called attention to the need for a method that could give a continuous measurement of compliance.

CORONARY DRUG PROJECT TRIAL

Funded by the United States National Institutes of Health, the Coronary Drug Project was a parallel trial of the effects of five lipid-lowering regimens and placebo on mortality and morbidity from coronary heart disease and other causes. Plans for feasibility began in 1960, funding occurred in 1965, and patients were recruited during 1966 to 1969. A total of 8,341 patients were enrolled by 55 collaborating centers, with 93 to 284 patients per center (31).

Unlike the Lipid Research trial and the Helsinki trial, both of which enrolled late-middle-aged men with high lipid levels but no evidence of coronary artery disease, the Coronary Drug Project enrolled men from a wider age range (30–64) who had had a prior myocardial infarction. At enrollment, 44% of the patients were taking nitroglycerin, 15% were taking digitalis, 14% were taking a diuretic, and many had evidence of other complications of coronary heart or peripheral vascular disease. Because of this serious morbidity, the all-cause mortality rate in the Coronary Drug Project trial was seven to nine times higher than in the Lipid Research and Helsinki trials (Table 24–3). Thus, the evaluation of events in this trial was complicated by, among many other things, variable compliance with treatment regimens for powerful nontrial medicines used to treat hypertension, myocardial ischemia, and/or heart failure.

TABLE 24–2. *Five-year mortality in Coronary Drug Project patients by treatment group, according to 5-year averages of estimated compliance*

Compliance (% of prescribed doses estimated to have been taken)	Treatment group			
	Clofibrate		Placebo	
	Patients (*n*)	Mortality (%)	Patients (*n*)	Mortality (%)
≥ 80	708	15.0	1,813	15.1
< 80	357	24.6	882	28.2
All patients	1,065	18.2	2,695	19.4

The agents compared in the Coronary Drug Project trial were conjugated equine estrogens at two dose levels, clofibrate, dextrothyroxine, nicotinic acid (niacin), and a lactose placebo (3.8 g/day) (31). The initial dosage for each treatment, one capsule three times daily, was increased during the next 2 months to two and then to three capsules three times daily. Thereafter, treatment was kept constant unless drug toxicity was evident. Patients were seen every 4 months.

About 1,100 patients were randomized to each of the drug groups, with 2,789 patients assigned to placebo. The two estrogen treatments and the dextrothyroxine treatment were discontinued early because of excessive numbers of adverse reactions (32–34). The clofibrate and niacin trials were completed and published in 1975 (12).

Compliance (termed *adherence* in the publications) was assessed in several ways at each follow-up visit. According to the published report of the trial design (31),

> clinic personnel also make an assessment of the patient's adherence to his CDP drug prescription for the past four months. This is done by counting (*or estimating*) the number of capsules returned by the patient at that visit and by questioning the patient [emphasis added].

In addition, laboratory measures of compliance with *d*-thyroxine, niacin, and clofibrate were based on samples collected at each visit for serum protein-bound iodine and urinary content of the pyridone of nicotinic acid and the glucuronide of clofibrate. Although neither these results nor results of cholesterol and triglyceride levels were reported back to the participating clinics, the Coordinating Center periodically distributed to the clinics "lists of patients for whom there is laboratory evidence of poor adherence, so that efforts may be made to improve adherence in these patients" (31).

This unusual procedure appears to have arisen from a concept that patient compliance is primarily an issue in the quality control of the study. The designers of the

TABLE 24–3. *Average annual mortality rate in the lipid-lowering trials*

Trial	Cumulative mortality (%)	Duration of trial (yrs)	Average annual mortality (%)
Lipid Research	3.7	7.4	0.5
Helsinki	2.2	5	0.4
Coronary Drug Project	19	5	3.8

trial regarded poor compliance in the same category as procedural mistakes by trial personnel (31). As discussed later, the decision to regard poor compliance as an issue in quality control is now as outmoded as the medicines studied in this large trial.

The policies regarding compliance had several other peculiarities. When clinics were informed about patients who appeared to be poorly compliant, the only patients who could be so described were recipients of *d*-thyroxine, niacin, or clofibrate, because there were no laboratory tests for the other agents or for placebo. These notifications thus violated the principle of applying similar procedures to all groups under study.

Another peculiar feature was the assessment of compliance by essentially subjective "estimates," rather than counts, of returned capsule numbers, by using interview results to modify the capsule counts or estimates for a final rating of compliance. These judgments might readily have been influenced by the knowledge that the patient was or was not on "the list" of poor compliers. The subjectivity of the compliance estimate is evident from the following item (#54) in the list of procedures that the clinic staff was to follow at each visit (31):

In your best judgment (based on a capsule count and/or any other information or impressions obtained from the patient at this visit), what percentage of the total prescribed number of capsules . . . has the patient actually taken?
At least 80% ....( )
At least 60% but less than 80%...( )
At least 40% but less than 60%...( )
At least 20% but less than 40%...( )
Less than 20% ....( )

Thus, although objective counts of returned, unused dosage forms can reliably indicate *poor* compliance, the one advantage of those counts may have been lost because of observer bias in the procedures used by the Coronary Drug Project.

Five-year results in estimated compliance with placebo, clofibrate, and niacin showed, relative to the placebo values, a downward shift that was modest among the clofibrate recipients and rather considerable among niacin recipients (12). The larger decline in estimated compliance for niacin is consistent with the wide array of adverse reactions in that group, including flushing and itching (experienced, respectively, by 92% and 47% of patients), gastrointestinal complaints, itching, decreased appetite, unexpected weight loss, various urinary symptoms, and excessive sweating. In contrast, the most common complaints in the clofibrate group (decreased libido or potency, difficulty in swallowing the dosage forms, and increased appetite) occurred with much lower incidence. The high incidence of characteristic niacin adverse reactions effectively unblinded that group.

The initial analysis of the clofibrate and niacin results led to the conclusion that neither agent reduced all-cause or coronary mortality. The niacin group, however, had the only positive result in this large trial: a small but statistically significant reduction in the incidence of nonfatal myocardial infarction (12). That result launched niacin as one of the recognized chemical interventions to modify lipids and reduce the risks of coronary heart disease.

In 1980, the Coronary Drug Project Research Group published a reanalysis of the clofibrate trial, with the data stratified by the estimated compliance (1). The crucial finding of that reassessment, shown in Table 24–2, was the compliance strata within treatments had significantly different differences in mortality, with p values on the order of 10^{-4}. However, the between-treatment, within-strata differences were not statistically significant. A further analysis of the baseline characteristics of the patients, stratified according to their later-estimated compliance, showed a notably higher incidence of ST-segment depression and of diuretic use, plus a modestly higher incidence of New York Heart Association Class 2 heart failure, among the less than 80% group than among the greater than or equal to 80% group. Adjustments for these baseline risk factors, however, seemed to account for only a small amount of the observed differences in mortality during the ensuing 5 years.

The results in Table 24–2 reinforce the view that clofibrate is ineffective, but the unexpected finding was a large reduction in mortality associated with compliance behavior. The obvious health and economic implications of this large difference might have triggered concerted efforts to learn its basis, but the authors chose to emphasize the following conclusion:

> Analyses of data from the Coronary Drug Project have demonstrated the great difficulty, if not impossibility, of drawing any valid conclusions from findings about mortality or morbidity in subgroups defined by patient responses—such as adherence or biochemical response—to a treatment.

Unless one ignores the placebo control data, there is certainly no possibility of this secondary analysis changing the conclusion of the primary analysis that the medicine was ineffective. Yet the strong association between placebo compliance and mortality in this trial indicates a difficulty that the trial analysts seem to have overlooked, as discussed below.

GENERAL REMARKS

The range of compliance was similar in all four studies. More recent data from electronic monitors reveal the same wide range, adding time-dependent aspects (e.g., periods of total cessation of dosing and previsit surges in compliance) (2–5,13,14,22). It underscores the remark of Haynes and Dantes (17): "No practitioner or researcher can afford to assume that patients or [trial] participants will follow prescribed treatments or follow-up procedures. Indeed, the opposite must be expected and planned for." A fair summary of what to expect and plan for is that 50 to 70% of patients will take greater than 80% of prescribed doses, 30 to 40% will take 40 to 80% of prescribed doses, and small percentages will take, respectively, 100 to 120% or less than 40% of prescribed doses. Patients' ability to take substantial numbers of extra doses may be limited by the dispensing policy, although overdosing may cluster at particular times. Low percentages of prescribed doses taken imply longer average intervals between doses, but averages often give a misleading impression of the actual patterns.

The earlier view that poor compliance means poor trial quality does not stand up to scrutiny in light of the experiences in the Lipid Research, Helsinki, and Oxford trials. These trials studied interventions robust enough to yield a positive primary test of efficacy by intention-to-treat analysis and then used the wide, dose-dependent range of responses to elucidate valuable additional information in secondary analyses.

A serious issue of trial quality, related to compliance, does arise when a trial's design allows a strong association to form between outcome and compliance with placebo, as occurred in the Coronary Drug Project clofibrate trial. Probably the most likely basis for this association is a linkage between compliance with placebo and compliance with important nontrial medications. There may be nonspecific behavioral influences as well, but they should be invoked only after careful assessment is made of the impact of variable compliance with pharmacological influences of proven strength.

Regardless of the origins of the association between placebo compliance and outcome, however, the stronger this association, the greater the burden placed on randomization to ensure precise balance between outcome-influencing factors in control and test groups. By analogy, one might regard the magnitude of the slope of the relation between placebo compliance and outcome as the counterpart of the problem of tare size in a weighing operation: Sensitivity diminishes as tare increases relative to the mass of the object being weighed. Thus, the slope(s) of the relation(s) between placebo compliance and outcome(s) stands in an inverse relation to one's confidence in the results of the primary analysis. In this light, the Coronary Drug Project clofibrate trial was poorly designed, because the strong association between placebo compliance and mortality jeopardizes the conclusion drawn from its primary analysis.

Figure 24–4 summarizes the three situations one may encounter in analyzing placebo-controlled trials results in relation to compliance. Case I is illustrated by the Oxford, Helsinki, and Lipid Research trials. The reassessment of the Stanford subset of the Lipid Research trial by Efron and Feldman (23) exemplifies case II, for there was a small but statistically significant slope in the relation between cholesterol reduction and placebo compliance. The Coronary Drug Project trial of clofibrate exemplifies case III. Statistical comparison of slopes between active and placebo is a test of efficacy, which becomes progressively more difficult as the slopes draw closer together.

Among the factors that can create strong associations between placebo compliance and outcome are (a) (mis)use of powerful nontrial medications and (b) strong dietary influences on outcome. There are probably others. Obviously this is an area that needs more research, but it is likely that compliance with a placebo is fairly predictive of compliance with nontrial medications and with compliance to dietary recommendations. Kruse et al. (14) described some surprising instances in which compliance differs markedly with two concomitantly taken medications, but these would seem to be exceptions. Rudd (35) predicted and Psaty et al. (6) found that misuse of some cardiovascular medicines includes abrupt stop–start patterns of dosing, which may be more hazardous than simple underdosing or even total nonuse.

Many circumstances require trial designs that involve powerful nontrial medications. In that case, a reasonable policy seems to be that followed in the Studies of Left Ventricular Dysfunction (SOLVD) trial of admitting only patients who meet a compliance criterion in a prerandomization screen (36), in hopes of minimizing the confounding effects of variable compliance with nontrial medications. When this prescreening maneuver is used, it is probably best done by taking dose timing into account and setting screening criteria in light of the pharmacodynamic properties of the medicines being taken. Regardless of the criteria used, however, more needs to be learned about the within-patient predictive power of a brief period of compliance data.

If clinical circumstances do not allow time for prescreening, one must accept the usual range of compliance and its impact on the actions of nontrial medications. The need to monitor compliance with all outcome-influencing medications should be

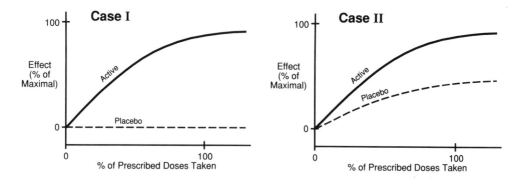

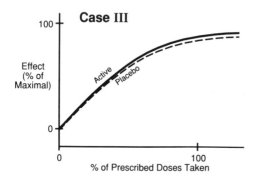

FIG. 24–4. Three types of relations between compliance and effect, as discussed in the text. (Copyright Aprex Corp., 1990, reproduced by permission.)

clear. The fact that it poses complex analytical problems only reflects the complexity of the design and the desirability of finding a simpler design.

When a medicine is tested in fully compliant patients, the results demonstrate "method-effectiveness," as it is termed in the oral contraceptive field. (See Chapter 16, *this volume,* for more on this subject.) When a drug is tested in some particular distribution of poorly, partially, and fully compliant patients, the results demonstrate "use-effectiveness," also a term from the contraceptive field. Because poor and partial compliance reduce statistical power (37) and because medicines do not work in patients who do not take them, an exceptionally large number of poor or partial compliers in a trial can make even high-dose oral contraceptives have a low use-effectiveness. In that light, a conceptual problem becomes evident with intent-to-treat analysis: What particular distribution of poor, partial, and full compliance is appropriate for the therapeutic situation being studied? The "luck of the draw" may not be a satisfactory answer because of the ancillary question: What draw? The Efron–Feldman method (23) may help resolve this vexing but usually ignored question.

Some authors (e.g., ref. 17) try to make the terms *efficacy* and *effectiveness* carry the distinction between method-effectiveness and use-effectiveness, but the latter terms seem preferable because their meaning is self-evident.

A policy for prescreening that may be useful in some instances is to select partially compliant patients. Extra-long-acting pharmaceuticals can be expected to find their greatest comparative advantages in patients who have extra-long intervals between doses (i.e., partially compliant patients). It seems sensible to test for comparative advantage in patients who have the problem that the product is designed to alleviate. A corollary of these considerations is that the boundaries between satisfactory and partial compliance are drug-specific, not fixed.

It is frequently said that "good" compliance is indicated by 80% or more of prescribed doses having been taken. There are several problems with this blanket approach. First, it ignores timing and classifies as a good complier a patient who, prescribed one tablet per day, takes two tablets per day for 15 days and none for the remaining 15, or any other pattern of variable daily dosing that results in the requisite number of tablets being ingested by the end of the interval. Second, it ignores the medicine's pharmacodynamics, which may permit unusually long intervals between doses without loss of efficacy. If that is possible without full compliers being at risk of overdosing or accumulation, the medicine can be judged "forgiving" of many dosing errors and well-suited to the special needs of patients who delay and omit many prescribed doses.

It is important to understand the reasons for partial compliance, particularly when it occurs more in the test group than in the control group. The information can help ascertain whether, for example, those who complied poorly have different drug responses than those who complied well, or whether, as in the Oxford trial, different levels of compliance were associated with different degrees of disease severity. These are, to be sure, biases, but having said that does not discharge one's scientific obligation to gain as much useful information as possible from the trial.

Trying to improve compliance in the midst of a blinded trial is problematic. Procedures used need to be examined carefully to make certain they do not inadvertently unblind the observers, as seems to have occurred in the Coronary Drug Project trial. Then there is the question of what methods are likely to be effective. The pioneering work of Inui et al. (38) and others (39,40) have shown that compliance can be improved by focusing efforts on improving the skills of caregivers. There is also evidence that partially compliant patients increase their compliance when motivated to do so, as occurs when a visit to the physician is imminent (2–5). Finding ways to strengthen these factors and bring them together is an important therapeutic challenge. Naturally, such methods should be properly tested and not simply adopted because of *a priori* appeal.

The Lipid Research and Helsinki trials show how compliance data can reveal a medicine's dose–response relations in a large number of patients during day-to-day outpatient drug usage. These dose-ranging "experiments of nature" cannot substitute for, but can complement, the usually highly contrived circumstances in which formal dose–response testing is done. Furthermore, developing placebo-controlled compliance-response curves in phase II to III trials may help avoid the occasional pitfall of overestimating optimal dosing requirements in premarket testing, as Temple (41) recently described.

With the Food and Drug Administration's policy of including salient trial findings directly in labeling, drug developers should carefully note the precedent set by the relabeling of cholestyramine. It makes four efficacy claims: all-patient average, full-dose, intermediate-dose, and low-dose. A parallel definition of dose-dependent adverse reactions would be a useful addition. If that were present, the label could be said to disclose the effects (good and bad) of actually following the recommended dose and of deviating from that dose in commonly occurring ways. The usual labeling of outpatient products discloses only the all-patient average effects associated with an average dose that was some unstated smaller amount of medicine than recommended. The cholestyramine label is a step forward in realization of full-disclosure labeling.

The major lessons from this review are

1. Widely variable patient compliance appears to be an inevitable attribute of outpatient prescription drug therapy in both trials and practice. It is almost all underdosing in various patterns. Simple negligence is responsible for much of the observed poor and partial compliance, as revealed by similar distributions of compliance with the active agent and with placebo. In some instances, compliance is further depressed as patients diminish their dosing in response to adverse reactions to active agents.

2. Compliance in clinical trials should be measured by objective means and used to help interpret the efficacy and safety results obtained. Subjective measures of compliance are notoriously unreliable and subject to bias if made by observers aware of the patient's health status. Trial protocols should include procedures for learning why patients have taken dosages different from the one prescribed.

3. The uses of compliance data in analysis of the trial's results should also be described in the protocol. Important secondary analyses are:
- estimation of the magnitudes of drug effects associated with full dosing and with the most commonly occurring patterns of partial dosing
- estimation of dose–response relations
- correlation of exceptional events, including rebound phenomena, with exceptional dosing patterns

Compliance data may be employed as an explanatory supplement to the primary analysis, as proposed by Efron and Feldman (23).

4. Measurement of compliance in the placebo group is no less important than in the active groups.

5. Concomitantly administered nontrial medications are also variably complied with, which may have major influence on trial outcomes. Such effects are likely to create correlation between placebo compliance and outcomes, because negligent partial compliance generally applies to all medications patients are supposed to take. For this reason, compliance with important, concomitantly prescribed nontrial medications should be monitored in both active and placebo groups and carefully examined for differences that might influence outcome of the primary analysis.

6. Careful consideration should be given to trial design features that are likely to create a strong correlation between placebo compliance and outcome; the stronger this correlation, the greater the difficulty to test efficacy and the greater the risk that randomization may fail to achieve precisely balanced groups, thus jeopardizing the validity of the primary analysis.

7. Certain clinically relevant questions can better be answered by trials involving patients selected for their demonstrated ability (or, in some instances, inability) to maintain a dosing schedule.

8. A program of intervention to improve compliance in the course of a trial should be carefully evaluated to be certain that it is effective and that it does not inadvertently unblind the study.

9. If partial or poor compliance is considered as a protocol violation (which is debatable), it is fundamentally different in nature than protocol violations by the investigational staff for two basic reasons. First, variable compliance is one of the patients' responses to the treatment situation and sometimes to the test agent itself.

Second, investigational staff have a professional responsibility to adhere to the protocol, with a management structure designed to minimize violations of the protocol. Patients' responsibilities are usually clear in respect to compliance with the schedule of visits but often ambiguous in respect to compliance with the prescribed drug regimen.

10. Accurate cost-benefit estimates depend on reliable data on compliance-related outcome and the distribution of compliance in a treated population.

These lessons are incomplete, for there are still many unknowns in this no-longer neglected area of therapeutics.

Note added in proof: Horwitz et al. have published a re-analysis of the results of the Beta Blocker Heart Attack Trial (BHAT) (*Lancet* 1990; 336: 524–8) showing an inverse association between placebo compliance and mortality akin to that found in the Coronary Drug Project clofibrate trial, summarized in Table 24–2. As in the Coronary Drug Project clofibrate trial, an inclusion criterion in the BHAT was a prior myocardial infarction, which brought with it extensive use of powerful nontrial cardiovascular medications and a substantially elevated in-trial mortality rate, relative to that in the Lipid Research and Helsinki trials. The points made in this chapter about the linkage between measured poor compliance with placebo, poor compliance with powerful nontrial medications, and adverse outcome apply as well to the findings of Horwitz et al.

ACKNOWLEDGMENTS

The author is indebted to Bradley Efron, Alvan R. Feinstein, Joerg Hasford, Frank Hurley, Louis Lasagna, and Lewis Sheiner for many discussions of the opportunities and problems of using compliance data as an explanatory variable in clinical trials analysis. The author is additionally indebted to Alvan Feinstein for critically reviewing the first draft of this chapter.

REFERENCES

1. Anonymous. Influence of adherence to treatment and response of cholesterol on mortality in the coronary drug project: the coronary drug project research group. *N Engl J Med* 1980;303:1038–1041.
2. Kass MA, Meltzer D, Gordon M, Cooper D, Goldberg J. Compliance with topical pilocarpine treatment. *Am J Ophthalmol* 1986;101:515–523.
3. Kass MA, Gordon M, Meltzer DW. Can ophthalmologists correctly identify patients defaulting from pilocarpine therapy? *Am J Ophthalmol* 1986;101:524–530.
4. Kass MA, Gordon M, Morley RE, Meltzer DW, Goldberg JJ. Compliance with topical timolol treatment. *Am J Ophthalmol* 1987;103:188–193.
5. Cramer JA, Scheyer RD, Mattson RH. Compliance declines between clinic visits. *Arch Intern Med* 1990;150:1509–1510.
6. Psaty BM, Koepsell TD, Wagner EH, LoGerfo JP, Inui TS. The relative risk of incident coronary heart disease associated with recently stopping the use of beta blockers. *JAMA* 1990;263:1653–1657.
7. Coats AJS, Adamopoulos S, Meyer TE, Conway J, Sleight P. Effects of physical training in chronic heart failure. *Lancet* 1990;335:63–66.
8. Anonymous. The lipid research clinics coronary primary prevention trial results: (I) reduction in incidence of coronary heart disease. *JAMA* 1984;251:351–364.
9. Anonymous. The lipid research clinics coronary primary prevention trial results: (II) the relationship of reduction in incidence or coronary heart disease to cholesterol lowering. *JAMA* 1984;251:365–374.

10. Frick MH, Elo O, Haapa K, et al. Helsinki heart study: primary-prevention trial with gemfibrozil in middle-aged men with dyslipidemia. *N Engl J Med* 1987;317:1237–1245.
11. Manninen V, Elo MO, Frick H, et al. Lipid alternations and decline in the incidence of coronary heart disease in the Helsinki Heart Study. *JAMA* 1988;260:641–651.
12. Anonymous. Clofibrate and niacin in coronary heart disease: the coronary drug project research group. *JAMA* 1975;231:360–381.
13. Cramer JA, Mattson RH, Prevey ML, Scheyer RD, Ouellette VL. How often is medication taken as prescribed? A novel assessment technique. *JAMA* 1989;261:3273–3277.
14. Kruse W, Weber E. Dynamics of drug regimen compliance—its assessment by microprocessor-based monitoring. *Eur J Clin Pharmacol* 1990;38:561–565.
15. Pullar T, Kumar S, Tindall H, Feely M. Time to stop counting the tablets? *Clin Pharmacol Ther* 1989;46:163–168.
16. Maenpaa H, Manninen V, Heinonen OP. Comparison of the digoxin marker with capsule counting and compliance questionnaire methods for measuring compliance to medication in a clinical trial. *Eur Heart J* 1987;8(suppl I):39–43.
17. Haynes RB, Dantes R. Patient compliance and the conduct and interpretation of therapeutic trials. *Controlled Clin Trials* 1987;8:12–19.
18. Detsky AS. Are clinical trials a cost-effective investment? *JAMA* 1989;262:1795–1800.
19. Anonymous. The lipid research clinics program. The coronary primary prevention trial: design and implementation. *J Chronic Dis* 1979;32:609–631.
20. QUESTRAN (cholestyramine). *Physicians' desk reference.* Oradell, New Jersey: Medical Economics Co., 1990;726–727.
21. Lasagna L. Hypercholesterolemia: whom and how to treat. (*letter*). *N Engl J Med* 1990;322:696.
22. Kruse W, Effert-Kruse W, Rampmaier J, Runnebaum B, Weber E. Compliance with short-term high-dose oestradiol in young patients with primary infertility—new insights from the use of electronic devices. *Agents Actions* 1990;(suppl 29):105–115.
23. Efron B, Feldman D. Compliance as an explanatory variable in clinical trials. Technical Report No. 129, Division of Biostatistics, Stanford University, March 1989. *J Am Stat Assoc* (*in press*).
24. Urquhart J. Pharmacopsychology—how the brain and behavior affect the way drugs act. In: Hindmarch I, Stonier P, eds. *Human psychopharmacology,* vol III. Chichester, United Kingdom: John Wiley, 1990;129–147.
25. Weinstein MC, Stason WB. Cost-effectiveness of interventions to prevent or treat coronary heart disease. *Annu Rev Public Health* 1985;6:41–63.
26. Oster G, Epstein AM. Cost-effectiveness of antihyperlipemic therapy in the prevention of coronary heart disease. *JAMA* 1987;258:2381–2387.
27. Himmelstein DU, Woolhandler S. Costs and effects: the lipid research trial and the Rand experiment. *N Engl J Med* 1985;311:1512–1513.
28. Maenpaa H, Javela K. Pikkarainen J, Malkonen M, Heinonen OP, Manninen V. Minimal doses of digoxin: a new marker for compliance to medication. *Eur Heart J* 1987;8(suppl I):31–37.
29. Rudd P, Byyny RL, Zachary V, et al. The natural history of medication compliance in a drug trial: limitations of pill counts. *Clin Pharmacol Ther* 1989;46:169–176.
30. LOPID (gemfibrozil). *Physicians' desk reference.* Oradell, New Jersey: Medical Economics Co., 1990;1626–1628.
31. Anonymous. The coronary drug project: design, methods and baseline results. *Circulation* 1973;47(suppl I):11–179.
32. Anonymous. Initial findings leading to modifications of its research protocol, coronary drug project research group. *JAMA* 1970;214:1303–1313.
33. Anonymous. Findings leading to further modifications of its protocol with respect to dextrothyroxine, coronary drug project research group. *JAMA* 1972;220:996–1008.
34. Anonymous. Findings leading to discontinuation of the 2.5-mg/day estrogen group, coronary drug project research group. *JAMA* 1973;226:652–657.
35. Rudd P. Blood pressure reduction and the risk of myocardial infarction. (*letter*). *JAMA* 1990;263:660.
36. Probstfield JL, Weiner DH, Bangdiwala SI, et al. The studies of left ventricular dysfunction (SOLVD) experience with a placebo run-phase (*abstr.*). *Controlled Clin Trials* 1989;10:334.
37. Goldsmith CH. The effect of compliance distributions on therapeutic trials. In: Haynes RB, Taylor DW, Sackett DL, eds. *Compliance in health care.* Baltimore, Maryland: Johns Hopkins University Press, 1979;297–308.
38. Inui TS, Yourtree EL, Williamson JW. Improved outcomes in hypertension after physician tutorials: a controlled trial. *Ann Intern Med* 1976;84:646–651.
39. Haynes RB, Sackett DL, Gibson ES, et al. Improvement of medication compliance in uncontrolled hypertension. *Lancet* 1976;1:1265–1268.
40. Foote A, Erfurt JC. Hypertension control at the work site: comparison of screening and referral alone, referral and follow-up, and on-site treatment. *N Engl J Med* 1983;308:809–813.
41. Temple R. Dose-response and registration of new drugs. In: Lasagna L, Erill S, Naranjo CA, eds. *Dose-response relationships in clinical pharmacology.* Amsterdam: Elsevier, 1989;145–167.

*Patient Compliance in Medical
Practice and Clinical Trials*
edited by J.A. Cramer and B. Spilker
Raven Press, Ltd., New York © 1991

25

Clinical Trial Prerandomization Compliance (Adherence) Screen

Jeffrey L. Probstfield

*Clinical Trials Branch, National Heart, Lung, Blood Institute,
Bethesda, Maryland 20892*

The patients' failure to comply with clinical trial interventions has profound impact on study power (1). Recognition of this phenomenon by investigators and compensation for it during the planning phase of a trial will cause study designers to increase a study's projected sample size accordingly (2). It is now recognized that the clinical trial participant frequently demonstrates early in the trial the compliance performance with the study interventions that he or she is likely to manifest during the remainder of the trial (3). This observation and practical experiences with prerandomization run-in (placebo administration to test for pill-taking behavior) and test-dosing (active drug administration to test for the more severe adverse reactions) have made the use of prerandomization compliance screening procedures increasingly common in trials in which the alteration of the natural history of disease is being investigated. These procedures are thought to eliminate patients during the prerandomization phase who would likely do poorly with study interventions during the randomized portion of the trial. This is critical if an "intention-to-treat analysis" of study results is to be done. This chapter will focus on a description of run-in and test-dosing periods and some practical examples of how these maneuvers have been used in clinical trials. It will further describe the indications, contraindications, limitations, and potential problems associated with the use of prerandomization compliance screening procedures. Finally, it will describe some aspects of research that should be done to validate and further develop the use of these procedures.

CHARACTERISTICS OF PRERANDOMIZATION COMPLIANCE SCREENING PROCEDURES

A prerandomization compliance screening procedure is an evaluation method done in the time period before randomization when clinical trial staff members observe how screenees (potential participants) respond to and comply with the selected elements of a clinical trial protocol. Staff may assess compliance in the broader sense of attendance to clinic visits or participation in study evaluation procedures, but more commonly the prerandomization compliance screening procedure is done to assess the screenee's ability to deal with study interventions. Usually these are medications, although assessment of compliance to diet would be useful and appropriate.

The assessment is usually done single-blind (screenee unaware of intervention assignment). Good indications exist for using either an active medicine, a placebo, or both.

DEFINITIONS

Compliance is the degree to which a patient is *willing* to carry out a set of procedures or practices (including interventions), with established guidelines or standards (as part of a clinical trial protocol) (4). This definition has the specific connotation of *passively* following orders.

Adherence is the degree to which a participant is willing to carry out the protocol procedures, or practices with established guidelines or standards and *actively* seeks to cooperate with a clinical trial protocol.

This is the term preferred over compliance by many working in this area especially those in cardiovascular clinical trials. Notwithstanding, compliance is used hereafter in this article for uniformity within this monograph.

Run-in procedure is a prerandomization compliance screening procedure that is used solely for the purpose of testing the prospective participant's pill-taking behavior.

Because this procedure tests a purely behavioral phenomenon, it is suggested that a placebo should be used. Thus the possibility of later unintentional unblinding in the study should be reduced.

Test-dosing procedure is a prerandomization compliance screening procedure that is used to test for adverse reactions to the medicine(s) that is to be used as an active agent in the clinical trial.

This procedure is particularly useful in the case in which early or severe reactions may occur with the intervention(s). The active agent(s) is obviously necessary for this procedure. This procedure should be distinguished from others that may be used during the prerandomization period to determine the efficacy or the correct dose of a medication (e.g., The Cardiac Arrhythmia Suppression Trial) (5).

Efficacy trial is a clinical trial with active medicines (e.g., phase 2 or 3), in which part of the testing procedure is to get information about acceptability or the proportion of patients who are able to tolerate the medicine as well as how much the agent may impact a biochemical or other clinical variable.

All patients who are generally willing and able to participate and who meet the inclusion–exclusion criteria should participate.

Alteration of natural history of disease trial is a clinical trial in which one is trying to impact the natural history of a disease, symptom, or sign.

Compliance to the intervention in this type of clinical trial is of paramount importance. In an attempt to answer the posed scientific question in the most rigorous fashion, the trial carries within an obligatory "intention-to-treat" primary analysis (6). Testing for acceptability of the medicine is not a priority in these trials. Those who are readily and efficiently identified as noncompliers or as having severe reactions to a trial's intervention(s) should be disqualified before randomization because of the potential substantial impact of noncompliance on study power and therefore sample size.

RATIONALE FOR USE OF A PRERANDOMIZATION COMPLIANCE SCREENING PROCEDURE

Compliance has been documented (1) to be a problem in clinical trials (Figure 25–1). In studies that are testing an alteration of natural history of disease reduced compliance can have a profound effect on study power. Although adjustment can be made (by increasing the sample size), a more efficient approach would be to disqualify as many as possible of those who are unable or unwilling to follow the intervention before randomization. This allows for a reduction in the recruitment goal and improved probability that the staff will be able to follow all those who have been enrolled.

In a pair of publications, Roth and Caron (7,8) have shown that physicians, regardless of training or experience, have no better than a chance probability of identifying those who will or will not comply with an intervention. Evidence suggests that the majority of those who will drop out of a trial will do so early (1,9) (Table 25–1) and that the compliance performance in the early postrandomization period is highly predictive of future compliance performance in a trial (3). Using a run-in or test-dosing period before randomization as a test of compliance performance and/or drug tolerance allows for the above-mentioned prerandomization disqualification using an objective method that has an empirical basis. However, comparing the number dropping out initially against the entire experience of trials that employed run-in as opposed to those that did not give a mixed picture. The number of examples is as yet small, but support for run-in as a measure of promoting efficiency in clinical trials is only presumptive.

The opposite situation may occur when a trial uses as its intervention a common medicine, even one that is widely available in many over-the-counter preparations. An example is aspirin and the Aspirin in Myocardial Infarction Study. During the

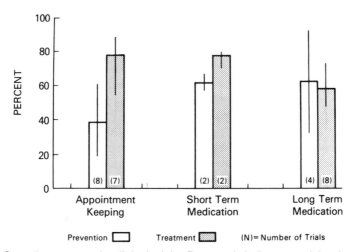

FIG. 25–1. Compliance rates in clinical trials. Bar graph indicates weighted averages and associated ranges of compliance to appointment-keeping, short-term medication-taking, and long-term medication-taking in clinical trials with prevention and treatment as primary goals. Numbers within bars in parenthesis indicate number of trials in each analysis.

TABLE 25–1. *Dropouts (%) at first and last visit postrandomization in long-term studies*

Study[a]	Dropouts (%)		Time of visits	
	First	Last	First	Last
BHAT	3.5	15	1 mo	36 mo
AMIS[b]	3	6	1 mo	36 mo
U.K. Physicians	18	30	6 mo	72 mo
CAPS	4	9	3 mo	12 mo
LRC—CPPT	1.8	6.1	1 mo	89 mo
U.S. Physicians[b]	4	17	6 mo	57 mo

[a]BHAT, beta-blocker heart attack trial; AMIS, aspirin in myocardial infarction study; U.K. Physicians, United Kingdom physicians study; CAPS, cardiac arrhythmia pilot study; LRC—CPPT, Lipid research clinics—coronary primary prevention trial; U.S. Physicians, United States physicians study.
[b]Run-in and/or test-dosing part of protocol.

prerandomization period for Aspirin in Myocardial Infarction Study, screenees were warned to avoid aspirin and aspirin-containing preparations (10). Urine samples were collected to check for salicylates; however, few screenees were excluded from Aspirin in Myocardial Infaction Study because of a positive urine salicylate prerandomization (6).

Limitations and problems associated with the use of prerandomization compliance screening procedures are summarized in Table 25–2. A potential problem with the use of the prerandomization compliance screening procedure is its impact on recruitment. Although, one would hope to eliminate noncompliers before randomization (11), for every screenee who is disqualified by one of these procedures, another must be brought to that point in the prerandomization cascade. Written information on previous experience with compliance screening is limited. However, with two exceptions (12,13), the number of screenees disqualified using either run-in or test-dosing is small (about 5–10%). Two recent examples of run-in periods have disqualified about 20 to 25% of potential participants (12,13). If the number disqualified is large, it may bring into question the use of the procedure, unless those being disqualified are truly those who will be noncompliers in the trial itself. The recent report of Blackwelder et al. (13), although not true validation of the run-in and despite a large disqualification percentage, is supportive of its use. Questions regarding generalizability of trial results could be raised if large numbers are disqualified by compliance screening. Agreement on what is "large" has not been reached.

Brittain and Wittes (14) addressed another aspect of the use of the procedure in a recent paper. The model they described simulates trial situations and uses some actual trial data. They demonstrated that there can be and is substantial misclassification of patients using the first month of compliance performance information and therefore by inference calls into question the use of the run-in period. Although the authors agreed that the run-in may have use, they urged care and thoughtful consid-

TABLE 25–2. *Limitations and problems with run-in and test-dosing*

Limitations on recruitment (reduced numbers of screenees)
Utility (correct identification of noncompliers and those with adverse reactions)
Added cost (e.g., additional visits)
Special packaging of medication(s)
Generalizability (special population recruited)
Late occurrence of adverse reactions from interventions

eration rather than automatic inclusion of the run-in procedure in every trial. Strong suggestion is made that in some instances the run-in may actually decrease the efficiency of a trial and produces little if any gain.

Prerandomization compliance screening procedures clearly add cost to the trial. Not only is the prerandomization period lengthened, appropriate materials must be available so that the procedure(s) can be carried out. Special packaging of medication may be necessary. Additional visits are also required. This cost must be balanced against the potential negatives for the study. Patients who are noncompliers with either the protocol schedule or interventions put substantial strain on the trial staff and frequently necessitate additional staff to ensure continued compliance or complete follow-up (9).

In circumstances in which the compliance screening procedures are used, the screenee may be given a single opportunity to repeat the procedure(s). This is left to the judgment of the clinician. If too many individuals are allowed to repeat and "pass" the procedure, its purpose is circumvented with potential future consequences.

In summary, the rationale for use of the prerandomization compliance screening procedure(s) is to disqualify screenees who have high potential for poor compliance from participation in the clinical trial. Specifically, the trials most at risk are those in which there is investigation of the alteration of the natural history of disease. The screenee at risk for poor compliance must be disqualified before participation in the trial, when actual poor compliance would adversely impact the primary analysis that includes all those randomized.

INDICATIONS AND CONTRAINDICATIONS FOR USING A PRERANDOMIZATION COMPLIANCE SCREENING PROCEDURE

Run-in

Indications for a run-in period have been discussed in part (15) and are expanded here (summarized in Table 25–3). Contact with the clinical trial staff promotes bonding or the development of loyalty to a clinical trial staff member or the project. Cost and logistics frequently dictate that the frequency of contact with staff during prerandomization may be limited, yet bonding or more particularly a constant caretaker relationship is thought to contribute to good compliance. Trials such as the Physicians' Health Study may have infrequent or nonexistent personal contact at anytime during a trial between clinic staff and trial patients (12). Run-in periods would appear

TABLE 25–3. *Indications and contraindications for run-in and test-dosing periods in a clinical trial*

	Indications	Contraindications
Run-in	Infrequent contact with staff	Short prerandomization period
	Complex or demanding protocol (e.g., multiple interventions or procedures, life-style changes)	Suboptimal placebo and trial blinding essential
Test-dosing	Early occurrence of increased frequency of adverse reactions to interventions	Benign study interventions
	Severe adverse reactions to interventions	Efficacy trials

to be especially important in those instances in which opportunities for the establishment or maintenance of bonding are limited. In trials in which the protocol requirements, especially the interventions, are complex or in which either a life-style intervention (e.g., exercise) or significant behavior change (e.g., dietary change) is associated with the intervention, use of the run-in to assess the screenees' potential for compliance with the intervention should be useful.

The general statement is made that compliance is more difficult to obtain and maintain in primary prevention studies (15) (the patients are at risk for developing the disease or a disease-related end point but at trial outset have not had an end point within the primary response variable). Figure 25–1 would not support this notion, because the data indicate that in both short- and long-term medication studies, the level of noncompliance for prevention and treatment studies is similar and substantially reduced from full compliance.

Contraindications for using the run-in are more difficult to identify clearly. There will be some trials that by nature of either the disease process or the logistics of the trial will require a short prerandomization period. Benefits of the short prerandomization period may obviate or substantially limit any efficiency gained from the run-in period. Secondly, if there is an unsatisfactory or even a less than optimal placebo, the use of the run-in may result in substantial subsequent unblinding during the postrandomization period depending on the remaining trial design (e.g., presence or absence of a blinded end points adjudication committee). Unblinding may be an intolerable situation for either the patients or staff. Obviously, in efficacy trials, the run-in should not be used. Here the widest participation possible is desired.

Test-Dosing

This procedure should be used when an intervention has the early occurrence of a high frequency or extreme severity of adverse reactions associated with it. Those who fit into this category may be at increased risk if they attempt to perform in the trial. These patients should be identified and disqualified before randomization. To put this procedure in the prerandomization period of a study with an intervention that is benign adds needlessly to the cost and complexity.

HISTORICAL DEVELOPMENT OF PRERANDOMIZATION COMPLIANCE SCREENING PROCEDURES

The trace of information regarding prerandomization compliance screening procedures is difficult at best. The words *run-in, faint of heart,* or *test-dosing* are not standard terminology used in either Medline or Index Medicus. However, the European computerized database on medical literature, EMBASE, will allow searches to be done under the heading of run-in. Searches under the Psychological Information and Mental Health abstracts databases produced references adding little.

The first clinical trial with information given about a run-in period was the Veterans Administration Cooperative Study on Hypertension published in 1967. There are general references to the use of the procedure mentioned in earlier sources, but no specific examples with evidence of implementation have been identified. A partial list of references discussing the use of run-in (10,13,16–23) and those for the use of test-dosing (12,13,21,23–26) is included in the Reference section of this chapter. Readers are urged to consult the original sources for details of logistics and format.

A CURRENT EXAMPLE OF A PRERANDOMIZATION COMPLIANCE SCREENING PROCEDURE: THE STUDIES OF LEFT VENTRICULAR DYSFUNCTION EXPERIENCE

The Studies of Left Ventricular Dysfunction is a parallel set of trials investigating whether or not treatment, using an angiotensin-converting enzyme inhibitor, in patients with left ventricular ejection fractions of 0.35 or less results in a reduced number of deaths in the treated group as compared with those given a placebo (23). The treatment trial is investigating those who have already had an episode of overt heart failure. The prevention trial enrolled patients who had a depressed ejection fraction as defined above but who had not had an episode of overt failure.

The Studies of Left Ventricular Dysfunction trials are using the angiotensin-converting enzyme inhibitor enalapril as the active agent. Angiotensin-converting enzyme inhibitors are known to produce severe adverse reactions in approximately 3 to 5% of patients. Most so-identified will be unable to continue with the medication (24–26). Hypotension, worsening renal failure, neutropenia, and angioedema are the commonest of the severe reactions observed. Premorbid clinical characteristics help to predict those patients who may experience hypotension or worsening renal failure but not angioedema (27,28). Beginning with small doses helps to reduce the number of patients who are unable to tolerate the medicine (29).

For the above reasons the Studies of Left Ventricular Dysfunction investigators elected to give potential patients small doses of the active agent enalapril in a single blind fashion from 2 to 7 days during the prerandomization period as a test-dosing of the medication (11). The period of exposure to the active drug during the prerandomization phase is purposefully short to minimize unblinding later in the study. A preliminary analysis of Studies of Left Ventricular Dysfunction data reveals that approximately 3% of the screenees are not able to tolerate (i.e., take at least 75% without adverse reaction) the active medicine during the prerandomization screen (30). These data along with the data from the three other trials of angiotensin-converting enzyme inhibitor would indicate that in some trials, in which interventions are associated with severe adverse reactions, the test-dosing procedure is useful for disqualifying screenees unable to use an intervention at the protocol-defined dose.

Because the test-dosing period was kept brief in Studies of Left Ventricular Dysfunction, this offered little opportunity to test the pill-taking behavior of potential participants. The protocol prescribes, therefore, that all screenees who remain eligible subsequently take the placebo for enalapril in a single-blind fashion for 14 to 17 days (23). The screenee must take at least 80% of the placebo during this prerandomization run-in period to remain eligible. Under extenuating circumstances, the screenee is allowed to repeat the run-in period once (31). Preliminary analyses of the data from about 5,000 eligible potential patients demonstrated that approximately 3% failed to meet the run-in placebo consumption criterion (32). Age, gender, and marital status appeared to have no predictive value in assessing compliance performance. The relative severity of disease as determined by ejection fraction and by the New York Heart Association Criteria had a modest impact on compliance performance in the run-in (32). The confirmation of these findings and an evaluation of the subsequent compliance performance of patients during the trials awaits the analysis of the complete data set of the full Studies of Left Ventricular Dysfunction cohort in the pre- and postrandomization periods.

The only conclusions regarding the Studies of Left Ventricular Dysfunction prerandomization compliance screening procedures that can be made at this juncture are that they did not appear to impact adversely recruitment or the potential generalizability of any trial results because small numbers were disqualified by the procedures.

RESEARCH THAT NEEDS TO BE DONE ON PRERANDOMIZATION COMPLIANCE SCREENING PROCEDURES

Research in the area of prerandomization compliance screening procedures has been minimal. Issues of sensitivity, specificity, and generalizability as previously mentioned are all yet to be resolved.

Run-in

The use of the run-in procedure in clinical trials has never been validated. It is known that some potential participants are eliminated during a run-in period. These patients are never randomized. It remains to be established, however, that the correct screenees (i.e., future poor compliers in the trial) have been excluded prerandomization. The assumptions are made that because these patients have failed to perform up to expectations during the run-in and that because patients who drop out or who do poorly with drug compliance during a study will demonstrate this early on, that the patients who might have been randomized and performed badly during the study have been eliminated. There is an appropriate logical sequence to this line of reasoning. However, several validation studies are needed using different populations and different types of run-in procedures. At minimum there would need to be randomization with continued follow-up of patients who do not meet the prerandomization compliance criterion in the same fashion as those randomized into the trial but qualify in all other regards. Whether or not those who fail to meet the prerandomization compliance criterion were truly those who would do badly with compliance after they are randomized should be clearly determined. Actual data from previous experience gives little information about the specificity of the procedure as described.

Data shows that the sensitivity of the run-in screening procedure, particularly, is inadequate. More than half of the patients who drop out of a trial and still more who ultimately do badly with the intervention in a trial would not be identified by the first month's compliance data (Table 25–1). Further, there is some indication that those who would drop out have more events (33,34) so that as a consequence there is a healthier population with fewer events among those randomized, making the trial less powerful for testing the question.

The entire issue of pill taking at regular intervals and the documentation of same as a measure of compliance has become an issue of substantial investigation. Because pill count is the usual assessment method of determining compliance but has many attendant problems, the method of doing pill counts becomes a critical issue with regard to the sensitivity of compliance screening.

A workshop was held in May 1982 at the National Heart, Lung, and Blood Institute, at which time the use of markers of compliance was surveyed (35). In a summary of the workshop, the plea was made for the development of adequate markers for the assessment of compliance in clinical trials.

Recently, Cramer et al. (36) described the efficacy of a new method of compliance assessment in a trial with antiepileptic agents. The Medication Event Monitor Systems (Aprex Corporation, Fremont, California) is described elsewhere in this volume. This computerized monitoring system, which uses the cap of the medication container to track compliance, satisfies five of the six criteria set up as the ideal for a marker or evaluation method of compliance (35). The only criterion not successfully met is that the evaluation method must be unknown to the patient. The monitoring device has more than trivial expense, and it must be returned for proper compliance assessment to be made. The criterion unmet would seem relatively inconsequential; however, a patient with malice aforethought could still defile this attempt at compliance monitoring. On balance, the sensitivity of the method of prerandomization compliance screening could be substantially enhanced with the use of this device, and its potential should be explored properly.

Davis (30), particularly, raised the issue of generalizability of trial results after the use of prerandomization compliance screening procedures. Although it can be inferred that low numbers of screenees disqualified by the procedure(s) would suggest no difficulty for generalizability of results, that conclusion would not necessarily follow. At minimum one would have to make a registry of all screenees disqualified by the prerandomization screening procedure(s) used and compare the prerandomization characteristics to those of all randomized patients. Further, the event rate of the primary outcome variable in the placebo group of the trial would need to be compared with the event rate observed at the end of the trial for the screenees not randomized. Although some difference would be expected because of the commonly observed reduction of primary end points occurring when patients are randomized into clinical trials, a large difference would be an important observation suggesting that a somewhat special population had been randomized into the study.

Test-Dosing

The use of the test-dose has other associated problems, which need to be carefully investigated. There are no data regarding rechallenge of those who have severe adverse reactions in the test-dosing situation. Rechallenge is an accepted form of establishing a firmer link of cause and effect between the pharmacologic agent and the response to the test. If rechallenge is done, it should be done during the prerandomization period. Further data would need to be collected on those who have adverse responses to the test-dose of the interventions. It is suggested that the patients identified by the test-dosing likely represent those who would have a therapeutic response at the low end of the dose–response curve. They would not only have better tolerance for a lower dose but likely would get an acceptable therapeutic response from the intervention at the lower dose. The rigidity of the protocol often precludes the possibility of these patients being randomized because multiple doses, especially those that are small, are not and cannot be included.

A partial list of research efforts has been proposed on run-in and test-dosing, which is needed but difficult and expensive to do in the course of the usual clinical trial. To date established clinical trials have been the only laboratory for those interested in compliance. Unless and until the validity, specificity, and sensitivity of the prerandomization compliance screening procedures and the indication for their use can be further defined, the appropriateness and use of the procedures will continue to be questioned.

REFERENCES

1. Probstfield JL, Russell ML, Insull W, Yusuf S: *Dropouts from a clinical trial, their recovery and characterization: a basis for dropout management and prevention. Health behavior change handbook.* New York: Springer Publishing Co., 1990;376–400.
2. Lachin JM. Introduction to sample size determinations and power analysis for clinical trials. *Controlled Clin Trials* 1981;1:13–27.
3. Dunbar J. *Predictors of patient adherence. Health behavior change handbook.* New York: Springer Publishing Co., 1990;348–360.
4. Meinert CL. *Clinical trials, design conduct and analysis.* New York: Oxford University Press, 1986;288.
5. Preliminary report: effect of eincainide and flecainide on mortality in a randomized trial of arrhythmia suppression after myocardial infarction. *N Engl J Med* 1989;321:406–412.
6. Friedman LM, Furberg CD, DeMets DL. *Fundamentals of clinical trials,* 2nd ed. Littleton, Massachusetts: PSG Publishing, 1985.
7. Caron HS, Roth HP. Patients' cooperation with a medical regimen. *JAMA* 1958;203:922–926.
8. Roth HP, Caron HS. Accuracy of doctors' estimates and patients' statements on adherence to a drug regimen. *Clin Pharmacol Ther* 1978;23:361–370.
9. Probstfield JL, Russell ML, Henske JC, Reardon R, Insull W Jr. A successful program for returning dropouts to a clinical trial. *Am J Med* 1986;80:777–784.
10. Aspirin Myocardial Infarction Study Research Group. *Aspirin myocardial infarction study: design, methods, and baseline results.* NIH Publication No. 80-2106, 1980.
11. Hunninghake DB. *Recruitment in clinical trials. Impact on adherence. Health behavior change handbook.* New York: Springer Publishing Co., 1990;335–341.
12. Buring JE, Hennekens CH. Cost and efficiency in clinical trials: the US Physicians' Health Study. *Stat Med* 1990;9:29–33.
13. Blackwelder WC, Hastings BK, Lee MLF, Deloria MA. For the vaginal infections and prematurity (VIP) study group. *Controlled Clin Trials* 1990;11:187–198.
14. Brittain E, Wittes J. The run-in period in clinical trials: the effect of misclassification on efficiency. *Controlled Clin Trials* 1990 (*in press*).
15. Lang JM. The use of a run-in to enhance compliance. *Stat Med* 1990;9:87–95.
16. Lachin JM, Marks JW, Schoenfeld LJ, the NCGS Protocol Committee. Design and methodologic considerations in the National Cooperative Gallstone Study: a multicenter clinical trial. *Controlled Clin Trials* 1981;2:177–229.
17. Coronary Drug Project Research Group. The coronary drug project: design, methods and baseline result. *Circulation* 1973;49(suppl I):II-150.
18. Veteran's Administration Cooperative Study Group on Antihypertensive Agents. Effects of treatment in morbidity in hypertension: results in patients with diastolic blood pressure averaging 115 through 129 monthly. *JAMA* 1967;202:116–122.
19. Li J, Taylor PR, Li G, et al. Intervention studies in Linxian, China: an update. *J Nutr Growth Cancer* 1986;3:199–206.
20. Albanes D, Virtamo J, Rautalahti M, et al. Pilot study the US–Finland lung cancer prevention trial. *J Nutr Growth Cancer* 1986;3:207–214.
21. The Post Coronary Artery Bypass Graft Protocol, 1988.
22. The Asymptomatic Carotid Artery Plaque Study Protocol, 1989.
23. Studies of left ventricular dysfunction (SOLVD), rationale, design and methods. Two trials that evaluate the effect of angiotensin converting enzyme inhibitor in patients with reduced ejection fraction. The SOLVD investigators. *Am J Cardiol* 1990;66:315–322.
24. Captopril multicenter research group. A placebo controlled trial of captopril in refractory chronic congestive heart failure. *J Am Coll Cardiol* 1983;2:755–763.
25. Long-term effects of enalapril in patients with congestive heart failure. A multicenter, placebo controlled study. *Heart Failure* 1987;3:102–107.
26. Comparative effects of captopril and digoxin in patients with moderate heart failure. *JAMA* 1988;259:539–544.
27. Edwards CRW, Padfield PL. Angiotensin-converting enzyme inhibition: past, present and bright future. *Lancet* 1985;1:30–34.
28. Packer M, Medine N, Yushak M. Relationship between serum sodium concentration and the hemodynamic and clinic responses to converting enzyme inhibition with captopril in severe heart failure. *J Am Coll Cardiol* 1984;3:1035–1043.
29. Webster J, Newnham DM, Petrie JC. Initial dose of enalapril in hypertension. *Br Med J* 1985;290:1623–1624.
30. Davis CE. *Prerandomization compliance screening in clinical trials. Health behavior change handbook.* New York: Springer Publishing Co., 1990;342–347.

31. The Studies of Left Ventricular Dysfunction Protocol, 1985.
32. Probstfield JL, Weiner DH, Bangdiwala SI, et al. The studies of left ventricular dysfunction (SOLVD), experience with a placebo run-phase. *Controlled Clin Trials* 1990;9:334.
33. Wilcox RG, Hampton JR, Rowley JM, Mitchell JRA, Roland JM, Banks DC. Randomized placebo-controlled trial comparing oxyprenol with dispopyramide phosphate in immediate treatment of suspected myocardial infarction. *Lancet* 1980;2:765–769.
34. Wilcox RG, Roland JM, Banks DC, Hampton JR, Mitchell JRA. Randomized trial comparing propranolol with atenolol in immediate treatment of suspected myocardial infarction. *Br Med J* 1980;1:885–888.
35. Insull W Jr. Workshop on the development of markers for use as adherence measures. Workshop summary. *Controlled Clin Trials* 1984;5:451–458.
36. Cramer JA, Mattson RH, Prevey ML, Schayer RD, Ouelette VL. How often is medication taken as prescribed. A novel assessment technique. *JAMA* 1989;261:3273–3277.

*Patient Compliance in Medical
Practice and Clinical Trials*
edited by J.A. Cramer and B. Spilker
Raven Press, Ltd., New York © 1991

26

Patient Selection Bias in Analyses Using Only Compliant Patients

*Joseph F. Collins and **Walter Dorus

*Cooperative Studies Program Coordinating Center, DVA Medical Center,
Perry Point, Maryland 21902; and **DVA Edward Hines Jr. Hospital,
Hines, Illinois 60141, and Department of Psychiatry, Loyola University of Chicago,
Maywood, Illinois 60153*

Most statisticians and clinical investigators believe that the proper statistical analyses for clinical trials are based on results of all patients who begin treatment and not on only those patients that actually adhered (i.e., were compliant) to the protocol. They feel that compliant patients are a self-selected population and are, thus, a biased population. Treating physicians and others, however, usually want to know the effect of a treatment on patients who actually receive it. This chapter explores the possible problems and biases that can arise when only compliant patients are used to report the results of a clinical trial. The results of a large clinical trial, the Department of Veterans Affairs Cooperative Study on Lithium Treatment in Alcohol Dependence (1), are used as an example.

At the time that the Department of Veterans Affairs cooperative study was nearing completion, the results of a similar study by Fawcett et al. (2) were published. The study of Fawcett et al. indicated that patients receiving lithium carbonate (lithium) who were highly compliant were less likely to drink again than lithium low-compliers, lithium noncompliers, placebo compliers, and placebo noncompliers. When the Department of Veteran Affairs study results showed no lithium treatment effect using a total sample and a sample of completer patients, the study's Executive Committee (study management committee) felt that it would be necessary to also do analyses of the compliant patients even though such analyses were not believed to be appropriate. Therefore, the final manuscript (1) included intention-to-treat analyses and analyses on patients who completed the study, as had originally been planned, as well as analyses of compliant patients.

STUDY BACKGROUND

The details of the study have been described elsewhere (1) and will only be briefly described here. The study was a double-blind, placebo-controlled clinical trial to evaluate the efficacy of maintenance treatment with lithium for alcohol-dependent patients with and without a history of depression. The depression group met DSM-III criteria (3) for major depression or dysthymic disorder sometime during their life.

Four hundred fifty-seven patients entered into the study; 286 had no history of depression, and 171 had a history of depression. Patients were seen weekly for the first 14 weeks and biweekly for the remainder of the 1-year study period. Major evaluations of outcome measures were done at 4-week intervals. Thus, each patient was scheduled for 33 clinic visits and 13 major evaluations. Seven Department of Veteran Affairs medical centers participated.

The patient sample consisted of male military service veterans, 60 years old or younger, who met DSM-III criteria for alcohol dependence, lived within 50 miles of their participating medical centers, and gave informed consent. Patients were excluded for certain psychiatric diagnoses, medical disorders that made lithium contraindicated, and marked instability. Patients with the following psychiatric diagnoses were excluded: schizophrenia, bipolar disorders, antisocial personality disorder, psychoactive substance use disorder (except alcoholism), agoraphobia, anorexia nervosa, and organic mental disease. Exclusion medical disorders were current renal disease, history of thyroid disease, current heart failure, and epilepsy. Instability was defined as a history of noncompliance in previous treatment episodes, no permanent address, or fewer than three people living in the vicinity who could be used to contact them. For the analyses that follow, the depressed and nondepressed groups were combined. Table 26–1 gives the demographic characteristics of the patients who entered the study.

COMPLIERS, NONCOMPLIERS, AND DROPOUTS

A definition was needed to specify compliance that could be applied identically and without bias to both lithium and placebo patients. Because there was no biochemical measure that could be used for both the lithium and placebo patients, pill counts and patient interviews were relied on, the traditional methods of assessing compliance. It was also required that for patients to be rated as compliant, they be reasonably compliant during the entire course of the 12-month treatment period. Thus, the definition for a compliant patient was:

TABLE 26–1. *Characteristics of 457 patients in "Lithium Treatment in Alcohol Dependence Study"*

Age (mean years)	41.6 ($\pm$ 9.0)
Race	
White	67.5%
Black	30.5%
Other	2.0
Marital status	
Married	31.8%
Divorced/separated	50.4%
Never married	16.0%
Widowed	1.8%
Education	
> High school	38.4%
High school	40.8%
< High school	20.8%
Employment	
Full-time	73.9%
Part-time	14.0%
Unemployed	7.9%
Retired	4.2%

1. The patient had to have had a 52-week interview (i.e., he had to be a completer).
2. The patient must have been rated by the study assistant as having taken at least 50% of his study medications on at least 20 clinic visits (60% of visits). Ratings were based on pill counts and patient interviews.
3. The patient had to be rated as compliant on at least one clinic visit in each quarter of the patient's treatment year.

It was found that this definition of compliance was appropriate. For lithium complier patients ($n = 82$) for whom it was possible to obtain drug serum levels, the mean lithium serum level was 0.71 mEq/liter (standard deviation = ± 0.25 mEq/liter). A level of 0.50 mEq/liter was considered adequate. Only four of the 82 lithium complier patients had mean levels less than 0.30 mEq/liter. For all the complier patients combined, 83.3% were rated at all 13 of the major rating periods, 92.2% had all but one of the major ratings, and 94.1% had all but two major ratings. When all clinic visits were considered, it was found that 18.1% of the complier patients attended all 33 of their visits, 56.1% attended at least 30 visits (90.9%), and 78.9% attended at least 27 visits (81.8%). Only four patients (2.3%) attended the minimum 20 visits.

To address some of our questions about compliance, two comparison groups were defined. They were called "noncompliers" and "dropouts." Noncompliers had a 52-week interview (and were thus study completers) but did not meet at least one of the other two complier criteria. That is, the patients either did not have 20 visits in which they were rated as compliant or they did not have at least one visit in each quarter-year in which they were rated as compliant. Dropouts were those patients who did not have a 52-week interview. They could be considered a more serious type of noncomplier because they did not complete the study, although it is likely that some dropouts left the study because they believed that they had resolved their problem and no longer needed treatment.

Patients were well-distributed between the three compliance-based groups. Of the 457 patients, 171 (37.4%) were classified as compliers, 109 (23.9%) as noncompliers, and 177 (38.7%) as dropouts. For the 228 lithium patients, 82 (36.0%) were compliers, 48 (21.1%) were noncompliers, and 98 (43.0%) were dropouts, whereas for the 229 placebo patients, 89 (38.9%) were compliers, 61 (26.6%) were noncompliers, and 79 (34.5%) were dropouts. The differences in compliance group distributions between lithium and placebo patients were not statistically significant.

COMPARISONS OF DEMOGRAPHIC AND CLINICAL BACKGROUND CHARACTERISTICS

The first question addressed was whether compliers, noncompliers, and dropouts differed on demographic and clinical background characteristics and whether there were differences between treatment groups (i.e., lithium and placebo) for these characteristics. Table 26–2 lists 21 of the 22 characteristics that were considered and gives the means or distributions of the characteristics by compliance group. The 22nd characteristic was medical center.

As given in Table 26–2, four of the 21 characteristics listed have statistically significant differences ($p < 0.05$) between the three compliance groups. These four characteristics are age, number of years drinking, marital status, and a history of job troubles caused by drinking. There was also a significant difference found for medical center ($p = 0.014$). Chi-square tests and analyses of variance were used to deter-

TABLE 26–2. Comparisons of compliers, noncompliers, and dropouts on demographic and clinical background characteristics

Characteristic	Compliers (N = 171)				Noncompliers[a] (N = 109)				Dropouts (N = 177)				Probability level[b]
	N	%	X̄	SE	N	%	X̄	SE	N	%	X̄	SE	
Means[c]													
Age			44.5	0.7A			39.5	0.8B			40.0	0.7B	< 0.001[d]
Times treated for alcoholism			2.5	0.3			2.6	0.3			2.7	0.3	0.923
Years drinking			25.9	0.7A			20.6	0.9B			21.7	0.7B	< 0.001[d]
Age alcoholism onset			26.4	0.6			25.0	0.8			25.4	0.6	0.323
Weight			167.2	2.2			167.5	2.7			164.3	2.2	0.549
Pre–Beck depression Inventory (5)			9.4	0.7			9.3	0.8			8.8	0.7	0.779
Pre–alcohol abuse rating (4)			7.2	0.2			7.3	0.3			7.3	0.2	0.985
Frequencies													
Race—white	127	74.3			75	69.4			106	59.9			0.058
Controlled environment—No	126	73.7			81	75.0			136	76.8			0.782
Education—some college +	72	42.1			43	39.8			60	33.9			0.399
High school	61	35.7			44	40.7			81	45.8			
< High school	38	22.2			21	19.4			36	20.3			
Employment—full	127	74.3			75	69.4			135	76.3			0.107

	n	%	n	%	n	%	p
Marital status—married	70	40.9A	32	29.6AB	43	24.3B	0.022[d]
Divorced/separated	77	45.0	59	54.6	102	57.6	
Never married	24	14.0	17	15.7	32	18.1	
Psychological treatment—yes	35	20.5	17	15.7	32	18.1	0.604
Drug use—yes	29	17.0	20	18.5	33	18.6	0.907
Chronic medical problem—yes	39	22.8	21	19.4	29	16.4	0.319
Taking prescription medicine—yes	34	19.9	19	17.6	29	16.4	0.692
Criminal conviction—yes	27	15.8	21	19.4	33	18.6	0.684
History of depression—yes	69	40.4	39	35.8	63	35.6	0.605
Job trouble caused by drinking—yes	109	63.7A	79	72.5AB	138	78.0B	0.013[d]
Driving trouble caused by drinking—yes	112	65.5	70	64.2	106	59.9	0.532
Other alcohol arrests—yes	114	66.7	71	65.1	123	69.5	0.723

[a]Most characteristics based on only 108 patients because most prestudy forms being lost on one patient.
[b]Probability level for either a compliance group by characteristic group χ^2 or a compliance group by drug group analysis of variance.
[c]Least square means and standard errors from a compliance group by drug group analysis of variance.
[d]Means or percents having same letter are not significantly different from each other.

mine these differences. To determine which compliance groups were significantly different from each other, Brunden's method of partitioning significance level (6) was used for the χ^2 tests, whereas Duncan's multiple range test was used for the analyses of variance.

For age, it is seen that compliers were significantly older than the noncompliers and the dropouts. When lithium and placebo patients were considered separately, similar significant findings were found for the placebo patients ($p<0.001$). Placebo compliers had a mean age of 45.4 (standard deviation = ±8.8) years, noncompliers had a mean age of 38.6 (±8.6) years, and dropouts had a mean age of 38.9 (±8.0) years. Although not quite statistically significant ($p=0.087$), lithium patients showed a similar trend with the mean age being 43.5 (±9.0) years for compliers, 40.4 (±8.2) years for noncompliers, and 41.1 (±9.1) years for dropouts. When lithium and placebo patients were compared for each of the three compliance groups separately, no significant differences were found.

The results for number of years drinking are similar to those seen for age, with compliers more likely to have been drinking for more years than either noncompliers or dropouts. That age and years drinking are similar is not surprising because these two characteristics are highly correlated ($r=0.80$). As with age, the differences were more pronounced in the placebo patients ($p<0.001$) than in the lithium patients ($p=0.093$). For the placebo patients, the mean number of years drinking was 26.9 (±9.9) years for the compliers, 20.1 (±8.6) years for the noncompliers, and 20.6 (±7.4) years for the dropouts, whereas for the lithium patients, it was 24.8 (±10.0) years for the compliers, 21.2 (±8.2) years for the noncompliers, and 22.8 (±9.3) years for the dropouts. As with age, there were no statistically significant results when lithium and placebo patients were compared for each of the compliance groups separately.

For the third significant characteristic, marital status, there is a statistically significant result with complier patients more likely to be married and less likely to be divorced or separated than either noncompliers or dropouts. Only the complier–dropout differences are significant, however. When the lithium and placebo patients are considered separately (Table 26–3), a different pattern emerges. For the lithium patients, there are no statistically significant differences between the three groups, and in fact, the percentages are similar. For the placebo patients, however, there is a significant difference between the three compliance groups. The compliers were

TABLE 26–3. *Comparisons of compliance groups by lithium and placebo patients separately for marital status*

Status	Compliers N	Compliers %	Noncompliers N	Noncompliers %	Dropouts N	Dropouts %	Probability level[a]
Lithium patients							
Married	24	29.3	14	29.2	25	25.5	0.493
Divorced/separated	45	54.9	31	64.6	57	58.2	
Never married	13	15.9	3	6.3	16	16.3	
Placebo patients							
Married	46	51.7A	18	30.0B	18	22.8B	0.002[b]
Divorced/separated	32	36.0	28	46.7	45	57.0	
Never married	11	12.4	14	23.3	16	20.3	

[a]Probability level for compliance group by marital status group χ^2 test.
[b]Percents with same letter are not significantly different from each other.

more likely to be married and less likely to be divorced or separated or to have never been married than were the noncompliers or dropouts. The differences between compliers and noncompliers and between compliers and dropouts are statistically significant.

When lithium and placebo patients were compared in Table 26–3 for the three compliance groups separately, a statistically significant difference ($p = 0.011$) was found between lithium and placebo compliant patients, with the placebo compliers more likely to be married. For the noncompliers, there is also a statistically significant difference ($p = 0.038$) between lithium and placebo patients, with lithium patients more likely to be divorced or separated and less likely to never have married.

For alcohol-related job problems, Table 26–2 shows an overall difference between the three compliance groups for all patients in which compliers were less likely to have experienced job problems than either noncompliers or dropouts. Only the complier–dropout difference is significant. For the placebo patients ($p = 0.005$), compliers experienced statistically fewer job problems (41.6%) than either the noncompliers (21.3%) or the dropouts (21.5%). For the lithium patients ($p = 0.217$), the noncompliers experienced the fewest alcohol-related job problems (35.4%), although not significantly different from either the compliers (30.5%) or the dropouts (22.4%). None of the differences between the lithium and placebo patients in the three compliance groups separately were statistically significant.

For the final significant characteristic, medical center, there were no significant differences between compliers and noncompliers, but there were between compliers and dropouts and between noncompliers and dropouts. The differences were due to one medical center having a low dropout rate (16.9%) compared with the other six centers (range 34.0–53.4%). When the lithium and placebo patients were considered separately, differences were found only for the lithium patients ($p = 0.023$). The same center had a low dropout rate (12.9%) in comparison with the other centers (range 34.5–58.3%). There were no significant differences between lithium and placebo patients for medical center when the three compliance groups were considered separately.

ADVERSE REACTION COMPARISONS

The next question addressed concerned whether noncompliers and dropouts experienced more adverse reactions than did complier patients. It was hypothesized that adverse reactions cause patients to be noncompliers or dropouts. In this study, the patients were questioned each time that they were seen in the clinic about 25 specific adverse reactions that have been reported for lithium. For 22 of these adverse reactions, significant differences (based on χ^2 tests) were found in the total sample between the three compliance groups for the number of patients reporting the adverse reaction at least once during their tenure in the study. For each of these 22 adverse reactions, there were no significant differences in the number of patients reporting symptoms between the compliant and noncompliant patients. The dropout group had significantly fewer patients reporting the adverse reaction than the compliant patients for 19 of the adverse reactions, significantly fewer than the noncompliers for 17 adverse reactions, and significantly fewer than both the compliers and noncompliers for 14 adverse reactions.

When lithium and placebo patients were compared separately for the 22 adverse

TABLE 26–4. Comparisons of compliance groups for the three adverse reactions having significant lithium effects for the total population of patients

Population	Compliers			Noncompliers			Dropouts			Probability level[a]
	N	Symptom	% Symptom	N	Symptom	% Symptom	N	Symptom	% Symptom	
Diarrhea										
Total	171	76	44.4A	108	37	34.3AB	162	52	32.1B	0.049
Lithium	82	44	53.7	48	19	39.6	88	33	37.5	0.082
Placebo	89	32	36.0	60	18	30.0	74	19	25.7	0.362
Shakiness										
Total	171	69	40.4A	108	52	48.1A	162	37	22.8B	< 0.001
Lithium	82	39	47.6A	48	29	60.4A	88	26	29.5B	0.001
Placebo	89	30	33.7A	60	23	38.3A	74	11	14.9B	0.005
Trouble walking										
Total	171	40	23.4A	108	28	25.9A	162	17	10.5B	0.002
Lithium	82	25	30.5A	48	15	31.3A	88	11	12.5B	0.008
Placebo	89	15	16.9	60	13	21.7	74	6	8.1	0.082

[a]Probability level for compliance group by adverse reaction–no adverse reaction χ^2 test; % with same letter are not significantly different from each other based on Brunden's method of partitioning significance level.

reactions having a significant overall difference between the three compliance groups, the only differences were again between compliant patients and dropouts and between noncompliant patients and dropouts, with dropouts always reporting fewer adverse reactions. For four of these adverse reactions, there were no statistically significant differences between the three compliance groups in the lithium or placebo patients separately; for seven adverse reactions, differences occurred for both lithium and placebo patients; for five adverse reactions, differences occurred in the lithium patients but not the placebo patients; and, for six adverse reactions, differences occurred in the placebo patients but not the lithium patients.

Table 26–4 gives the number of patients reporting diarrhea, shakiness, and trouble walking at least once; these adverse reactions were the only ones for which significant differences between lithium and placebo patients were found for the entire sample of patients. For diarrhea, there was a significant result only for the total sample. Only the complier–dropout comparison is significant, with fewer dropouts reporting diarrhea. For shakiness, significant differences were found for both the lithium and placebo patients, as well as for the total sample. Dropouts had significantly fewer patients reporting shakiness than for either the compliers or the noncompliers. In the case of trouble walking, significant differences were seen only for the total sample and the lithium patients. Dropouts had significantly fewer patients reporting the symptom than either the compliers or the noncompliers.

COMPARISONS OF OUTCOME MEASURES

The third question addressed was whether there were differences between the three compliance groups on the study's four outcome measures: abstinence, average number of days drinking per 4-week period, hospitalization for alcohol-related reasons, and ratings of alcohol abuse at 12, 24, 36, and 52 weeks. Abstinence was defined as no reports of drinking by the patient or his significant other, usually a relative or friend, at any of the 4-week major evaluation periods and no positive breath alcohol tests at any clinic visit. Reports by the patient or his significant other of alcohol-related hospitalizations were also obtained at the 4-week major evaluations. At each of the 4-week evaluations, the patient and his significant other were asked how many days the patient had at least one drink during the past 4 weeks. When discrepancies arose, the larger number of days was used. The mean number of days drinking during all the 4-week periods was used as the outcome measure to account for missing rating periods. The use of these means assumes that patients' drinking patterns during missing rating periods was the same as at those rating periods in which data were actually collected. The final outcome measure was a rating by the patient interviewer, usually a study assistant, which was made after the patient's interview was concluded. The Addiction Severity Index (4) global assessment of alcoholism severity was used to make these ratings. The scores for this rating ranged from 0 (no problem) to 9 (extreme problem requiring immediate attention). Ratings obtained at the 12-, 24-, 36-, and 52-week evaluations were used in the analyses.

For abstinence, statistically significant differences between the three compliance groups were found for the lithium ($p = 0.039$) and placebo ($p = 0.012$) patients separately as well as for all patients combined ($p < 0.001$). The percent patients abstinent for the total sample was 40.4% for the compliers, 18.3% for the noncompliers, and 36.5% for the dropouts, whereas for the lithium patients, these percents were 42.7%,

20.8%, and 37.7%, respectively, and, for the placebo patients, they were 38.2%, 16.4%, and 35.2%, respectively. In each case, the noncompliers did significantly worse than either the compliers or the dropouts, and there were no differences between compliers and dropouts. That there were no differences between compliers and dropouts may be an artifact of the outcome measure. Abstinence was only determined for the time that the patient was in the study. If renewed drinking was the cause of dropping out, this lack of abstinence would not be detected or counted. When lithium and placebo patients were compared within each of the three compliance groups separately, no significant differences were found.

For average days drinking per 4-week period, there were again statistically significant results for all patients combined ($p<0.001$) and for the lithium ($p=0.001$) and placebo ($p=0.005$) patients separately. For the total patient sample, compliers drank fewer average days per 4-week period [2.9 (±5.6) days] than either noncompliers [6.3 (±6.4) days] or dropouts [5.9 (±7.9) days]. The same was true for the lithium patients in whom compliers drank 2.5 (±5.3) days per 4-week period whereas noncompliers and dropouts drank 5.5 (±5.7) and 6.3 (±8.3) days per 4-week period, respectively. For the placebo patients, a similar pattern is seen except that the difference between compliers and dropouts is not quite statistically significant. Here, compliers drank an average 3.3 (±5.9) days per 4-week period whereas noncompliers and dropouts drank 6.9 (±7.0) and 5.4 (±7.5) days per 4-week period, respectively, on average. Once again, there were no differences between lithium and placebo patients within any of the three compliance groups.

For alcohol-related hospitalizations, the only significant difference found was for the placebo patients ($p=0.030$). Noncompliers were more likely to have been hospitalized (38.3% hospitalized) for alcohol-related reasons than were dropouts (19.1%). Except for the placebo noncompliers, the remaining five lithium–placebo compliance groups all had similar rates of hospitalization (19.1–23.7% hospitalized).

For the alcohol abuse rating, differences between the compliance groups were seen only at the 24-week rating for placebo patients only ($p=0.023$) and at 52 weeks for both lithium ($p=0.011$) and placebo patients ($p=0.007$), as well as the combined sample ($p<0.001$). These analyses were performed as analyses of covariance using prescores as covariates. The mean scores below are given as least square means and least square standard errors to account for the effect of the covariate. For the placebo patients at 24 weeks, complier patients had better (lower) scores (2.0 ± 0.3) than noncomplier patients (3.6 ± 0.5). For the 52-week rating, compliers again did better than noncompliers. For the total sample, the compliers had a least square mean of 1.8 (±0.2) in comparison with 3.2 (±0.3) for noncompliers. For the lithium patients, compliers had a mean score of 1.7 (±0.3) to noncompliers mean score of 3.1 (±0.4), whereas for placebo patients, compliers had a mean score of 1.9 (±0.3) and noncompliers had a mean score of 3.4 (±0.4). By definition, there were no dropouts at 52 weeks. When lithium and placebo patients were compared within compliance groups, there were no statistically significant differences.

COMPLIER-ONLY ANALYSES

The final question investigated was whether the use of only compliant patients to report results of the study would have changed our original conclusions based on the total patient sample that lithium was not an effective treatment for alcoholism. To

TABLE 26–5. Comparisons of drug groups on the major outcome measures for all patients while in study and compliant patients only

Outcome measure	Population	Lithium			Placebo			Probability level[a]	Lithium			Placebo			Probability[b]
		N	n	%	N	n	%		N	X̄	SE	N	X̄	SE	
Abstinence	All patients	207	74	35.7	221	69	31.2	0.247							
	Compliers	82	35	42.7	89	34	38.2	0.553							
Alcohol-related hospitalizations	All patients	205	43	21.0	217	56	25.8	0.257							
	Compliers	82	16	19.5	89	20	22.5	0.862							
Days drinking (4 weeks)[c]	All patients								204	4.6	(0.5)	219	5.0	(0.5)	0.496
	Compliers								82	2.4	(0.6)	89	3.3	(0.6)	0.287
Alcohol abuse (24 weeks)[d]	All patients								114	2.5	(0.3)	131	2.4	(0.3)	0.742
	Compliers								77	2.2	(0.4)	83	2.1	(0.3)	0.837
Alcohol abuse (52 weeks)[d]	All patients								123	2.1	(0.3)	147	2.5	(0.3)	0.253
	Compliers								80	1.6	(0.3)	89	2.0	(0.3)	0.310

[a] Probability level of Mantel-Haenszel χ^2-test stratified by medical center.
[b] Probability based on treatment by medical center analysis of variance (average number of days drinking) or analysis of covariance using premedication scores as covariates (alcohol abuse scores).
[c] Adjusted mean scores and SEs are treatment main effect least square means and SEs from a treatment by medical center analysis of variance.
[d] Adjusted mean scores and SEs are treatment main effect least square means and SEs from a treatment by medical center analyses of covariance using premedication scores as covariates.

do this, the same analyses used for the four major outcome variables (i.e., abstinence, alcohol-related hospitalizations, average number of days drinking per 4-week period, and alcohol abuse ratings at 24 and 52 weeks) in the original report (1) were used for compliant patients only. Abstinence and alcohol-related hospitalizations stratified by medical center were analyzed using Mantel-Haenszel χ^2 tests, whereas the mean number of days drinking per 4-week period was analyzed using a two-way (drug treatment by medical center) analysis of variance, and the alcohol abuse ratings were analyzed using a two-way analysis of covariance with prescore as a covariate. These latter results are reported as least square means and least square standard deviations to account for the effects of medical center and the medical center by drug group interaction on the drug group means as well as for the covariate in the analyses of covariance.

Table 26–5 gives the results for these analyses. As can be seen from this table, there are no statistically significant results for either the total population of patients or for the compliant patients only. Thus, the results for the compliant patients indicate the same conclusion as originally reported (i.e., lithium is not an effective treatment for alcoholism). The only difference between the total patient analyses and the compliant patient analyses for each outcome measure was in the estimate of the outcome measure. As expected from the previous section, which showed that compliers had better outcomes than noncompliers and dropouts, the compliant patient analyses reported better outcomes than did the analyses for all patients.

CONCLUSIONS

Based on the results of this study, there are a number of observations about compliant patients that show the potential biases and problems that can occur with an analysis based only on compliant patients.

1. *Compliant patients may be a different population than either noncompliant patients or dropouts.* In this study, compliers were older, more likely to have been married, more likely to have been drinking for more years, and less likely to have had job-related problems caused by drinking. This description suggests that compliant patients are more stable in their life-style and may be better able to resolve their drinking problems. Thus, generalizing results from compliant patients only analyses to the entire population of alcoholic patients is unwarranted. Knowing to whom such results would generalize would be difficult.

2. *Patients compliant on lithium and those compliant on placebo may represent different populations.* In this study, placebo compliers were more likely to have been married and less likely to have had alcohol-related job problems than placebo noncompliers and dropouts in contrast to lithium compliers in whom these differences were not seen. When lithium and placebo compliers were compared, placebo compliers were more likely to be married than lithium compliers. The Coronary Drug Project Group (7) also found differences in baseline characteristics between patients taking their active drug and placebo. This indicates that analyses of compliant patients only may not be analyzing similar patients in their treatment groups and, therefore, could make such analyses invalid.

3. *Compliant patients do not report fewer adverse reactions than noncompliant*

patients or dropouts. Dropouts had fewer reports of adverse reactions than either compliers or noncompliers, and there were no differences between compliers or noncompliers for the number of patients reporting any of the 25 adverse reactions. This was interpreted as indicating that adverse reactions are not related to noncompliance or dropping out. However, it is possible that noncompliers and dropouts are less tolerant of adverse reactions, which causes them to be noncompliant or to drop out. It is also possible that some dropouts are just doing better and having no adverse reactions, which leads them to drop out because they no longer feel in need of treatment. If the latter two cases are true, it would represent another argument for noncompliers and dropouts being a different population than compliers. The differences between dropouts and the compliers and noncompliers could also be due to compliers and noncompliers having been followed for the entire 1 year, with the result that they had a longer opportunity to develop and report adverse reactions.

4. *Patients compliant on lithium and those compliant on placebo do better on outcome measures than noncompliant patients or dropouts.* That the lithium patients who are compliant do better than noncompliers or dropouts would be expected if lithium were an effective treatment. However, similar results were seen for the placebo patients for whom a treatment effect is not expected. This is additional evidence that compliant patients are different than noncompliant patients and dropouts. This conclusion supports the Coronary Drug Project Group (7) in which similar results were reported in their study, and the same conclusion was reached.

5. *The use of compliant patients only would not have altered the conclusions of this particular study.* This is not unexpected because the group of compliant patients is smaller than either the total sample or the completers, and, therefore, there is less statistical power in the analyses. However, this outcome may not always be the case, and when compliant patients' results and the total sample results differ, the results may be misleading. For example, Baekeland and Lundwall (8) in an alcoholism study of oxazepamprotriptyline versus placebo found a significant difference in their compliant-patient-only analysis but not their total sample. Review of their data indicated that the noncompliant placebo patients they excluded did far better than either the compliant placebo patients or even the compliant drug patients, whereas the noncompliant drug patients they excluded did far worse than the compliant drug patients and the compliant placebo patients. Thus, the patients excluded were not the same for each treatment group, a situation that calls to question the validity of the conclusions.

Our results indicate that caution should be used when using or reviewing study results based only on compliant patients. Demographic characteristics and reports of adverse reactions can be different in the group of compliant patients compared with either noncompliant or dropout groups, and these differences may vary by treatment group. Analyses based only on compliant patients may either be inconsequential because of decreased statistical power or invalid because of biased patient selection. Clinicians should, therefore, base their clinical decisions primarily on the results of intention-to-treat analyses in clinical trials and not on conclusions based *only* on compliant patient analyses. Additional analyses or subgroup analyses may be added to support or extend intention to treat results, but these should never replace them. Additional research needs to be done to determine why patients comply to treatment and what characteristics define these patients.

ACKNOWLEDGMENTS

This study was supported by the Cooperative Studies Program of the Department of Veterans Affairs, Veterans Health Services and Research Administration. Lithium carbonate and placebo were donated by CIBA-Geigy Corporation, Summit, New Jersey.

Participating investigators for the study were Raymond Anton, M.D., Charleston, South Carolina, DVA Medical Center; Paul Cushman, M.D., Richmond DVA Medical Center; H.L. Charles, M.D., Dallas DVA Medical Center; Pradip Desai, M.D., DVA Edward Hines Jr. Hospital; Usha Malkerneker, M.D., DVA Edward Hines Jr. Hospital; Young Nam Park, M.D. (past investigator), DVA Edward Hines Jr. Hospital; Motoi Hayashida, M.D., Philadelphia DVA Medical Center; Mark Willenbring, M.D., Minneapolis DVA Medical Center; Robert Fiscella, M.D., Baltimore DVA Medical Center; and Frank L. Iber, M.D. (past investigator), Baltimore DVA Medical Center. The participating investigator at the central laboratory was David G. Ostrow, M.D., Ph.D., Ann Arbor DVA Medical Center. Mike R. Sather, R.Ph., M.S., and Cindy Colling, R.Ph., M.S., of the Cooperative Studies Program Clinical Research Pharmacy Coordinating Center, Albuquerque, New Mexico, DVA Medical Center provided pharmacy support. The project director in the chairman's (Dr. Dorus) office was Melodie Schaefer, M.S. Programming and data management support at the Perry Point, Maryland, Cooperative Studies Program Coordinating Center was provided by Debra Davis, George Medairy, Dorothy Morson, and Hong-Jen Yu, M.S. DVA Central Office administrative support was provided by Ping Huang, Ph.D., and James A. Hagans, M.D.

REFERENCES

1. Dorus W, Ostrow DG, Anton R, et al. Lithium treatment of depressed and nondepressed alcoholics. *JAMA* 1989;262:1646–1652.
2. Fawcett J, Clark DC, Aagesen DO, et al. A double-blind, placebo-controlled trial of lithium carbonate therapy for alcoholism. *Arch Gen Psychiatry* 1987;44:248–256.
3. *Diagnostic and Statistical Manual of Mental Disorders,* 3rd ed. Washington, DC: The American Psychiatric Association, 1980.
4. *Guide to the Addiction Severity Index: Background, Administration, and Field Testing Results.* Rockville, MD: National Institute on Drug Abuse, 1985.
5. Beck AT, Ward CH, Mendelson M, Mock J, Erbauch J. An inventory for measuring depression. *Arch Gen Psychiatry* 1961;4:561–571.
6. Brunden MN. The analysis of non-independent 2×2 tables using rank sums. *Biometrics* 1972;28:603–607.
7. Coronary Drug Project Research Group. Influence of adherence to treatment and response of cholesterol on mortality in Coronary Drug Project. *N Engl J Med* 1980;303:1038–1041.
8. Baekeland F, Lundwall LK. Effects of discontinuity of medication on the results of a double-blind drug study in outpatient alcoholics. *J Stud Alcohol* 1975;36:1268–1272.

Patient Compliance in Medical
Practice and Clinical Trials
edited by J.A. Cramer and B. Spilker
Raven Press, Ltd., New York © 1991

27

Variability of Antiepileptic Medication Concentrations and Compliance

Ilo E. Leppik

University of Minnesota, and Minnesota Comprehensive Epilepsy Program,
Minneapolis, Minnesota 55416

During the treatment of epilepsy, it is extremely important to maintain stable concentrations of antiepileptic medication at the active receptor site. Unlike many other conditions (e.g., treatment of pain or infections) in which intermittent attainment of analgesic or bacteriocidal concentrations is acceptable, control of epilepsy is best-achieved with as little variation as possible of medication concentrations during the course of treatment. This arises from two factors. Epilepsy is an active process, requiring constant modulation of excitatory and inhibitory processes. A patient with epilepsy has a population of hyperexcitable neurons, which may, at any time, develop into a clinical seizure. Also, the range between effective and toxic concentrations is narrow for all antiepileptic medications. The therapeutic range for most medications is narrow, with only a two- or threefold difference between the lowest effective concentration and toxic levels. For example, the usually quoted therapeutic range for phenytoin is 10 to 20 μg/ml; for carbamazepine it is 4 to 12 μg/ml; and valproate 50 to 100 μg/ml. Although some patients can tolerate concentrations somewhat higher than these, the ranges are still much narrower than for most other classes of compounds. One of the most common precipitants of a seizure is a lowering of medication concentrations. This may occur because of missed medications (1) or be associated with an illness in which metabolism increases, causing a drop in levels (2). Thus, the issue of variability of drug concentrations in the treatment of epilepsy is critical, and although some variability in medication levels can be expected from pharmacokinetic factors, compliance is the major determinant of whether stable antiepileptic medication concentrations are maintained.

As many as one-third to one-half of patients with epilepsy are noncompliant to a degree that interferes with optimal treatment (3–9). Noncompliant behavior may significantly increase health care costs at many levels. A poorly compliant patient may increase medical costs directly by having an increase in the number of seizures, resulting in ambulance rides, emergency room visits, and hospitalizations. In addition, this patient may suffer direct physical injury as a result of seizures. Also, social and economic costs may result from the adverse consequences of having seizures while at work or in social settings. Patients whose seizures are poorly controlled because of noncompliance may injure others (e.g., a woman with epilepsy who is poorly compliant during her pregnancy, causing injury to the unborn child as a consequence of her seizures).

Compliance can be measured in many ways. The most commonly used direct measurement of compliant behavior is measurement of antiepileptic medication levels. Many studies have used this measure and describe patients who are in the "therapeutic range" as being compliant and those whose levels fall outside this range as being noncompliant. Indirect measurements of compliance rely on patient interviews (10–13). Measures of physician assessment (14) or outcome of therapy may be inaccurate or biased (11). Two clinically useful and relatively easy to apply methods are the absolute measurement of medication concentrations and an open patient interview regarding compliant behavior (3,15).

Compliance is not necessarily stable and may change over time. The type of noncompliant behavior in which medication ingestion is irregular creates the possibility of measuring compliant behavior through serial blood level determinations. Thus, fluctuations of medication concentrations during constant prescribed dose conditions may reflect noncompliance with the prescribed regimens.

DIMENSIONS OF COMPLIANCE

Compliance has usually been treated as an either/or situation (16). This simplistic approach does not reflect reality. The view that divides the population into patients who are compliant and those that are not ignores the fact that an all-inclusive "noncompliance category" makes noncompliant behavior difficult to describe. In reality, compliance is a multidimensional attribute that can be classified by three dimensions: type of behavior, extent of compliance, and degree of intentionality (Table 27–1).

The first dimension is *behavior* (Table 27–1). The most readily identified, and usually of the most concern to clinicians, is compliance with medication ingestion. A patient can be consistently overcompliant or consistently undercompliant. Three patterns of irregularity exist: Irregular ingestion patterns can be present at all times, or a patient can be sporadically irregular or cyclically irregular.

An area of behavior less well-studied but important is that of compliance with prescribed life-style. There are many habits that may precipitate seizures. These include irregular sleep patterns, alcohol abuse, exposure to psychological stress, or exposure to light for patients who are photosensitive.

The second dimension, *intentionality,* can be described as patient-controlled or structural (Table 27–1). Patient control can be rational or irrational. Rational noncompliance usually arises from a well-defined, logical, and consistent belief system (e.g., a woman who may decide not to comply with antiepileptic drug treatment because of fear of injury to the fetus). Although the accuracy of the risk–benefit calculation might be questioned, the decision is based on a logical process. An example of an irrational belief system is one in which the patient believes that seizures are caused by phases of the moon, and thus medications are not needed during some of the lunar phases. Structural reasons for noncompliance are outside of a patient's control. For example, a patient with epilepsy after head trauma that damaged the temporal lobes would have memory dysfunction, making it difficult to remember to take medications.

The third dimension of compliance, that of *extent,* must be viewed as a continuum of behavior. Extent of compliance ranges from that rare patient who takes every prescribed dose precisely as directed to those who never comply. Most patients have behaviors that are between these extremes.

TABLE 27–1. *Dimensions of compliance*

Behavior
  Medical
    Medication ingestion
      Consistent overcomplier
      Consistent undercomplier
      Irregular
        irregularly irregular
        sporadically irregular
        cyclically irregular
    Prescription filling
    Medical appointments
  Life-style
    Sleep patterns
    Alcohol use
    Psychological stress
    Exposure to music, strobe lights
    Drug abuse
    Adhering to regulations
Intentionality
  Patient controlled
    Completely rational
      Pregnant women afraid of teratogenicity
      Compensation related
    Irrational
      Fear of medicine; superstitious
  Structural
    Memory deficit
    Financial problems
Degree
  Complete compliance
  Compliant some of the time
  Never compliant

METHODS OF MEASUREMENT

The calculation of the coefficient of variation can describe the degree of fluctuation of medication concentrations over time. The coefficient of variation is calculated by using Equation 1.

$$\text{Coefficient of variation } (\%) = \frac{\text{Standard deviation}}{X} \times 100$$

where X = number of plasma concentration measurements.

Much of the variability in antiepileptic medication concentrations not accounted for by small fluctuations caused by pharmacokinetic factors can be attributable to noncompliance (17). In the remainder of this chapter, data from studies involving antiepileptic medicines will be reviewed to explore the amount of variability that can be expected from four major sources: laboratory variability, pharmacokinetic factors, timing of sampling related to dose, and patient compliance.

A number of devices exist today for the measurement of antiepileptic medication concentrations in plasma, serum, saliva, and other biological samples. These include gas liquid chromatography introduced in the late 1960s (18). This method is generally accurate with coefficients of variation of less than 5% for standard antiepileptic medications (18). High-performance liquid chromatography is often used in laboratory settings, and its accuracy is the same as gas liquid chromatography (19). These methods have the advantage of being able to measure a number of the commonly used antiepileptic medicines simultaneously. Also, by inspection of the chromatographic tracing, errors of assay performance can often be detected. Both of the chromatographic techniques, however, require highly skilled personnel along with laboratory support systems and thus have not gained widespread use in the clinical settings. In the clinical setting, methods that rely on immunoassays have gained widespread acceptance. These include the Syva EMIT, Abbott TDx, Ames Seralyzer, and Syntex Acculevel systems. A number of studies comparing the accuracy of these techniques of analyzing antiepileptic medicines have been published (20–24). These studies generally report only small differences in accuracy between these methods. For a device to be approved by the Food and Drug Administration for therapeutic drug monitoring, it must be able to perform with a coefficient of variance of less than 5%. Although all these devices perform to these standards under strict testing conditions, the potential for error in clinical settings has been a major problem (25). Laboratory standards have improved, and thus today it is reasonable to assume that less than 5% of the variability in serial antiepileptic drug determinations can be ascribed to measurement error if testing is done by a certified laboratory.

A number of pharmacokinetic factors can influence the absorption and elimination of antiepileptic medications. Changes in product formulation may markedly alter the absorption, especially of phenytoin, to the degree that toxicity can occur (26). In the situation of permissible or mandated generic substitution, product formulation changes may play a larger role in creating variability of medication concentrations than was the case in the past. Alteration of gastric or intestinal absorption related to food or other medicines may influence the time of extent of absorption (27). Changes in hepatic blood flow or renal blood flow may modify the rate of clearance and influence the concentrations of medications to a small degree (28).

Sampling time may contribute to variability. Phenytoin has a relatively long absorption time (T_{max} of 6–10 hr) because of its absorption in the small intestine. Its elimination half-life ranges from 18 to 36 hr because of its nonlinear kinetics. Times between peak and trough concentrations are thus in the order of 24 to 46 hr, and with more than once-a-day dosing, the variability of peak and trough levels is small. Carbamazepine and valproate both have shorter absorption times and, during chronic therapy, elimination half-lives of 6 to 14 hr. Timing of sample to dose may be more important for these medications to reduce fluctuations.

PATIENT STUDIES

The variability of antiepileptic medication concentrations over time has been determined in various settings. In all these studies, three or more samples were obtained while the patient was prescribed the same dose. Laboratories of the University of Minnesota or St. Paul Ramsey Medical Center were used. The first series of studies involved phenytoin (17). A total of 174 "steady-state" conditions from 74 patients were analyzed. These patients had been prescribed the same dose for periods long enough to meet the definition of steady state. They came from three samples (Fig. 27–1). The supervised patients were residing in a complete-care facility, and their medications were given by attendants. Meals and activities were regulated. Coefficients of variance for these patients all were 10% or less. A second group in this study consisted of clinic patients at St. Paul Ramsey Medical Center, who had

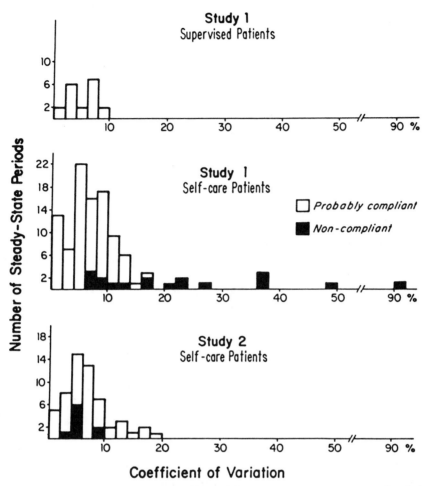

FIG. 27–1. Coefficient of variation as a measure of extent of noncompliance. Coefficient of variation was greater than 20% in all noncompliant patients. Some patients with coefficient of variations of less than 20% reported missing only occasional doses a few days before sampling, reflecting only minor deviations from absolute compliance. Thus, coefficient of variation may be used as a measure of the extent of noncompliance, and all persons with coefficient of variations of less than 20%, even if noncompliant, have an extent of noncompliance that is not clinically significant. (From ref. 17, with permission.)

three or more serial phenytoin concentrations obtained during the course of clinical treatment and were then interviewed to determine extent of compliance. In these patients, blood drawings were done within 1 hr of each other to minimize fluctuations induced by differences in relation of sampling to dosing. The last group was patients who had participated in a bioavailability study. Coefficients of variation of less than 20% were associated with compliant behavior. Some patients with coefficients of variation of less than 20% who reported noncompliance usually had minimal deviation from prescribed dosing, usually one missed dose a few days before sampling. Thus, for phenytoin, a coefficient of variation of less than 20% is indicative of clinically acceptable compliant behavior. Furthermore, the extent of noncompliance can be inferred from the magnitude of the coefficient of variation.

The second series consisted of patients who had participated in carefully controlled clinical trials of two experimental medications, progabide and felbamate (29). Compliance was enhanced by removing many of the barriers that lead to noncompliance. The primary method used to foster absolute compliance was the packaging of all medicines (phenytoin, carbamazepine, and study medicine) in a single "unit-of-use" container, which patients were required to return at each clinic visit. As close to complete compliance as can be expected in an outpatient setting was attained. The database of phenytoin and carbamazepine serum concentrations generated by these studies was evaluated to determine the variability in concentrations of these medicines that can be expected under ideal conditions.

Data from 58 patients were evaluated, 32 from progabide and 26 from felbamate. A randomized, double-blind, cross-over, placebo-controlled design was used. Patients were seen in the clinic every 2 weeks throughout the entire study for evaluation of seizure control, adverse reactions, and determination of serum antiepileptic drug concentrations. The time between dose and blood collection was held as constant as possible for each patient throughout the study and ranged from 1 to 4 hr among all patients.

The range of coefficients of variation for phenytoin was 4.3 to 28% during felbamate and 4.5 to 42% during progabide (Fig. 27–2). Mean coefficients of variation did not vary significantly among baseline placebo treatment periods. During both studies, 83% of coefficients of variation were less than 20%. The range of coefficients of variation during felbamate was 4.7 to 36.1% and during progabide 3.5 to 42% (Fig. 27–2). Mean coefficients of variation did not vary significantly among baseline or placebo treatment periods. During both studies, 69% of all coefficients of variation were less than 20%.

The third series involved a review of the computerized patient database (30). During 5 years, data regarding antiepileptic drug doses, concentrations, seizure types and frequency, and other information obtained from patients at the Comprehensive Epilepsy Program's clinic were entered into the CLINFO database system. During each visit the physician or nurse clinician filled out a data gathering sheet. Blood samples for antiepileptic medication concentrations were obtained. An attempt was made to have stable clinic appointment times for each patient to decrease variability from fluctuations due to peak and trough sampling. The database was searched to identify all patients receiving phenytoin, carbamazepine, and/or valproate. Then all patients who had three or more clinic visits with no change in dose were identified. To simplify the analysis, each medicine was evaluated without considering other medications. Many of the patients were on more than one medication because of the severity of their seizures. The intervals between the visits ranged from a few weeks to many months.

The database included information from 793 outpatients. Ages ranged from 1.7 years to 85.7, with a mean age of 32 years. The vast majority of patients were between 18 and 65. A total of 579 patients had three or more visits with no dose changes for at least one of the antiepileptic medicines. A total of 283 coefficients of variation from 192 patients (97 male, 95 female) was available for phenytoin. There were more coefficients of variation than patients because some patients were included more than once because each three-visits-or-more block after a dose change had been made was included. Figure 27–3 contains a histogram of the frequency distribution for phenytoin. Approximately 34% of the serial visits had a coefficient of variation of less than 20%, and 52% had a coefficient of variation less than 26%. The mode coefficient of variation was 25.2%. For carbamazepine, 290 coefficients of variation

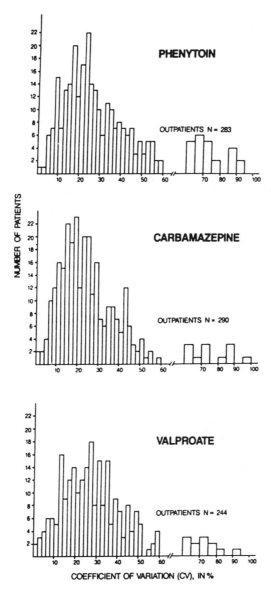

FIG. 27–2. Coefficient of variation values from patients participating in studies of felbamate (FBM) and progabide (PGB). (From ref. 29, with permission.)

from 206 patients (92 male, 89 female) were available. Thirty percent of the coefficients of variation were less than 20%, and 61% had a coefficient of variation of less than 26%. The mode coefficient of variation was 23.2% (Fig. 27–3). For valproate, 244 visits from 181 patients (92 male, 89 female) were analyzed. Thrity-one percent of the visits had a coefficient of variation of less than 20%, and 46% had a value of less than 26%. The mode coefficient of variation was 27.1% (Fig. 27–3). This last series had, in addition to compliance, the variables of sample timing and drug interactions. However, it is representative of the variability that can be expected in an epilepsy clinic setting.

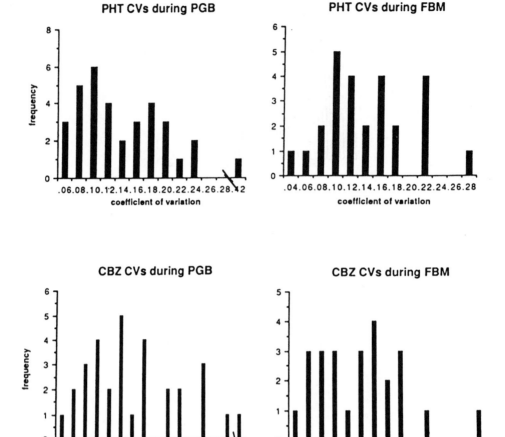

FIG. 27–3. Coefficient of variation values from an epilepsy clinic using three measurements. Time of sampling and changes in doses of other medication were not controlled. (From ref. 30, with permission.)

COMMENT

It is apparent from the data presented in this chapter that the greatest source of variability in antiepileptic medication concentrations is caused by noncompliance. In patient populations in which compliance is strictly monitored and enforced and time of sampling is strictly adhered to, variability can be expected to be small, with coefficients of variation of less than 20% for most patients receiving phenytoin and 25% for patients receiving carbamazepine and valproate. The larger values for carbamazepine and valproate are likely related to the fact that these two medications have shorter half-lives and larger fluctuations between peak and trough concentrations than is the case for phenytoin. Data presented here define the biological variability that may be expected in patients receiving antiepileptic medicines and who are compliant. Designs for antiepileptic medication trials should recognize the attainable limits for allowable fluctuations in phenytoin and carbamazepine concentrations, and enforcement of compliance can increase the statistical power of these studies (31). In clinical settings, careful monitoring of blood levels to bring concentrations into the effective ranges and maintaining compliance can reduce seizure frequency.

Measuring serial concentrations of medicines used to treat disorders other than epilepsy may be helpful in determining compliance. The coefficient of variation would be most meaningful for medicines with long half-lives (12–24 hr or more). Antipsychotic medication compliance could be evaluated by this means. However, using coefficients of variation for medications with half-lives of less than 6 to 8 hr could be misleading. Using the coefficient of variation will give a measurement of compliance over time, but it is not sensitive to abrupt, short-term noncompliance, which may occur more than a week or two before sampling. In this situation, the decrease in blood concentration would go undetected if a patient resumed medication five to six half-lives before sampling. Under these circumstances, steady-state concentrations would have been reestablished by sampling time. Thus, the usefulness of the coefficient of variation approach is dependent on the pharmacokinetic properties of the medicine being evaluated and the interval between samplings.

ACKNOWLEDGMENTS

This work was supported by the National Institute of Neurological and Communicative Disorders and Stroke (P50 NS1-16308). Word processing by Diane Rider is gratefully acknowledged.

REFERENCES

1. Stanaway L, Lambie DG, Johnson RH. Noncompliance with anticonvulsant therapy as a cause for seizures. *NZ Med* 1985;98:150–152.
2. Leppik IE, Ramani V, Sawchuk RJ, Gumnit RJ. Increased clearance of phenytoin during infectious mononucleosis. *N Engl J Med* 1979;300:481–482.
3. Leppik IE, Schmidt D, eds. Summary of the First International Workshop on Compliance in Epilepsy. *Epilepsy Res* 1988;S1:179–182.
4. Mucklow JC, Dollery CT. Compliance with anticonvulsant therapy in a hospital clinic and in the community. *Br J Clin Pharmacol* 1978;6:75–79.
5. Shope J. Intervention to improve compliance with pediatric anticonvulsant therapy. *Patient Counsel Health Educ* 1980;21:135–141.
6. Wannamaker BB, Morton WA Jr, Gross AJ, Saunders S. Improvement in antiepileptic drug levels following reduction of intervals between clinic visits. *Epilepsia* 1980;21:155–162.
7. Peterson GM, McLean S, Millingen KS. A randomized trial of strategies to improve patient compliance with anticonvulsant therapy. *Epilepsia* 1984;25:412–417.
8. Takaki S, Kurokawa T, Aoyama T. Monitoring drug noncompliance in epileptic patients: assessing phenobarbital plasma levels. *Ther Drug Monit* 1985;7:87–91.
9. Driessen O, Hoppener R. Plasma levels of phenobarbital and phenytoin in epileptic outpatients. *Eur Neurol* 1977;15:135–142.
10. Francis V, Korsch BM, Morris MJ. Gaps in doctor–patient communication: patients' response to medical advice. *N Engl J Med* 1969;280:535–540.
11. Gordis L. Methodological issues in the measurement of patient compliance. In: Sackett DL, Haynes RD, eds. *Compliance with therapeutic regimens*. Baltimore: University Press, 1976;51–66.
12. Park KC, Lipman RS. A comparison of patient dosage deviation reports with pill counts. *Psychopharmacology* 1964;6:299–302.
13. Sackett DL. The magnitude of compliance and noncompliance. In: Sackett DL, Haynes RB, eds. *Compliance with therapeutic regimens*. Baltimore: University Press, 1976;9–25.
14. Mushlin AI, Appel FA. Diagnosing potential noncompliance. Physicians' ability in a behavioral dimension of medical care. *Arch Intern Med* 1977;137:318–321.

15. Trostle J. Doctors' orders and patients' self-interest: two views of medication usage? *Epilepsy Res* 1988;S1:57–69.
16. Green LW, Simons-Morton D. Denial, delay and disappointment: discovering and overcoming the causes of drug errors and missed appointments. *Epilepsy Res* 1988;S1:7–22.
17. Leppik IE, Cloyd JC, Sawchuk RJ, Pepin SM. Compliance and variability of plasma phenytoin levels in epileptic patients. *Ther Drug Monit* 1979;1:475–483.
18. Kupferberg HF. Quantitative estimation of diphenylhydantoin, primidone, and phenobarbital in plasma by gas-liquid chromatography. *Clin Chim Acta* 1970;29:282–288.
19. Wad N. Simultaneous determination of 11 antiepileptic compounds in serum by high-performance liquid chromatography. *J Chromatogr* 1984;305:127–133.
20. Wilson JF, Tsanaclis LM, Williams J, Tedstone JE, Richens A. Evaluation of assay techniques for the measurement of antiepileptic drugs in serum: a study based on external quality assurance measurements. *Ther Drug Monit* 1989;11:185–195.
21. Leppik IE, Oles KS, Sheehan ML, et al. Phenytoin and phenobarbital concentrations in serum: a comparison of Ames Seralyzer with GLC, TDX, and EMIT. *Ther Drug Monit* 1989;11:73–78.
22. McGovern EM, MacRobbie A, Thomson AH, Whiting B. Evaluation of a new Seralyzer assay for carbamazepine. *Ther Drug Monit* 1988;10:355–358.
23. Brettfeld C, Gobrogge R, Massoud N, Munzenberger P, Migro M, Sarnaik A. Evaluation of Ames Seralyzer for the therapeutic drug monitoring of phenobarbital and phenytoin. *Ther Drug Monit* 1989;11:612–615.
24. Graves NM, Holmes GB, Leppik IE, Gallagher TK, Parker DR. Quantitative determination of phenytoin and phenobarbital in capillary blood by Ames Seralyzer. *Epilepsia* 1987;28:713–716.
25. Pippenger CE, Penry JK, White BG, et al. Interlaboratory variability in determination of plasma antiepileptic drug concentrations. *Arch Neurol* 1976;33:351–355.
26. Tyrer JH, Eadie MJ, Sutherland JM, Hooper WD. Outbreak of anticonvulsant intoxication in an Australian city. *Br Med J* 1970;4:271–273.
27. Levy RH, Unadkat JD. General principles: drug absorption, distribution and elimination. In: Levy RH, et al., eds. *Antiepileptic drugs,* 3rd ed. New York: Raven Press, 1989;1–22.
28. Dosing M. Effect of acute and chronic exercise on hepatic drug metabolism. *Clin Pharmacokinet* 1985;10:426–431.
29. Graves NM, Holmes GB, Leppik IE. Compliant populations: variability in serum concentrations. *Epilepsy Res* 1988;S1:91–99.
30. Leppik IE. Variability of phenytoin, carbamazepine and valproate concentrations in a clinic population. *Epilepsy Res* 1988;S1:85–90.
31. Pledger GW. Compliance in clinical trials: impact on design, analysis and interpretation. *Epilepsy Res* 1988;S1:125–134.

Patient Compliance in Medical
Practice and Clinical Trials
edited by J.A. Cramer and B. Spilker
Raven Press, Ltd., New York © 1991

28

Intent-to-Treat Policy for Analyzing Randomized Trials

Statistical Distortions and Neglected Clinical Challenges

Alvan R. Feinstein

*Clinical Epidemiology Unit, Yale University School of Medicine, New Haven,
Connecticut 06510; and Cooperative Studies Program Coordinating Center, Veterans
Administration Medical Center, West Haven, Connecticut 06516*

When the medical community began to accept the idea of evaluating therapy with randomized trials, the design of the trials became a prime challenge in biostatistical creativity. After the trials came into common usage, however, events that occurred after randomization created a new set of challenges in the analysis of results. This symposium is concerned with the challenges that arise from patients' noncompliance or partial compliance with the planned protocol. This chapter will discuss three sets of problems: those that randomization was intended to solve, those produced by less-than-full compliance, and those created by the intent-to-treat analysis that has been proposed as a solution for problems in compliance.

When randomization was introduced to assign the treatments compared in clinical trials, investigators thought they had solved the basic statistical challenges of evaluating therapy. Randomization would eliminate the susceptibility bias with which treatments were often assigned in ordinary clinical practice and would allow the results to be analyzed with stochastic principles of probability.

Unfortunately, clinical therapy is not as simple as the agricultural treatments for which randomization had been developed so successfully. As randomized trials were applied to diverse clinical situations, the investigators soon discovered many other sources of problems. One prominent problem was in the generalization of results. The admission criteria used to improve efficiency within the trial often led to a limited spectrum of investigated patients, whose results might not be pertinent for the larger spectrum of the outside world. Another problem arose from distinctions in therapy itself. The fixed dosage schedule of the new active agent or the particular agent used as the comparison treatment might be satisfactory for the trial but might not answer clinical questions thereafter about flexible dosage schedules or comparisons with other treatments. A third problem that could not be managed merely with randomization was the evaluation of outcome events. Unless double-blind or other objective procedures were used, the outcomes might be affected by detection bias.

Although these problems could be prevented or reduced with suitable adaptations in designing a trial, a more striking set of problems became apparent in analyzing the results for the complexity of patients, treatments, and clinical events in a completed trial.

COUNTING AND ATTRIBUTING EVENTS

Some of the analytic problems can be cited under the title of "counting and attributing events" (1).

Problems in Counting

Problems in deciding what to count arise because most trials are aimed at determining the effect of treatment on a "responsive event" such as the recurrent myocardial infarction that is to be prevented by therapy with beta blockers or anticoagulants. If a responsive event occurs with the wrong timing—before or after the assigned treatment has had a chance to act—should its occurrence be counted among the events associated with the treatment?

What about an "unresponsive" or "inappropriate" event such as the unanticipated development of a cancer, cataract, or death from an apparently unrelated cause? Should these entities be included or excluded when the total events are counted? What should be done about precluding events such as an automobile accident that kills a patient early in the trial before any responsive events have had a chance to occur? Should this person be included in a count of those who have had no responsive events?

Problems in Attributing

Another fundamental problem arises because the randomly assigned treatments are not always properly maintained. If a treatment was assigned but never taken, should it be blamed or credited for subsequent events? What should get the blame or credit if the assigned treatment was taken in an improper manner, or supplemented with other potentially active agents, or completely replaced either by some other agent or by the "rival" agent under comparison in the trial?

The Intent-to-Treat Principle

Regardless of the decisions about what events to count, the principle called *intent-to-treat analysis* has been offered as the statistical answer to questions of attribution (i.e., which treatment to credit or blame for the events). All counted events would be attributed to the originally assigned treatment and analyzed as though the intended treatment had been given in the intended manner, regardless of what had actually happened. Behind this principle is the idea that randomization itself produces an unbiased distribution of the patients before treatment begins and that any changes in treatment thereafter may be affected by unrecognized sources of bias. To avoid those biases, and with the hope that they occur randomly for each of the compared treatments, the results would be analyzed according to the randomized groups of treatment to which the patients were originally assigned.

Although a simple solution is always appealing for a complex problem, the intent-to-treat analysis has brought many scientific and clinical distresses in exchange for its statistical comforts. The distresses arise because the intent-to-treat proposal is too simple for the diverse ways in which treatment can be used and in which plans for treatment can be violated. This chapter will classify the different types of violation, consider their different impacts on the results of a trial, and discuss what can be lost or gained by analyzing the violations.

COMPONENTS, GOALS, AND PROFICIENCY OF TREATMENT

One obvious major problem in evaluating therapy is deciding what to regard as treatment. Each treatment has different components, goals, and proficiency that will be affected differently if the therapeutic plan is violated.

Components

Almost every mode of therapy can be divided into at least two components: a specified agent and an inherent accompaniment. An oral pharmaceutical substance contains an active chemical and many excipients. The treatment of diabetes mellitus, hypertension, or hyperlipidemia may involve an active pharmaceutical agent as well as a particular diet. Treatment with oxygen involves the oxygen itself and a suitable delivery system. Surgical operations require anesthesia and postoperative care as well as the operation itself, which is a combination of anatomic maneuvers and the tactical skill of the surgeon.

The combination of agent and accompaniment constitutes a regimen, but most analyses of "treatment" usually consider only the agent, not the rest of the regimen. Thus, when a particular event is attributed to a "treatment," how carefully should the specified agent be separated from the inherent accompaniment? Are the results of a radical operation by Surgeon A better than those of a simple operation by Surgeon B because the operation itself is superior, because Surgeon A is a better technical operator, or because of differences in the anesthetic and postoperative facilities at the institution where the radical operation is done?

This type of problem is particularly difficult to manage, even if the assigned therapeutic regimen is perfectly maintained. The problem has led to difficulties in evaluating new surgical procedures (if the surgeons were still in the "learning phase" and not suitably experienced), in appraising the effects of new pharmaceutical agents (if the best dosage schedule had not yet been identified), and in testing different schools of psychotherapy (if the other professional skills of the practicing therapist were more important than the Freudian, Jungian, or other "school" used as principles for the practice).

Goals and Duration of Treatment

A separate problem in evaluation is produced by the different goals and durations of treatment. These differences will affect the types of events to be counted and the length of the observation period that permits intervening phenomena to occur and complicate the analyses.

Remedial treatment (i.e., the classical form of clinical therapy) is aimed at a manifestation that exists when the treatment begins. As the main goal of treatment, the relief or cure of this manifestation is the principal target to be observed, measured, and "counted." The course of treatment is usually short, as with analgesics for headache or muscular strain or with antibiotics for respiratory or urinary tract infections. The efficacy of most pharmaceutical agents has usually been demonstrated with relatively short courses of remedial therapy. Remedial treatment, however, can sometimes have a long course when oral iron therapy is given for anemia, nonsteroidal anti-inflammatory drugs for arthritic pain or dysfunction, caloric restriction for weight reduction, or repeated dialyses for uremia.

Prophylactic treatment of individual patients has become a prominent tactic in modern medicine. The treatment is intended to prevent a target that is not yet present. A classical example of such "primary-prevention" treatment is vaccination against poliomyelitis or the use of antimalarial prophylaxis for persons entering a region of high exposure.

Prophylactic treatment, however, can also be aimed at preventing a subsequent target by giving remedial therapy to an existing target. This type of double-targeted treatment has become frequently used in clinical practice and often tested in randomized trials. The first (remedial) target might be to remove or shrink an existing cancer; to bypass an occluded coronary artery; to lower elevated blood pressure, sugar, or lipids; to alter existing mechanisms of bleeding or clotting. The subsequent (prophylactic) target, measured as the main outcome event, is to prevent or retard the occurrence of death, metastasis, recurrent myocardial infarction, or diverse vascular complications.

In these situations, the successful prevention of the main second target depends on how well (or proficiently) the first target has been achieved or regulated (2). Because both phenomena occur after randomization but because proficiency itself is not randomized, inevitable problems will occur in evaluating the results. The main second target cannot be adequately appraised without considering the proficient remedial effect on the first target, but the achievement of proficiency may involve biases that were not eliminated by the randomization.

Prophylactic therapy is usually classified according to its main goal in relation to the baseline state of the patient. Thus, primary prevention is aimed at avoiding the inception of a disease such as poliomyelitis or stroke in someone who has not yet manifested that disease. Secondary prophylaxis is aimed at preventing adverse progression of an established disease (e.g., cancer, diabetes mellitus, myocardial infarction, or transient cerebrovascular ischemic attacks). A third form of prophylaxis, which might be called *interposed* or *antiepisodic,* is aimed at preventing recurrences of episodic phenomena such as seizures, asthma attacks, or severe dysmenorrhea.

Prophylactic treatment can also be classified as *single-targeted* or *double-targeted.* In single-targeted prophylaxis, the only target is prevention of the main outcome event. The treatment is given in a standard manner, without specific measurement of an intervening target. This type of prophylaxis occurs with vaccination against poliomyelitis, antimalarial drug regimens, or daily aspirin therapy to prevent vascular complications. The single-targeted treatment is given without specific efforts to measure its proficiency in changing antibodies, achieving specified blood levels, or altering hematologic variables.

In double-targeted prophylaxis, the prime goal is still to prevent the main outcome event, but it is a subsequent target. The treatment is more directly aimed at an existing first target, which is measured for a response that is often used to regulate the treatment. With this approach, a blood level of the medicine itself may be the target that guides the appropriate dosage of lithium or anticonvulsant agents. A different type of blood level (i.e., for targets such as prothrombin time or values of sugar, lipids, or pressure) will guide the appropriate dosage of anticoagulants or hypoglycemic, hypotensive, or hypolipidemic agents. The first target may sometimes be measured in an anatomic structure rather than in a blood level. Thus, radiotherapy or chemotherapy may be curtailed or extended according to the response of the tumor mass; a surgical procedure may be repeated if adequate patency is not found postoperatively in the affected vessel.

For double-targeted prophylaxis, the evaluation of efficacy is a particularly tricky problem because it involves two appraisals: the proficiency with which the first target was regulated, and the occurrence or nonoccurrence of the subsequent target. For example, we might determine the occurrence of diabetic vascular complications in relation to the degree of control with which normal blood sugar was maintained.

A course of primary prophylactic therapy can be short or long. Examples of short courses are vaccination or antibiotics to eradicate streptococcal infections for the goal of preventing rheumatic fever. Long courses are used in lowering elevated blood pressures or lipids to prevent cardiovascular disease. Secondary and interposed prophylaxis usually consist of a long, continuous course of treatment, particularly when antiplatelet, hypoglycemic, hypolipidemic, or hypotensive agents are given to patients who have had myocardial infarction, stroke, or diabetes mellitus. Occasionally, a course of secondary prophylaxis can be relatively short, in a surgical operation or when radiotherapy or chemotherapy is used to retard or prevent death in patients with cancer.

Proficiency of Treatment

A treatment is given proficiently if the agent (or regimen) has had an adequate opportunity to carry out its anticipated action on the target. One requirement is a suitable patient, who should be appropriately susceptible to the anticipated outcome and responsive to the treatment. For example, in a trial of oral contraceptive agents, we would not enroll men or postmenopausal women. In a study of over-the-counter analgesic agents, we would not enroll patients whose pain was too mild (from a pin prick) or too severe (from a thoracotomy).

A second requirement is that the agent be given with suitable timing, dosage, and regulation. If given too late after the onset of the chest-pain signal, lidocaine prophylaxis would not be expected to prevent arrhythmias in the first 24 hr after acute myocardial infarction, nor would antibiotics prevent rheumatic fever if given too long after onset of the etiologic streptococcal sore throat. A medicine that must be injected or absorbed through appropriate mucosa will not work if swallowed orally. A medicine that requires a specified magnitude of dosage and reinforcement at regular time intervals would not be expected to work well if the schedule is improperly maintained. A medicine that prevents a subsequent target such as vascular complications by regulating an existing target (e.g., elevations in blood pressure, sugar, or lipids) would not be expected to work well unless the desired regulations are actually achieved.

A third requirement for proficiency is that the agent be given with suitable inherent accompaniment. The surgical procedure must be done by a competent surgeon working with a suitable environment before, during, and after the operation. The accompanying diet, if needed for success of the pharmaceutical agent, must be effectively maintained. The oxygen treatment must be given with an appropriate delivery system.

ADDITIONAL POST-TRIAL CONCLUSIONS

After a randomized trial has been analyzed (with or without an intent-to-treat arrangement of data), the main statistical conclusion refers to the comparison of the treated agents. Is one of them better or worse than the other for the action of the agents in both efficacy for the selected main target and safety in avoiding adverse phenomena? This comparison contains the "internal" events of the trial itself. Because an unbiased comparison is the prime goal of the trial, its "internal validity" is the main reason for randomization, double-blinding, and other precautions (including intent-to-treat analyses) used to prevent bias.

The results of the trial will also be used, however, for three additional types of conclusions. One set of conclusions refers to the effect of the individual agents. These results will contribute to the "history" of experience with that agent, to meta-analyses in which results are pooled from several trials involving that agent, or to other types of appraisals for individual agents.

Another set of conclusions refers to the external generalizability of the results beyond the trial itself. The "external validity" of this generalization will depend on how closely the selected patients, treatments, outcomes, and analyses approximate the conditions of conventional clinical practice. A problem in all randomized trials, the external generalization usually depends on the basic elements of each trial's structure. If substantially biased, the results may be difficult or impossible to generalize externally, but their external validity may sometimes be affected by the efforts made to avoid bias in internal validity (2).

A final set of conclusions refers to the direct application of the results in clinical practice. For this purpose, clinicians are seldom satisfied with the overall statistical appraisal of comparative efficacy. They want to know about results in specific clinical subgroups of "responsive" or "unresponsive" patients, so that decisions can be made about what treatments are best for which kinds of patients and what kind of outcomes can be expected in these patients. These issues are not the main purpose of randomized trials but can be a highly desirable byproduct of the work if the results are suitably arranged and presented.

For subsequent discussion, these four types of conclusions can be called *direct comparison, individual effects, generalizability,* and *clinical application.*

VIOLATIONS OF REGIMEN

All the foregoing discussion becomes pertinent when the ways in which a planned regimen can be violated are considered, as well as the impact of the violations on conclusions drawn from the trial. Different types of violation will be produced by different types of treatment and will have different effects on the corresponding results, analyses, and conclusions. Thus, the key questions to be answered are what kind of violations will produce distorted results if they are either specifically analyzed or deliberately ignored in an intent-to-treat analysis.

The two main types of violation consist of inadequate performance and contamination. The performance is inadequate if the agent, accompaniment, or both were not given or received in a proficient manner. The regimen is contaminated if it is improperly augmented or substituted. Augmentation occurs if the patient receives unscheduled additional agents or regimens that may have active effects. For example, the control group in the Multiple Risk Factor Intervention Trial study (3) became contaminated when many of the patients received multiple risk factor interventions that had not been anticipated in the original design of the trial. Substitution occurs if the patient is transferred (by self-selection or with consent of the supervising clinician) to a rival regimen under comparison in the same trial. This substituted type of contamination arises when patients assigned to receive either insulin or oral hypoglycemic agents transfer to the "opposing" regimen or when patients assigned to receive medical therapy decide to have the competing surgical operation.

Unless the patient's status is regarded as a "terminal" outcome at the time of contamination, contaminated regimens are particularly difficult to evaluate. No unanimity of agreement has been developed about whether the original or the subsequent treatment should be held responsible for the ultimate outcome. In the absence of contamination, however, regimens that are inadequately performed might be classified and analyzed according to the relative proficiency of the performance. Thus, uncontaminated patients could be categorized as *good, fair, poor* (or in some other suitable rating scale) for compliance with prescribed treatment or for their proficiency in regulating an existing target such as prothrombin time, blood sugar, or blood pressure.

REASONS AND ANALYTIC CONSEQUENCES FOR VIOLATIONS OF COMPLIANCE

The reasons for violating a regimen are particularly important because they determine whether an intent-to-treat analysis will help avoid bias or produce it. The reasons are either unrelated or related to the events that occurred after the regimen was imposed. The four main reasons for violation are provoked by negligence, nuisance, intervening outcomes, and difficult regimens. Each reason has its own sources and consequences.

Negligence

Simple negligence occurs if the patient is forgetful, noncompulsive, or otherwise uninterested in carefully maintaining an assigned regimen. It is taken in a suboptimal dosage or schedule, or perhaps not at all, but the patient has had no particular problems arising from the regimen itself and no distinctively bad or good outcome events after the start of treatment.

In this situation, the patient is untreated or inadequately treated for personal reasons unrelated to postrandomization phenomena. The individual treatment will be falsely credited or blamed for whatever events are attributed to it, but the comparison of treatments in the trial will be unbiased if the negligent patients are equally distributed in the compared groups. Conclusions about generalizability and clinical application will be quantitatively altered unless the number of negligent patients is relatively small. The inclusion of negligent patients in an intent-to-treat analysis will not distort "internal validity" but will reduce the statistical efficiency of the trial by lowering the opportunity to find a "significant" difference (if it exists) between the treatments.

Analysis of negligent patients offers an opportunity to use dose–response curves for checking or confirming efficacy. An appropriate pattern would occur if efficacy rises progressively with better maintenance for the active treatment but not for the placebo group. This type of "dose–response" analysis can also be applied to negligent patients if a trial contains two (or more) active agents but no placebo. For example, when placebo treatment was omitted for ethical reasons in randomized trials of antimicrobial prophylaxis against recurrent streptococcal infections (4), the investigators were surprised to find essentially equal efficacy for oral penicillin and sulfadiazine. Because the results might have been explained by relatively low virulence of streptococci in the community, the investigators were worried about whether the antimicrobial agents were indeed efficacious. Because poor compliance in the study seemed readily explained by negligence alone, the investigators concluded that the drugs were indeed efficacious when the attack rate of streptococcal infections was found to be substantially lower in the groups of patients with good rather than poor compliance.

Nuisance

An individual agent may have inherent properties that make it unpleasant to maintain. It may have a bad taste, be hard to swallow, require injections, or need frequent daily dosage. In this situation, the therapeutic schedule is violated because the agent is regarded as a nuisance, not because of any outcome effects or other clinical difficulties in maintaining the total regimen.

The effects of nuisance-violation patients are essentially similar to those in patients who are negligent. If the trial is truly double-blind, its internal validity will not be affected by the nuisance violations. In trials that compare an oral against an injectible regimen, however, or treatment once a day versus treatment five times daily, the comparative agents may not be arranged in a symmetrical, double-blind manner. For example, the investigators may be reluctant for ethical reasons to give placebo injections to patients receiving an active oral agent.

In an asymmetrical comparison of agents with high and low nuisance capacities, the true efficacy of the high-nuisance agent will be unfairly evaluated in an intent-to-treat analysis. The results will show what might happen in actual practice: Many patients will have no effect because they fail to take the nuisance treatment. Nevertheless, its true efficacy will be obscured, and the investigators may not discover that the treatment is indeed potent and that its efficacy might be better revealed if appropriate improvements were possible in the packaging, method, or schedule of administration to reduce the nuisance factors.

The conclusions about generalizability and clinical application of the medicine will also be misleading if the nuisance violators are not analyzed separately. A clinician whose charisma or communication can persuade patients to maintain the treatment, despite its nuisance features, may be surprised at getting results that differ substantially from what is reported in the intent-to-treat analysis.

Because the effects on the trial outcome are basically similar for nuisance violators and for negligent violators, the results for different degrees of maintenance can be analyzed with dose–response curves in the same manner described previously for the negligence group.

Intervening Outcomes

In contrast to violations produced by a patient's negligence or a treatment's nuisance, the two other types of violation arise from events that have specific clinical connotations. In one of these violations, treatment is altered because of intervening outcome events.

Treatment aimed at a remedial target may be discontinued because the target manifestation was promptly "cured" (e.g., cessation of pain). Conversely, the remedial treatment may be stopped or contaminated with some other "active" treatment because the expected relief did not occur (e.g., the pain persisted or worsened). Another source of violation for either remedial or prophylactic therapy is the occurrence of an untoward adverse reaction. These adverse reactions, which are especially likely when agents are given for a long course, have been a common reason for violating treatments prescribed for such conditions as epilepsy, hypertension, or chronic arthritis.

The intervening-outcome-dependent violations can occur for treatment that is wholly remedial or for the first (remedial) phase of a double-target prophylactic treatment. Thus, a patient whose acute low back pain is not promptly relieved may transfer from an unknown randomized analgesic agent to some other known active agent. A patient whose severity of angina pectoris is not adequately reduced by the randomized medical therapy may decide to have surgery.

If the patient's clinical state is noted at the time of the violation and is analyzed as the main outcome event, the results will not be misleading. The associated randomized treatment will be properly classified as successful or unsuccessful at that time. A substantial problem will arise, however, if two-target prophylactic treatment is altered by a short-term outcome (e.g., failure to relieve angina pectoris or regulate blood sugar) but if the main counted event is the long-term outcome. At the time of the long-term outcome, the patient will have been receiving a treatment different from the one assigned by randomization.

The management of these altered regimens is a particularly striking dilemma. A strategy that is both statistically and clinically acceptable has not yet been developed for analyzing the complexities of what really happened in the trial. Furthermore, the crucial information about reasons for therapeutic changes may not have been collected or made available for analysis with whatever alternative strategies may be proposed. Consequently, an intent-to-treat analysis is commonly applied for lack of anything better. If many patients have been contaminated, however, the results of an intent-to-treat analysis will often be greeted with derision by clincial practitioners and patients, regardless of the merits of the statistical argument about avoiding postrandomization bias. Even if relatively few patients were contaminated, most people would claim that simple common sense has been violated if patients who received surgery are analyzed as though it had not been done. The common-sense viewpoint could readily accept the idea of "charging" the surgical cohort for deaths that occurred before the surgery could be carried out but not the idea of counting as "surgical" a patient who refused the randomly assigned operation and who was followed thereafter on long-term medical therapy.

This chapter is not the place to discuss alternative strategies for analyzing the results of randomized trials that contain many violations caused by distinctive early outcome events. Some of the most controversial results of the past two decades, however, have occurred in randomized trials in which an intent-to-treat analysis was used for treatments that had been highly contaminated. The results have often been interpreted according to ideologic preconceptions. For example, according to the intent-to-treat analyses, tolbutamide was a cardiovascular killer in the University Group Diabetes Program trial (5), and multiple risk factor intervention was a useless treatment in the Multiple Risk Factor Intervention Trial (3). Nevertheless, many clinicians have refused to accept the University Group Diabetes Program results, and many clinicians and epidemiologists have rejected the Multiple Risk Factor Intervention Trial results.

The main point to be noted now is that when intervening outcomes and contaminations are ignored, an intent-to-treat analysis is neither statistically nor clinically satisfactory. Substantial bias can be introduced statistically if the good and bad intervening outcomes are not equally distributed among the compared treatments, and the results will lack "common sense" for all four types of clinical conclusions (i.e., individual regimens, comparisons, generalizability, and applicability).

Difficult Regimens

A more subtle, clinically important violation occurs if maintenance of a regimen rather than an agent alone requires strong personal resolution or difficult medical adjustments. Most forms of treatment involve adding something to a patient's lifestyle: an oral medication, an injection, or a surgical procedure and its subsequent consequences. Other forms of treatment, however, take something away. The patient may have to forego cigarettes, reduce caloric intake, or be deprived of certain foods. The deprivation regimens often accompany a pharmaceutical agent given for two-target prophylaxis, and maintenance of the regimen may require a psychic resolution that is difficult for many patients. They may then comply poorly with both the pharmaceutical agent and the accompanying diet or other treatment.

A difficult but analogous problem occurs if a patient must regulate an intervening target (e.g., blood sugar or blood pressure) but cannot achieve the desired goal without the discomfort of frequent excessive effects. This type of problem occurs when "brittle" diabetic or "resistant" hypertensive patients, trying to prevent long-term vascular complications, get frequent episodes of hypoglycemia or hypotension while attempting to regulate the intervening target blood sugar or blood pressure.

Problems in compliance or regulation may sometimes be the best (or only) way to show important features of differential prognostic susceptibility to the long-term outcome event. For example, patients who are able to maintain an unappealing diet, stop smoking, or engage in vigorous daily exercise may also have general life-styles or psychic states that make them less likely to develop coronary or other vascular diseases. In the absence of effective methods for measuring the appropriate psychic distinctions, the inability (or unwillingness) to comply with difficult regimens may be the best available prognostic marker for denoting a heightened susceptibility to cardiovascular disease.

Among insulin-requiring diabetic patients, it is generally well-accepted (although seldom documented) that vascular complications are particularly likely to occur in the brittle group. Thus, the reasons for inadequate regulation of a difficult regimen may also denote important prognostic distinctions that may otherwise be overlooked.

The subsequent analytic problems could be avoided or reduced if patients entering a randomized trial were first checked in a "qualification period" (6) that determined how well they could regulate or comply with the potentially difficult regimen. The patients could then be randomized within strata of good or poor regulation (or compliance), and the subsequent results could be analyzed appropriately within strata. In the absence of such prerandomization preparations, however, the prognostic susceptibility denoted by good or poor compliance (or regulation) may not be determined until after the trial has begun.

The results may then produce an intriguing problem in intent-to-treat analysis. For example, in the Coronary Drug Project (7), the mortality rates in an intent-to-treat analysis were 18% for the clofibrate group and 19% for the placebo group. When requested to analyze the results according to lowering of serum lipids during the trial, the investigators responded by analyzing compliance rather than regulation. Nevertheless, the mortality rates for clofibrate were 15% in the good compliance group and 25% in the poor compliance group. This significant difference would have suggested that clofibrate was efficacious except that a similarly significant mortality distinction was found in patients receiving placebo: 15% mortality rate in the good compliance group and 28% in the poor compliance group.

The results have been correctly hailed as convincing evidence that an intent-to-treat analysis prevented a false claim of efficacy for clofibrate. An additional conclusion, however, is that the investigators failed to suitably investigate the most powerful "agent" noted in the study: compliance. The psychic factors that induced people to comply with the total regimen (which included diet) in that trial are obviously powerful agents in reducing mortality. Yet this major clue to prognostic susceptibility was given no further attention. A unique opportunity was missed to study the personality or other features that affected compliance in that trial, to use the information for delineating "risk factors," and to help improve the design and analysis of future studies of analogous agents and similar outcome events.

Furthermore, the intent-to-treat analysis—if unquestioned and unextended into the appraisal of compliance—would have failed to identify a crucial prognostic attribute that is probably the most important result emerging from the entire trial. Contrary to the claims of intent-to-treat advocates, an analysis according to compliance can *always* be done in any trial if the compared groups were treated in a symmetrical manner, so that the results can be compared for the good and poor compliance groups for each treatment. A differential response in the compliance groups for both the active and placebo treatments will denote the important susceptibility factor of compliance. A differential response for compliance in the actively treated group but not for placebo will help indicate efficacy for the active agent. A differential response for compliance with two active treatments will require separate considerations according to the reasons for noncompliance.

An analysis according to degree of regulation of a target rather than mere compliance with a prescribed dosage schedule is also worth doing when pertinent. Because the problems of regulation may not be symmetrical in the compared treatments, the results could not be used for decisions about comparative efficacy of the treatments. Nevertheless, the results can be highly worthwhile for the information they may provide about prognostic factors or about the impact of regulation itself. Thus, it is generally contended that normalization of blood pressure, sugar, or lipids is highly desirable, but little documentary evidence has been obtained to support the contention. In most randomized trials devoted to those subjects, the results have been analyzed with intent-to-treat arrangements and sometimes for different degrees of compliance. The results have seldom been analyzed, however, for the different degrees of regulation achieved by the patients. Such analyses might not be statistically important for evaluating efficacy of the compared treatment, but the results could be clinically invaluable for supporting (or refuting) the idea that normalization or regulation is desirable for the intervening target events. For example, the merits of anticoagulant therapy after myocardial infarction or stroke might require major reevaluation if the same results were found in groups of patients who did or did not maintain properly regulated prothrombin times.

By avoiding these additional analyses, the intent-to-treat policy deprives the investigators (and the public) of valuable information that is contained but analytically ignored in the data of randomized trials. Such information might even help justify the money and effort that were expended in trials now regarded as "wasteful" because they yielded "negative" or "controversial" results.

CONCLUSIONS

An intent-to-treat analysis has the desirable statistical virtue of possibly avoiding biases that occur after randomization. Because of this virtue and because the analytic method has become so popular, an intent-to-treat analysis can be done as one of various analyses on data from a randomized trial. Several other analyses should also be done, however, to be sure that the intent-to-treat process does not produce deceptive or misleading results and to learn important clinical, therapeutic, and prognostic distinctions that will otherwise be lost, neglected, or overlooked. The additional analyses should make appropriate use of the reasons for violations of the intended treatment. With the clinical information and clarifications gained from those additional analyses, randomized trials can improve the effectiveness of their clinical contributions to the evaluation of treatment.

ACKNOWLEDGMENTS

This work was supported in part by grants from the Andrew W. Mellon Foundation and The Council for Tobacco Research-U.S.A., Inc., as a special project.

REFERENCES

1. Sackett DL, Gent M. Controversy in counting and attributing events in clinical trials. *N Engl J Med* 1979;301:1410–1412.
2. Feinstein AR. *Clinical epidemiology. The architecture of clinical research*. Philadelphia: WB Saunders, 1985.
3. MRFIT Research Group. Multiple risk factor intervention trial. *JAMA* 1982;248:1465–1477.
4. Feinstein AR, Wood HF, Epstein JA, Taranta A, Simpson R, Tursky E. A controlled study of three methods of prophylaxis against streptococcal infection in a population of rheumatic children. II. Results of the first three years of the study, including methods for evaluating the maintenance of oral prophylaxis. *N Engl J Med* 1959;260:697–702.
5. University Group Diabetes Program. A study of the effects of hypoglycemic agents on vascular complications in patients with adult-onset diabetes. Part I. Design, methods, and baseline characteristics. Part II. Mortality results. *Diabetes* 1970;19(suppl 2):747–830.
6. Knipschild P, Leffers P, Feinstein AR. The qualification period. *J Clin Epidemiol* (in press).
7. Coronary Drug Project Research Group. Influence of adherence to treatment and response of cholesterol on mortality in the Coronary Drug Project. *N Engl J Med* 1980;303:1038.

PART V

Perspectives on Health Care
and Research

Patient Compliance in Medical
Practice and Clinical Trials
edited by J.A. Cramer and B. Spilker
Raven Press, Ltd., New York © 1991

29

Epidemiological and Community Approaches to Patient Compliance

*Lawrence W. Green, **Patricia Dolan Mullen, and
†Rhonda B. Friedman

*Henry J. Kaiser Family Foundation, Menlo Park, California 94025; **Center for
Health Promotion Research and Development, The University of Texas Health Science
Center at Houston, Houston, Texas 77225; and †SysteMetrics/McGraw–Hill,
Washington, DC 20008

The changing epidemiology of diseases calls for a shift in medical interventions within the epidemiologic triad of host-agent-environment from a primary emphasis on the agent to a greater emphasis on the host (patient) and the environment. Most efforts to maximize the benefits and to minimize the risks of medical interventions have concentrated on the regulation of the "agent"—the invading organism or pathology. With the decline in acute communicable diseases and the increasing frequency of chronic conditions in the population, more patients must manage their own often complex, long-term regimens of medicines and life-style modifications. This requires a refocusing of attention to environments and patients outside hospitals and other clinical settings.

Most studies of patient "compliance" begin with the medical care setting as the locus of patient identification and intervention. A community approach to the problems of patient compliance with medical recommendations begins with a population in which many of the potential benefactors of medical advice are in varying degrees of contact with medical practitioners, some with no contact. The purpose of this chapter is to present a rationale and framework for analysis of medical compliance that considers the total population at risk, including those who should be but are not receiving medical care, as well as those who are misusing their prescribed medicines or recommended self-care practices.

The following four questions will be addressed in developing the framework:

1. What groups of potential patients have illnesses, conditions, or risk factors that would benefit from medical interventions the patients are not receiving?
2. What patients have illnesses or conditions that would benefit from more appropriate use of the medications or self-care procedures prescribed for them?
3. What types of patients, conditions, medical settings, medicines, and self-care regimens most likely result in error and would benefit from improved compliance?
4. What means of intervention for each group of patients and type of regimen appears most effective when (a) a condition is either diagnosed or undiagnosed,

(b) a regimen is either prescribed or not prescribed, (c) a drug is either dispensed or not dispensed, and (d) medical regimens are either followed or not followed?

EPIDEMIOLOGY OF HEALTH CARE COMPLIANCE ERRORS[1]

A health care error may be an error of commission or an error of omission. A medical compliance error is committed when a patient misuses a prescribed regimen or uses a medicine prescribed for another patient. An error of omission occurs when a patient fails to receive or apply a clinically important medication or procedure as needed.

Figure 29–1 identifies the circumstances under which patients would benefit from receiving medical information: (a) to inform them about treatable signs and conditions; (b) to inform them about the risks and benefits of a medicine and alternative nonpharmacologic therapies or self-care procedures; and (c) to inform them about the proper use of a medication or procedure. The figure identifies needs for patient education and broader public health education both to prevent errors of omission (in categories A, B, and C_2) and to prevent errors of commission (in category C).

Compliance Errors of Omission

Potential patients can be classified into two groups, each of which could be the target of different health education programs to reduce compliance errors of omission:

1. Those who are not currently seeking or receiving medical care for their illness or condition (the undiagnosed), or a symptom or risk factor that could warrant examination and health counseling (the unscreened).
2. Those who received a medical diagnosis but did not receive, fill, or use a prescription or recommendation for a procedure or medicine that could benefit them (the nonusers). (See Fig. 29–1.)

The Undiagnosed

The purpose of health education for people with undiagnosed conditions is to predispose and enable them to obtain screening or medical diagnosis and treatment, assuming that one or more tests, medications, or procedures would help prevent or treat their condition and would be prescribed for them (1). General communications targeted to these people would advise them that if they had certain high-risk characteristics or were experiencing specified symptoms, they should obtain periodic screening tests or consult a physician because medical advice or treatment may be needed.

Health education of this kind has long been part of public health programs to induce high-risk populations to seek prenatal care, immunizations, contraceptives,

---

[1]The terms *compliance* and *patient* are used for convenience and convention, even though several of the types of error discussed here are not patient errors of failing to follow physicians' directions, but rather are errors sometimes of physicians themselves or of patients who have not yet received appropriate directions from a physician or other health care provider.

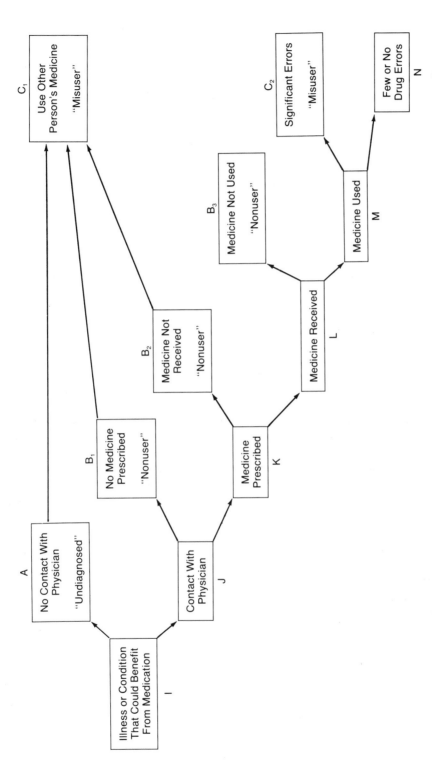

FIG. 29–1. Flow of patients into target groups for drug information: the undiagnosed (A), the nonusers (B), and the misusers (C).

blood pressure screening, and a variety of other preventive measures (2). The effectiveness of such efforts has been documented in primary prevention and communicable disease control (3) (accounting for the dramatic reductions in infant mortality, congenital defects, and the near eradication of some childhood diseases) (4), high blood pressure control (5) (accounting for dramatic reductions in the incidence of strokes and cerebrovascular death rates) (6), family planning (7), cancer control (8), mental health care (9), and other areas of secondary prevention and early diagnosis (10). Those suffering overt symptoms and the "worried well" (11) will be most responsive to media messages that encourage them to seek medical care to alleviate their symptoms or worries. Those with risk factors considered normal in their family, culture, or experience (12) will require more intensive case finding (13), outreach (14), and screening programs (15).

Nonusers

The first class of nonusers (B_1) consists of patients with preventable or treatable conditions, but who do not receive self-care or medical recommendations or education from their physicians or who receive a prescription or recommendation for the wrong therapy or self-care regimen. These patients might benefit from some of the same information as directed to the undiagnosed even though these errors of omission are made by their health care providers (16,17). A more appropriate remedy, however, is improved quality assurance activity with prescribers (18).

In another category of nonusers are those patients who do not obtain recommended self-care devices (e.g., a blood pressure cuff), medications, or who fail to fill their prescriptions (B_2). This occurs more frequently when patients cannot get to pharmacies, when they are exceptionally fearful of adverse reactions, and when the price of devices or medicines is perceived to exceed the value of the therapy (19).

Where the medical conditions are not life-threatening, the purpose of educational communications would be to increase awareness that the patient's condition may lead to complications, spread, or recurrences if untreated. Education for patients with symptoms that cannot consistently be seen or felt (e.g., high blood pressure) would attempt to strengthen the belief that the conditions may nevertheless be serious (20). For those who cannot afford the cost of medicines, information about less expensive medicines and sources of financial aid would be most useful. In particular, the degree of benefit from palliative regimens should be clarified so that the user is able to weigh potential benefits against financial and other costs, including possible adverse reactions (21).

Compliance Errors of Commission

Two types of possible errors of compliance commission are (a) those made by physicians, pharmacists, or others recommending or prescribing medications or self-care procedures and (b) those made by patients.

Professional Errors

The first type of compliance error of commission can occur when a diagnosis is applied without adequate confirmation, when medicines are prescribed in lieu of more appropriate nonpharmacologic therapies, when a new medicine's potential interaction with other regimens has not been evaluated, or when the proper medicine is prescribed in the wrong dosage. Such errors are arguably amenable to professional media communication and continuing education or quality assurance for physicians and others who care for patients (22), although general messages to high-risk subpopulations of the public may be helpful in shaping patients' expectations (23). Physician errors of commission are not considered further in this framework.

Patient Errors

Patients who are screened or diagnosed and receive self-care instructions or medications are at risk of misunderstanding and making errors in the use of procedures or medicines (24). The amount of information provided about a particular product to prevent these errors of commission does not always correspond to the amount needed by the patient or, indeed, to what the patient can understand (25). In the debate over patient package inserts, some proponents argued that full disclosure in a consistently available written format would at least give patients access to all the information they needed (26). In fact, however, some patients received a great deal of unnecessary information with patient package inserts, whereas some others may have received but failed to notice, comprehend, or recall the specific information they needed (27).

An alternate to the universal, uniform patient information strategy, but necessarily more complicated, is to carry out systematic surveys of the behavioral and educational needs of each demographic or epidemiologic grouping of patients. This should be less complicated and burdensome on practitioners than attempting to do a systematic educational diagnosis on each patient. A simplification of this approach is to develop synthetic estimates of the probabilities of drug use errors in each group or subpopulation of patients and the severity of consequences associated with each potential error. A specific group's relative need for drug education or counseling may be defined mathematically and estimated from a combination of national survey data (28) and local census data. Formulas for estimating drug information needs in local populations have been proposed (29).

Special Groups

Two groups present special problems of compliance errors of commission: pregnant women and those patients who medicate themselves by using prescription medicines obtained for another illness or by another person. For women who are—or intend to become—pregnant or are breast-feeding, more active health education campaigns need to be launched through the mass media or through fertility clinics (30,31). The campaigns need to urge them to report fully their use of medicines, tobacco, and alcohol to their physician or to a drug information service for evaluation, even before other needs for prenatal care arise (32). Formulas and software for synthetic estimates of women at risk of poor pregnancy outcomes caused by smoking have been developed (33).

Patients who use medicines obtained for previous illnesses or from other persons risk making a variety of mistakes, including use of an inappropriate medicine, the wrong dosage of the right medicine, or the right medicine at the wrong time. A survey conducted by the CBS Television Network found that at least one person in 45% of the United States households reported borrowing medicines or using old prescriptions to treat a medical condition (34). Only education through nonmedical channels can reach most of these consumers to warn them about these potential hazards (35).

PATIENT CONSIDERATIONS IN TARGETING INTERVENTIONS

Two conclusions follow: (a) Broad-scale patient educational programs must reach beyond the clinical setting, but they can be contained and targeted to demographic groups in which the prevalence of risk factors, undiagnosed conditions, or untreated illnesses are high, and (b) the remaining patient education and counseling resources can be concentrated on clinical and self-help group settings. Based on estimates of a 50% prevalence of compliance in patients (36), the potential of preventing a potentially harmful error per patient per encounter could be as high as 0.50 if methods of patient education and counseling were 100% effective. To maximize their effectiveness, educational and counseling resources must be conserved and concentrated on those patient encounters that represent the greatest need and opportunity to improve or protect health. The first task, then, is to determine what patients are in these target groups, and what kinds of compliance errors could be prevented by educating and counseling them effectively.

The Undiagnosed

Who are the undiagnosed? National statistics can be used to identify groups or types of would-be patients who are most likely not to seek help or to receive medicines for various conditions. The prevalence of those types in a local area or population can then be estimated from census data. National statistics indicate, for instance, that women experience (or acknowledge) more symptoms than men within most broad classifications of illness (37), and women also are more likely to seek diagnosis, medical care, and prescription therapy for the same symptoms than men, who are more likely to prefer home remedies (38).

When they do seek care, men account for 40% of the total number of patient visits to office-based physicians and 40% of drug "mentions" (39). [By convention, the National Disease and Therapeutic Index employs the term *mentions* (including refills or renewal of prescriptions) to reflect usage, which should not be interpreted as equivalent to number of patients or prescriptions.] The same bias in underrepresentation of men can be found in preventive care visits as in symptomatic care (40).

In addition, lower socioeconomic and nonwhite groups have higher incidence rates for most illnesses and lower medical and preventive care utilization rates relative to their greater need (41). White patients tend to receive more information from physicians than do blacks and Hispanics (42). Low income patients receive less than more affluent patients (43).

Patients older than 65 years of age are more often ill and require more visits and medicines than those in younger age groups. Patients 65 years and older purchase almost 25% of all prescription and nonprescription medicines (44). The elderly require more medication than younger patients for the management of acute disease (45), and they have a higher incidence of chronic disease (46).

Although the elderly may not make more drug compliance errors than younger patients with the same prescriptions, the deleterious consequences may be more serious (47), less easily detected, and less easily resolved than in younger patients (48). In addition, their complex medical regimens place the elderly at greater risk of compliance errors (49).

The best indicators, then, for targeting broad patient education and counseling programs to reduce compliance errors of omission are male sex, lower socioeconomic status, and older age. The following are the most prevalent illnesses and conditions of older men in lower socioeconomic groups (listed in order from highest to lowest): high blood pressure; respiratory, mental, nervous, digestive, skin, urinary, eye, and ear conditions; arthritis; and pain in bones and joints (50).

Diagnosed Nonusers Who Received Inappropriate Medical Recommendations

Those patients who received no prescription or the wrong medical advice cannot be considered noncompliant, in the strictest sense, especially if they followed the wrong advice. Nevertheless, their compliance error puts them at risk, and this class of compliance errors must be prevented or corrected. Continuing medical education of physicians and other health care providers is expected to prevent diagnostic and prescribing errors in individual practitioners and to build a level of knowledge and skill in the medical community that might detect and correct many of the individual errors that continue. Only weak and inconsistent evidence supports this expectation of traditional forms of continuing medical education (51). Innovative modalities of continuing education involving patients (52) and more comprehensive quality assurance methods combining educational with behavioral, economic, and environmental approaches to physicians' and other professionals' practices show greater promise but also mixed results (53).

The evidence that prescribing can be influenced through the mass media also seems conflicted. During 1973–1981, the national media aided a campaign by the National Institute of Mental Health targeted prominently to physicians who were "over-prescribing" barbiturate sedatives and minor tranquilizers. Prescriptions for these medicines declined substantially (54). A Canadian study suggested, moreover, that some physicians have overreacted to this publicity and as a result may have under-prescribed these medicines (55). Media events such as news of Nancy Reagan's breast cancer diagnosis tend to result in exaggerated increases in the demand for selected medical or screening procedures such as mammography (56). Thus, it appears that certain mass communications can influence clinical behavior, prescribing patterns and public demand for certain procedures.

Nonusers Who Did Not Obtain Medicine or Device Recommended

For nonusers who fail to fill prescriptions, to purchase nonprescription medicines or devices, or to adopt recommended procedures, two further strategies of targeting health education and communications can be considered. One is direct-to-public advertising of the price advantage of one product or pharmacy over another. The second is patient education directed at patients in medical care settings including pharmacies, especially for illnesses in which the cost of medicines most frequently discourages the filling or refilling of prescriptions. Such discouragement most often occurs when the illness or condition is not life-threatening, the symptoms are not very painful or noticeable, the patient is averse to taking medicines generally, or the patient simply cannot afford the cost of the medicine (57). A survey of the American Association of Retired Persons, for example, found that 20% of older patients never filled their prescriptions (58).

Misusers

Misusers provide a more efficient target for compliance-improving strategies than do nonusers for several reasons. They can be reached more readily—through providers of medical care—than the nonpatient and nonuser (B_3) groups. Patient education can be tailored more closely to their information needs and learning capacities (59). Misusers also can be assumed to be more highly motivated, on average, to respond more readily to drug information than nonpatients and nonusers, because they have made the effort to obtain medical care and to fill their prescription or to purchase recommended nonprescription medications or devices. The cumulative evidence from 102 published evaluations of patient education directed at drug misuse indicates that drug errors are reduced by an average of 40% to 72% and clinical outcomes are improved by 23% to 47% (60).

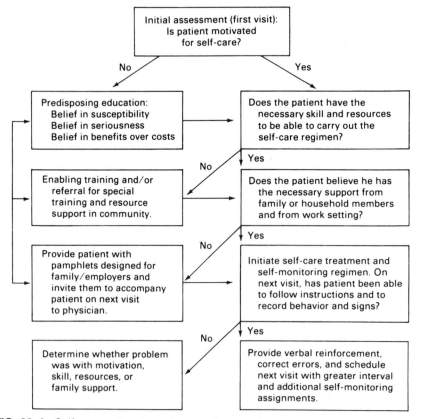

FIG. 29–2. Self-care protocol—a triage and stepped protocol for self-care education.

The same meta-analysis of the 72 studies of patient education directed at drug compliance specifically in chronic disease treatment showed that the medium, channel, or technique of communication mattered less than the appropriate application of learning principles such as individualization, relevance, facilitation, feedback, and reinforcement (61). A subsequent meta-analysis of patient education for preventive recommendations found a similar pattern (62). These principles can be applied more efficiently, systematically, and strategically with an algorithm that sorts or "triages" patients into educational groupings according to their educational needs (63). Figures 29–2 and 29–3 suggest such an algorithm for patient drug information, based on our

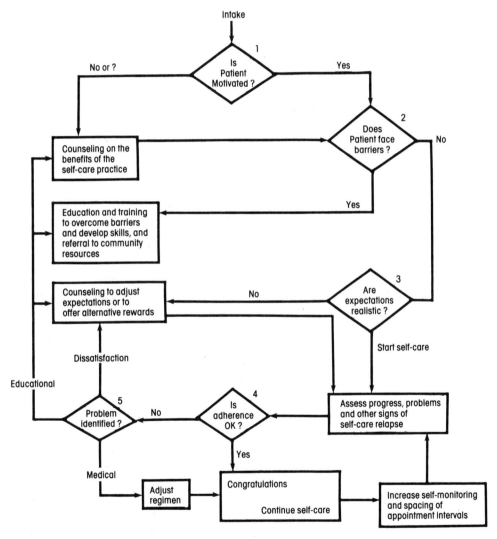

FIG. 29–3. Steps in diagnosing patient educational needs for specific self-care behavior. ◇, decision mode; ▢, recommended intervention.

retrospective analysis of randomized triage of patients with high blood pressure (64). Nevertheless, the principles of relevance (predisposing factors), facilitating (enabling factors), and feedback combined with social support (reinforcing factors) were tested prospectively in this study (65). The combined interventions yielded significant improvements in compliance and blood pressure control after 3 years (66) and a 50% reduction in mortality after 5 years (67).

A more refined model of patient decisions in accepting influenza vaccination has been derived from patient questionnaires and tested prospectively with correct prediction of vaccination behavior for 82% of high-risk patients (68). This hierarchical utility model questionnaire could provide the source of more specific answers to the initial questions in Fig. 29–2.

Allocation Decisions

Despite the efficiencies and cost-effectiveness of interventions directed at patients classified as misusers or potential misusers of medical advice and prescriptions, the cost-benefit potential of reaching the undiagnosed and dropouts from treatment could be much greater in the long run. These nonusers represent new markets for the pharmaceutical companies who should find it beneficial to support public health agencies in their efforts to reach these patients and to reduce the extent of untreated illness in the poorest populations. Recently, pharmaceutical companies, the Food and Drug Administration, consumers, and advertising firms have experimented with bringing medication information directly to the general public. Several attempts have been made by individual companies to educate consumers on signs and symptoms of certain diseases (e.g., hypertension, diabetes, depression) without mentioning products by name. These ads are referred to as "institutional advertising" and have been applauded by both consumers and the Food and Drug Administration. Institutional advertising could be an efficient and profitable method of reaching the undiagnosed and nonuser groups.

Efforts to bring more of the nonusers (i.e., the undiagnosed, the dropouts, the uninsured) into the medical care system will be frustrated if the burden on the system only makes the problems of compliance worse because of overworked staff spending too little time with patients. More widespread and more effective patient education and professional education related to the compliance problems, combined with organizational, economic, and environmental reforms of the system itself, will make the efforts to reach the nonusers worthwhile.

SUMMARY AND CONCLUSION

The opportunities and needs for patient education and counseling exceed the current supply, not so much in quantity available as in quality, willingness, and distribution. Much of the available energy devoted to patient education and counseling fails to reach the patients who need it most, when they need it, and in ways that would be most helpful to them. This chapter describes compliance problems in terms of errors of omission and errors of commission. An epidemiological assessment of needs for intervention on the various categories of compliance errors would segment the potential patient population in five high-risk groups: (a) nonusers who are not under medical care but have a condition that would benefit from use of a prescription or other medical or life-style regimen; (b) nonuser patients whose medical care provider has not recommended or prescribed a needed medicine, device, or life-style regimen; (c) nonuser patients who did not purchase a recommended medicine or device or adopt a recommended life-style modification; (d) misusers who are using someone else's medicine or a medication or procedure previously recommended or prescribed for another problem; and (e) misusers who are not following the schedule or dosage recommended. The environments, channels, and methods for communicating effectively with each of these groups vary systematically in ways that recommend new strategies for the support of public health education, professional education, and patient education.

Pharmaceutical companies and third-party payers could play a more active role in direct mass communications to the public about the risk factors, signs, and symptoms of diseases and conditions for which medical or self-care measures are available. Encouraging and enabling patients who have such risk factors, signs, or symptoms to seek screening or medical advice would improve the public health more in the long run than increased efforts to eliminate "noncompliance" for those already under care. However, burdening the medical system with more patients when it is failing to deal effectively with patient compliance problems because staff has too little time to spend understanding and interacting with patients will only make the problems worse.

The efficiency of patient education for those under care could be improved by systematic analyses of compliance error rates in various subpopulations of patients. This would lead in most settings to a greater allocation of patient education and counseling effort directed at men, lower socioeconomic, and older patients relative to women, higher income, and younger patients. A similar epidemiologic analysis of relative rates of compliance error for specific pathologies or symptomatologies could segment the patient population for effective educational triage within demographic groups.

Medical schools and other continuing education and quality assurance resources could be targeted more sharply to those physicians who are prescribing medicines incorrectly or who are unconvinced about the efficacy or benefit–risk ratio of underused medicines or procedures. Physicians, for example, do not have as much conviction and belief in their ability to modify dietary practices in their patients as they do to control blood pressure. Similarly, these educational resources could give greater emphasis to patient education and counseling skills required by physicians in educating and strengthening the motivation of their patients to fill prescriptions and to adhere to the prescribed regimens. Such an investment, according to the net results of 102 published evaluations of patient education related to errors with drug regimens, would reduce drug errors by 40% to 72% and improve clinical outcomes such as blood pressure control and reduced emergency room visits by 23% to 47%.

ACKNOWLEDGMENTS

This chapter is adapted from *Patient Education and Counseling* 1986;8:225–268, with permission from Elsevier Science Publishers. Support for this chapter was provided by a contract from the Pharmaceutical Manufacturers Association to the University of Texas Center for Health Promotion Research and Development. The authors gratefully acknowledge the research assistance of Janet Quillian, Ph.D., and Lorraine J. Lucas, M.S.P.H., and the statistical advice of Gary Persinger, M.S.

REFERENCES

1. Goldbloom R, Battista RN. The periodic health examination: 1. Introduction. *Can Med Assoc J* 1986;134:721–723.
2. Green LW. *Community health*, 6th ed. St. Louis: C.V. Mosby, 1990.
3. U.S. Preventive Services Task Force. *Guide to clinical preventive services: an assessment of the effectiveness of 169 interventions*. Baltimore, Maryland: Williams & Wilkins, 1989.
4. National Center for Health Statistics. *Health, United States, and prevention profile, 1989*. Hyattsville, Maryland: DHHS Pub. No. (PHS) 90-1232, 1990.
5. Lenfant C, Roccella EJ. Trends in hypertension control in the United States. *Chest* 1984;86:459–462.
6. Garraway WM, Whisnant JP. The changing pattern of hypertension and the declining incidence of stroke. *JAMA* 1987;258:214–217.
7. Udry J, Clark L, Chase C, et al. Can mass media advertising increase contraceptive use? *Fam Plann Perspect* 1972;4:37–44.
8. Butler M, Paisley W. Communicating cancer control to the public. *Health Educ Monographs* 1977;5:5–24.
9. Hersey JC, Klibanoff LS, Lam DJ, Taylor RL. Promoting social support: the impact of California's "Friends Can be Good Medicine" campaign. *Health Educ Q* 1984;11:293–311.
10. Lau R, Kane R, Berry S, et al. Channeling health: a review of the evaluation of televised health campaigns. *Health Educ Q* 1980;7:56–89.
11. Garfield SR. The delivery of medical care. *Sci Am* 1970;222:15–18.
12. Zapka JG, Stoddard A, Barth R, et al. Breast cancer screening utilization by Latina community health center clients. *Health Educ Res* 1989;4:461–468.
13. German PS, Shapiro S, Skinner EA, et al. Detection and management of mental-health problems of older patients by primary care providers. *JAMA* 1987;257:489–493.
14. Brimberry R. Vaccination of high-risk patients for influenza. A comparison of telephone and mail reminder methods. *J Fam Pract* 1988;26:397–400.
15. Fried LP, Bush TL. Morbidity as the focus of prevention in the elderly. *Epidemiol Rev* 1988;103:48–64.
16. Lewis CE. Disease prevention and health promotion practices of primary care physicians in the United States. *Am J Prev Med* 1988;4(suppl 4):9–16.
17. Mullen PD, Tabak ER. Patterns of family physicians' counseling practices for health habit modification. *Med Care* 1989;27(7):694–704. (Presented at the International Communication Association Health Communication Conference, Monterey, CVA, February 1989).
18. Pels RJ, Bor DH, Lawrence RS. Decision making for introducing clinical preventive services. *Annu Rev Public Health* 1989;10:363–383.
19. *Patient information and prescription drugs: parallel surveys of physicians and pharmacists*. New York: Louis Harris and Associates, 1983.
20. King AC, Martin JE, Morrell EM, et al. Highlighting specific patient education needs in an aging cardiac population. *Health Educ Q* 1986;13:29–38.
21. DeTullio PL, Eraker SA, Jepson C, et al. Patient medication instruction and provider interactions: effects on knowledge and attitudes. *Health Educ Q* 1986;13:51–60.
22. Lomas J, Haynes RB. A taxonomy and critical review of tested strategies for the application of clinical practice recommendations: from "official" to "individual" clinical policy. *Am J Prev Med* 1988;4(suppl 4):77–94.
23. *Prescription drug information for patients and direct-to-consumer advertising*. Boston: Medicine In the Public Interest, 1984.
24. Roter DL, Hall JA, Katz NR. Patient–physician communication: a descriptive summary of the literature. *Patient Educ Couns* 1988;12:99–119.
25. Tuckett DA, Boulton M, Olson M. A new approach to the measurement of patients' understanding of what they are told in medical consultations. *J Health Soc Behav* 1985;26:27–38.
26. Green LW, Faden R. Potential effects of patient package inserts on patients and drug consumers. *Drug Infor J* 1977;2(suppl):64–70.
27. Fisher S, Mansbridge B, Lankford DA. Public judgments of information in a diazepam patient package insert. *Arch Gen Psychiatry* 1982;39:707–711.
28. Lawrence L, McLemore T. National ambulatory medical care survey. In: *Vital and health statistics series*, No. 88. Washington, DC: National Center for Health Statistics, 1983.
29. Green LW, Mullen PD, Friedman RB. An epidemiological approach to targeting drug information. *Patient Educ Couns* 1986;8:255–268.
30. Hill IT. *Reaching women who need prenatal care*. Washington, DC: National Governors Association, 1988.
31. Department of Health and Human Services: *Caring for our future: the content of prenatal care*. A report of the Public Health Service Expert Panel on the Content of Prenatal Care, 1989.

32. Committeee to Study Outreach for Prenatal Care, Institute of Medicine. *Prenatal care: reaching infants.* Washington, DC: National Academy Press, 1988.
33. Green LW, Hogan P, Deutsch M. *Estimating need: manual for estimating prevalence of women at risk of poor pregnancy outcomes due to smoking.* Houston: Center for Health Promotion Research and Development, University of Texas Health Science Center, 1987.
34. CBS Television Network. *A study of attitudes, concerns and information needs for prescription drugs and related illnesses.* New York: CBS Television Network, 1984.
35. National Research Council. *Improving risk communication.* Washington, DC: National Academy Press, 1989.
36. Sackett DL, Snow JC. The magnitude of compliance and noncompliance. In: Haynes RB, Taylor DW, Sackett DL, eds. *Compliance in health care.* Baltimore: The Johns Hopkins University Press, 1979.
37. Glynn TJ, ed. *Women and drugs: research issues,* No. 31. Washington, DC: Govt Printing Office, DHHS Pub. No. 271-80-3720, 1983.
38. Povar GJ, Mantell M, Morris LA. Patients' therapeutic preferences in an ambulatory care setting. *Am J Public Health* 1984;74:1395–1397.
39. Baum C, Kennedy DL, Forbes MB, Jones JK. *Drug utilization in the U.S.* Rockville, Maryland: Food and Drug Administration, 1983.
40. Stephens T, Schoenborn CA. Adult health practices in the United States and Canada. In: *National Center for Health Statistics, Vital and Health Statistics series 5,* No. 3. Washington, DC: Government Printing Office, DHHS Pub. No. (PHS) 88-1479, 1988.
41. Woolhandler S, Himmelstein DU. Reverse targeting of preventive care due to lack of health insurance. *JAMA* 1988;259:2872–2874.
42. Hall JA, Roter DL, Katz NR. Meta-analysis of correlates of provider behavior in medical encounters. *Med Care* 1988;26:657–675.
43. Waitzkin H. Information giving in medical care. *J Health Soc Behav* 1985;26:81–101.
44. Kayne R, ed. *Drugs and the elderly.* Los Angeles: University of Southern California Press, 1984.
45. German P, Klein L, McPhee S, Smith C. Knowledge of and compliance with drug regimens in the elderly. *J Am Geriatr Soc* 1982;9:568–571.
46. National Center for Health Statistics, Moss AJ, Parsons VL. Current estimates from the National Health Interview Survey, United States, 1985. In: *Vital and health statistics series 10,* No. 160. Washington, DC: Government Printing Office, DHHS Publ. No. (PHS) 86-1588, 1986.
47. Lamy P, Beardsley RS. The older adult and the pharmacist educator. *Am Pharm* 1982;22(5):40.
48. Williamson J, Chapin JM. Adverse reactions to prescribed drugs in the elderly: a multicare investigation. *Age Aging* 1980;9:73–80.
49. Green LW, Mullen PD, Stainbrook GL. Programs to reduce drug errors in the elderly: direct and indirect evidence from patient education. *J Geriatr Drug Ther* 1986;1:3–16.
50. National Center for Health Statistics, McLemore T, DeLozier J. 1985 Summary: National Ambulatory Medical Care Survey. In: *Advance data from vital and health statistics,* No. 128, Washington, DC: DHHS Publ. No. (PHS) 87-1250, Government Printing Office, 1987.
51. Haynes RB, Davis DA, McKibbon A, Tugwell P. A critical appraisal of the efficacy of continuing medical education. *JAMA* 1984;251:61–64.
52. Avorn J, Soumerai SB. Improving drug-therapy decisions through educational outreach: a randomized controlled trial of academically based detailing. *N Engl J Med* 1983;308:1457–1463.
53. Davis DA, Haynes RB, Chambers LW, et al. The impact of CME. A methodologic review of the continuing medical education literature. *Eval Health Professions* 1984;7:251–283.
54. Baum C, Kennedy DL, Forbes MB, Jones JK. *Drug utilization in the U.S.—1981: third annual review.* Rockville, Maryland: Food and Drug Administration, 1982.
55. Rosser WW. Benzodiapazine use in a family medicine center. *Drug Protocol* 1987;2(10):9–15.
56. *Morbidity and Mortality Weekly Report* 1989;38:137.
57. Green LW, Fedder D. Drug information: the pharmacist, and the community. *Am J Pharm Educ* 1977;41:444–448.
58. Green LW. Some challenges to health services research on children and elderly. *Health Serv Res* 1985;19:793–815.
59. Inui TS, Carter WB, Pecoraro RE, et al. Variations in patient compliance with common long-term drugs. *Med Care* 1980;17:986–993.
60. Mullen PD, Green LW. Educating patients about drugs. *Promoting Health* 1985;6(6):6–8.
61. Mullen PD, Green LW, Persinger GS. Clinical trials of patient education for chronic conditions: a comparative meta-analysis of intervention types. *Prev Med* 1985;14:753–781.
62. Mullen PD, Green LW, Tabak E, et al. *Meta-analysis of studies evaluating patient education.* Report submitted to the National Center for Health Services Research and Health Care Technology Assessment.
63. Green LW. How physicians can improve patients' participation and maintenance in self-care. *West J Med* 1987;147:346–349.

64. Hatcher MW, Green LW, Levine DM, Flagel CE. Validation of a decision model for triaging hypertensive patients to alternate health education interventions. *Soc Sci Med* 1986;22:813–819.
65. Green LW, Levine DM, Deeds SG. Clinical trials of health education for hypertensive outpatients: design and baseline data. *Prev Med* 1975;4:417–425.
66. Levine DM, Green LW, Deeds SG, et al. Health education for hypertensive outpatients. *JAMA* 1979;241:1700–1703.
67. Morisky DE, Levine DM, Green LW, et al. Five-year blood pressure control and mortality following health education for hypertensive patients. *Am J Public Health* 1983;73:153–162.
68. Carter WB, Beach LR, Inui TS, et al. Developing and testing a decision model for predicting influenza vaccination compliance. *Health Serv Res* 1986;20:897–932.

Patient Compliance in Medical
Practice and Clinical Trials
edited by J.A. Cramer and B. Spilker
Raven Press, Ltd., New York © 1991

30

Identifying and Improving Compliance Patterns

A Composite Plan for Health Care Providers

Joyce A. Cramer

*Epilepsy Center, Department of Veterans Affairs Medical Center, West Haven,
Connecticut 06516; and Yale University School of Medicine, Department of Neurology,
New Haven, Connecticut 06510*

Identification of the range of patients who do not take their medication as prescribed leads health care providers to the issue of how to improve compliance. This process has two essential elements: Why is the patient a poor complier? What can be offered to enhance compliance with the recommended medical plan? This chapter reviews ways in which consideration of these two basic questions can be used by anyone interacting with patients in medical practice or clinical trials.

A health behavioral counseling process was designed by Russell (1) for the Lipid Research Clinics cholestyramine study using an 11-step process: (a) identify the problems; (b) select the short-term and long-term goals of treatment; (c) collect information; (d) develop a behavioral diagnosis; (e) generate an intervention plan; (f) intervene; (g) reassess the behavioral diagnosis; (h) generate a revised intervention plan, if necessary; (i) reintervene; (j) develop a maintenance program; and (k) review the behavior change program. This system can be adapted for use in most medical practice settings by the health care team and in many types of clinical trials in which research staff are trained to work closely with study patients.

COMPLIANCE CHECKLIST

A systematic compliance documentation checklist was developed for the Epilepsy Cooperative Study (sponsored by the Department of Veterans Affairs) to address the major compliance problems and the primary strategies used to resolve these problems. The purpose of the compliance documentation checklist is to obtain a comprehensive, prospective record of the nature and frequency of the primary compliance problems experienced by each patient as well as the strategies used by the clinic staff to resolve these problems. The project has three specific aims: (a) to document the types of primary compliance problems presented by patients at specific points throughout their treatment; (b) to document the types of strategies used by clinic staff to resolve the compliance problems at specific points throughout the program; and (c) to examine whether patients' compliance with medication regimens is associated with either the type of compliance problem or the strategy used to resolve it. The counseling program should be generally applicable to all types of health care issues because it concentrates on the individual rather than the disease state.

The compliance documentation checklist contains a list of 14 specific compliance problems. The physician and research assistant select the best description of the patients' primary compliance problem. This the problem that causes the patient to miss the greatest number of doses. Secondary compliance problems also may be indicated. Only problems with a 5% or greater effect on compliance are checked (i.e., three or more doses per month). Compliance problems are defined as follows:

Psychological problems
  1. Nonacceptance: Patient has not accepted the drug regimen or diagnosis of epilepsy.
  2. Emotions: Patient did not take medication because of strong emotional reactions, (e.g., angry, depressed, anxious).
  3. Other priorities: Patient decided not to take medication because other events had higher priorities (e.g., family, legal problems, job).
  4. Social criticism: Patient decided not to take medication because of possible criticism from others (e.g., friends, co-workers, family).
  5. Decision to omit dose: Patient decided not to take medication; no specific reason was identifiable.
  6. Negative thoughts: Patient decided not to take medication because thoughts about the regimen or the disease were upsetting.

Planning problems
  7. Forgot on regular schedule: Patient forgot to take the medication while on a usual schedule.
  8. Forgot on disrupted schedule: Patient forgot to take the medication because of an unusual, disrupted schedule.
  9. No medication: Patient ran out of medication; medication was lost or destroyed.
  10. Lacked information: Patient was given inadequate information or incorrect information about the treatment regimen.
  11. Flexible hours to schedule appointments: Patient needed a special time for clinic appointments.

Medical problems
  12. Adverse reactions: Patient decided not to take medication because of adverse reactions.
  13. Illness: Patient did not take medication because of illness, incapacity, or hospitalization.
  14. Testing efficacy: Patient omitted doses to determine whether problems would recur without medicine.

Other problems
  15. Not yet known: Nature of the problem was unable to be determined in this session.
  16. No compliance problem: Patient had no compliance problem (e.g., takes 100% of medication as prescribed).

The *compliance documentation checklist* contains 23 specific strategies to resolve compliance problems. These strategies are grouped into seven categories (Table

TABLE 30–1. *Strategies to enhance patient compliance[a]*

Provide information
    Education about treatment for this disease
    Education about the study
    Understand the compliance problem: Review the self-debate factors to improve the patient's
       understanding of the problem
Increase motivation
    Use persuasion to promote motivation and the decision to take the medication
    Help the patient resolve a nonstudy problem (e.g., personal, work, family, disability)
    Use general or social reinforcement for overall patient behavior
Collect information
    Obtain additional information from the patient about the problem during the session
    Plan to collect data by asking the patient to use a formal daily collection procedure (e.g., a log or
       diary)
    Plan a telephone contact with the patient before the next visit
Modify regimen administration
    Plan a cue to remind the patient when to take a dose
    Plan how to cope with an unusual schedule in the future
    Change the regimen schedule or method of administration
    Use a stepwise dose increase program (i.e., shaping) to approach the full prescribed regimen
       gradually
Change contingencies
    Discuss compliance failure: Identify and discuss how the patient failed to follow the regimen
    Reduce negative consequence: Remove or reduce a negative social consequence (e.g.,
       embarrassment, criticism)
    Reduce or remove an adverse reaction
    Use a contract: Use a formal contract with the patient
    Use specific social reinforcement for a specific patient behavior
    Arrange a positive consequence
Refer patient for extra help
    Arrange for a physician to discuss the disease, treatment, or study with the patient
    Arrange an appointment for the patient to receive additional medical treatment in another
       program or from another medical clinic
    Arrange an appointment for the patient with a psychologist or psychiatrist
    Arrange for the patient to obtain help for a personal welfare problem from another person or
       social services agency
Other items
    Other strategies not listed: Describe briefly
    Did not use any intervention strategy during this session

[a]Developed for the Department of Veterans Affairs Epilepsy Cooperative Study #264.

30–1). The physician and research assistant indicate the primary strategy that is being used to solve the patient's primary compliance problem. Additional secondary strategies used for the primary problem also may be indicated. It would not be unusual for individual research assistants to prefer a few types of intervention strategies and to use them repeatedly. However, the broad scope of strategies listed serves as a reminder of other techniques that might be useful.

A preliminary assessment of compliance problems and strategies demonstrates that forgetfulness is the single most common problem (Table 30–2). Information and motivation are the most commonly used strategies, encompassing almost half of the problems (Table 30–3).

Categorization by age shows fewer problems in those older than 55 years (74% none) than in those younger than 34 years and in the 35-to-54-years age groups (59% and 62% none). The oldest patients need few strategies other than increasing their education about the disorder and need for regular medication, and motivation to follow the medical plan. Employed patients need less education and motivation and more of other strategies for similar types of problems than unemployed patients.

TABLE 30–2. *Frequency of 309 reported problems*

Forgot, disrupted schedule	18%
Other priorities	16%
Forgot, regular schedule	12%
Decision to omit doses	11%
Lack of information	9%
Emotions	7%
(None)	(27%)

COMMENT

The core of the compliance counseling process is the engagement of patients in discussion. Didactic education about the diagnosis and the need for medication to control their disease often is not absorbed during the brief visit with a physician. Long-term follow-up tends to focus on current adverse reactions and problems that have occurred during the last interval. Thus, when the patient reports no adverse events, the interview often is over quickly without using the opportunity to refocus on the therapeutic goal. Specific questioning about medication-taking habits, reasons for missed doses, and discussion of drug serum concentrations reengages the patient in the process of his or her own treatment plan. Planning follow-up care, convenient appointments, pill boxes for medications, and other techniques as described in various chapters in this book are helpful tools for patients who want to use these as cues for their habits. However, patients may choose not to use any of the suggestions offered. The amount of time needed to discuss compliance problems and attempt to provide assistance aimed at these specific problems may not be feasible for many physicians.

In a Health Maintenance Organization, the cost of physician or staff time must be weighed against the value of compliance counseling to reduce the need for extra care. Physicians are trained to explain diagnoses and the need for medication or other treatment to patients but often do not convey this information in a manner that is easily understandable, acceptable, or remembered by the patient. Further explanations by other medical staff including nurses, physician's assistants, dieticians, and clinic assistants often are used by Health Maintenance Organizations to increase patient education to avoid misunderstandings and misapprehensions that lead to poor compliance. All staff easily could be trained to use specific compliance strategies to address particular needs of individual patients in a modest amount of time. Specialty clinics, particularly those dealing with chronic diseases, often use unique strategies for their patients. For example, a program for systematic training of research teams has been developed by Russell and Insull (2). Staff at Lipid Research Clinics counseled patients about compliance with low-fat diets and administration of medication.

TABLE 30–3. *Frequency of use of 805 strategies*

General reinforcement	30%
Education about the medical disorder	17%
Help with other problems	12%
Education about the study	7%
Psychological support	6%
(None)	(28%)

Once the diagnosis of a chronic disorder has been made, it is particularly advantageous for Health Maintenance Organizations and providers of free care (e.g., government programs) to give as much education and assistance as possible to enhance the patient's understanding of his or her medical problem. The patient who drops out of the medical care system today and reappears in the emergency room after another acute event often requires yet another full work-up and reintroduction to the system, at great expense. Assuming that the physician has recommended an optimum course for prevention, control, or cure of a chronic medical problem, the burden of acceptance and fulfillment falls to the patient. Lack of fulfillment of this responsibility puts the patient in the position of increasing the cost of the nation's medical care if he or she has to return for repeated evaluations of the same problems or develops a disorder that might have been prevented or diminished with appropriate precautions. The economy and potential savings to the country by using extensive compliance counseling are apparent. It should be used whenever possible to reduce overall health care cost by avoiding repeated assessment for known disorders.

Future Research

Future research into compliance should focus on several issues, such as

- What types of strategies work best to enhance compliance?
- Are specific strategies optimal for certain types of patients?
- Are specific types of patients particularly attentive to the details of medication dosing with special counseling?
- Are the conscientious, attentive patients more likely to seek or readily accept advice on how to use cues or to establish routines that enhance compliance?
- Are patients who are less conscientiously attentive to details more likely to have lower compliance rates because of a less systematic approach to medication-taking habits?
- Are the schedules of less conscientiously attentive patients more easily disrupted, leading to forgetfulness despite good intentions to take medication?
- Are the less conscientiously attentive patients those who decline to use counseling or compliance aids?

Unfortunately, no psychological test exists that will predict or discriminate between fully compliant and partially compliant types. At this time, every patient must be considered a potential noncomplier.

"Compliance lies within the patient" (3). Understanding the complex issues and providing patients with the knowledge and skills that will improve their willingness and ability to take medication appropriately will help solve the problem of under-compliance. There are no easy-to-memorize rules that will make a patient a good complier or a health care provider a good counselor. Effective compliance counseling depends on interactional skills, and these depend on understanding, insight, and practice, rather than on formulas. Until an ideal intervention technique is discovered, physicians and other health care providers should attempt to offer a variety of strategies in the hope that the individual patient will be attracted to use at least one technique. Current research is focusing on methods to monitor and measure individual rates and patterns of compliance to assist physicians and clinical trials staff to know actual drug usage. Health behavior research is needed to assess the value of various interventions as documented by the new electronic monitoring devices.

ACKNOWLEDGMENTS

This work was supported by the Department of Veterans Affairs Medical Research Service. Michael L. Russell, Ph.D., (deceased) collaborated in the development of this program. This chapter is adapted from a report previously published in *Epilepsy Research* (suppl 1): Compliance in Epilepsy, 1988;163–175, eds. D. Schmidt and I.E. Leppik, by permission of Elsevier Science Publishers BV, Amsterdam.

REFERENCES

1. Russell ML. Behavioral aspects of the use of medical markers in clinical trials. *Controlled Clin Trials* 1984;5:526–534.
2. Russell ML, Insull W. Evaluation and training of medication adherence counselors in a clinical trial: application of a skill inventory to video-recorded interviews. *Controlled Clin Trials* 1981;2:133–148.
3. Rehder TL, McCoy LK, Blackwell B, Whitehead W, Robinson A. Improving medication compliance by counseling and special prescription container. *Am J Hosp Pharm* 1980;37:379–385.

*Patient Compliance in Medical
Practice and Clinical Trials*
edited by J.A. Cramer and B. Spilker
Raven Press, Ltd., New York © 1991

31

Health Care, Research, and Regulatory Impact of Noncompliance

*Louis Lasagna and **Peter Barton Hutt

*Sackler School of Graduate Biomedical Sciences, Center for the Study of Drug
Development, Tufts University, Boston, Massachusetts 02111; and **Covington and
Burling, Washington, DC 20044

The introduction of increasingly more sophisticated prescription medicines in the past 50 years has produced profound changes in the ability of physicians to control human disease. Even for those diseases for which effective medicines are available, however, two significant limitations continue to reduce their overall use. First, there is a paucity of information about the dose–response relation of many medicines in humans. This requires practicing physicians to either treat patients with an average dose or to titrate doses in individual patients. Second, there is no effective way to ensure that patients follow the physician's directions for using prescription medicines. Consequently, the failure of a patient to improve as expected could result from noncompliance as well as from failure of the medicine itself.

Both of these limitations are caused by one of the best-documented problems in medical practice—patient noncompliance with directions for using prescription medicines.

NATURE AND EXTENT OF PATIENT NONCOMPLIANCE WITH PRESCRIPTION DRUG DIRECTIONS FOR USE

Few problems in daily medical practice are better documented than patient noncompliance with the physician's directions for use of prescription medicines. Noncompliance can take four different forms: (a) taking more medicine than has been prescribed, (b) taking less medicine than has been prescribed (or none at all), (c) taking the medicine at different times, or at different intervals, than specified in the directions for use, or (d) taking the medicine under conditions that were contraindicated by the physician (e.g., at the time of a meal or in conjunction with a particular type of food).

Two general circumstances in which patient noncompliance with prescription drug directions for use has major regulatory and therapeutic implications are (a) during clinical investigation of the medicine to determine its safety and effectiveness and (b) during therapeutic use of a marketed medicine after regulatory approval, when therapeutic failure or adverse reactions may occur.

The literature demonstrates wide variation in patient compliance with directions for use of prescription medicines. This occurs both during drug investigation and during routine medical use. There are many possible reasons for failure to follow directions, including forgetfulness, confusion, adverse reactions, apprehension about drug-related hazards, and the belief that medication has either failed or is no longer needed. Even within an inpatient setting, compliance issues may arise in terms of errors in timing, errors in dose, or patient refusal. Any of these events can perturb the patient's clinical response.

Noncompliance can either be the cause of a therapeutic failure or the result of a failure. Similarly, the failure of a patient to follow prescribing directions can either cause toxicity (e.g., by overdosage) or result from toxicity. Hence, one needs both to measure compliance and to seek to explain lapses from the prescribed regimen. The impact of noncompliance on the expected results of a medicine depends on such factors as the direction of noncompliance (i.e., overdosing or underdosing), the shape of the dose–response curve, the position of the prescribed dose on the curves for benefit and toxicity, and the need for constant drug levels as opposed to discontinuous therapy. In some situations a few missed doses have no clinical consequences, whereas in other situations such lapses may be of great significance. Several dose–response relations must be considered because these relations are different for benefit and toxicity. Moreover, multiple end points are involved in the evaluation of toxicity and often with regard to benefits.

Although the majority of patients usually achieve a substantial degree of compliance, a large minority—usually between 25 and 50%—do not comply with prescribed directions for drug use. As a result, there is no absolute means of assuring that a particular patient has complied with directions for a medicine's use. Some experts assume that all patients are noncompliant unless proven otherwise. As discussed below, this rate of noncompliance can have a major impact on the reported safety and effectiveness of a medicine.

Numerous studies have attempted to isolate the characteristics that determine individual patient compliance or noncompliance. Some of the more important ones in addition to those already described include

- Perceived and actual severity of the illness
- Whether the disease is acute or chronic
- Patient's age at onset of illness
- Ease of communication with health professionals
- Attitude of health professionals
- Follow-up care by health professionals
- Knowledge of the patient about the illness
- Participation of the patient in devising the treatment plan
- Convenience of treatment for the patient
- Complexity of the prescribing directions
- Number of medicines prescribed
- Patient's confidence in the physician
- Patient's confidence in the diagnosis
- Patient's confidence in the treatment
- Whether the medicine provides symptomatic relief
- Adverse reactions of treatment
- Whether the patient feels sick or well
- Economic status of the patient

- Support of family and friends
- Social acceptability of the disease
- Psychological stability of the patient
- Educational status of the patient

This list illustrates the variety of factors involved. Not surprisingly, the ability of a physician to assess compliance on clinical grounds alone has been shown to be poor.

Social scientists have developed models to account for and thus to predict patient compliance and noncompliance. Based on these models, which attempt to account for the multiple factors involved, various strategies for improving compliance have been developed and tested. These strategies include such techniques as

- Patient education
- Home follow-up programs
- Increased supervision
- Simplification of dosing regimens
- Alternative methods of treatment
- Greater pharmacist involvement
- Greater nurse involvement
- Written directions for use
- Special counseling
- Special labels on medicine containers
- Memory aids

These intervention techniques have met with varying degrees of success, but it is clear that none of these techniques has reduced patient noncompliance to an acceptable level.

WAYS TO MONITOR AND CONTROL PATIENT NONCOMPLIANCE WITH PRESCRIPTION DRUG DIRECTIONS FOR USE

Faced with serious rates of noncompliance and important public health consequences resulting from this noncompliance, a number of techniques have been used in the past to monitor and thus potentially to increase compliance. This has traditionally been done by such measures as

- Direct patient observation
- Periodic counting of pills
- Chemical monitoring of drug levels or markers in body fluids
- Radioactive tracer studies
- Patient interviews
- Review of pharmacy records

All these techniques, however, are subject to serious deficiencies. Most do not pinpoint the time at which or the circumstances under which the medicine is taken.

Novel microelectronic monitors, described in other chapters, have altered the ability to measure and understand issues that are affected by noncompliance. Although it is possible for a compulsive cheater to trick a microelectronic monitoring system, it is certainly difficult. To circumvent a pill count, the patient need only discard the requisite number of pills at any time before a clinic visit. To circumvent a microelectronic monitoring system, the container must be opened on the regular schedule and the requisite number of pills discarded—a far more demanding requirement.

Like many of the other previously available means of monitoring and controlling patient compliance, an electronic monitoring system cannot guarantee that the medicine, once removed from its container, is in fact ingested, or guarantee that a patient has not removed several doses at one time. Indeed, even a check of body fluids for the medicine or a marker is subject to the timing of the sample, interference by other substances, the half-life of the medicine or marker, the limits and variability of detection methods, and the vagaries of testing procedures. Chemical checks of body fluids for the medicine or a marker are often distorted by the strong tendency of patients to improve their compliance just before scheduled visits to a physician or laboratory. Moreover, detection of substances in body fluids does not provide accurate information about the actual dose consumed or the time at which or circumstances under which that dose was consumed, and provides no information about the compliance with directions at times other than those reflected in the biological sample.

IMPORTANCE OF ACCURATE MONITORING OF PRESCRIPTION DRUG USE DURING CLINICAL TRIALS OF INVESTIGATIONAL NEW MEDICINES

Clinical trial analysis has rarely accounted for patient noncompliance. Instead, it has usually been assumed, for data analysis, that either all patients comply with the directions for use or that the distribution of compliance and noncompliance among trial subjects corresponds to that in routine clinical practice. Some protocols make no attempt even to approximate the degree of compliance. Pill counts of the contents in returned containers are commonly made, and drug levels in biological fluids are sometimes measured, but these data are usually not used to stratify responses or to elucidate dose–response relations. Thus, statistical analysis of the effect of noncompliance on results is rarely performed.

The assumption that all investigational patients are completely compliant is invalid for most outpatient studies. It has been estimated that generally somewhere between 25 and 50% of such subjects are in fact noncompliant. Customary investigational techniques cannot detect reliably which patients have not complied or the detailed and specific nature of their noncompliance. It is also often assumed that the level of safety and effectiveness observed in a clinical trial is a direct reflection of the specified conditions of use. In fact, the results are the average of results in those who undercomply, those who overcomply, and those who accurately comply with the directions for use. This has a major impact on the determinations that regulatory authorities are required to make for a medicine.

One of the well-documented variations of noncompliance with directions for use is the patient-initiated "drug holiday"—an interruption in drug therapy of at least one 24–hr period, undertaken by the patient without the knowledge of the physician. Many patients resume correct dosing just before any scheduled visit to the physician or a laboratory. Unless the physician observes clinical deterioration in the patient and discovers the cause or chemical or electronic monitoring catches the "holiday," it can easily pass unrecognized.

IMPACT OF NONCOMPLIANCE ON A REGULATORY AUTHORITY'S
DETERMINATION OF DRUG EFFECTIVENESS

Based on past experience, most clinical trials should be assumed to involve patients who overdose, patients who underdose, and patients who accurately dose. Those evaluating the results of a clinical trial, however, have heretofore assumed (with some exceptions) that all patients accurately dose. This aspect of the intention to treat analysis[1] provides an average rate of effectiveness, not the rate of effectiveness that would occur were the medicines taken by all patients as prescribed.

Adjusting for compliance is diametrically opposed to the concept of intention-to-treat analysis. This latter approach is lauded by some as unbiased, but in fact it is itself biased by its failure to use information related to compliance to protocol. No one can defend the manipulation of data by *post hoc* dropping of patients to make a medicine look better than it deserves, but there is no merit in an obsessive mystification of data by counting patients who never received the medicine, or who received the wrong medicine, or who received the medicine in amounts inadequate to produce either harm or benefit. Increasing type II errors (concluding erroneously that no difference exists between treatments) is predictably the result. Type II errors are no more desirable than are type I errors (concluding that a difference exists when, in fact, it does not). Indeed, a conspicuous consequence of type II errors is an overestimate of the medicine's optimal dose—a common outcome of clinical trials that can lead to unnecessary adverse reactions. Only if a reliable dose–response relation is available can one determine an optimal dose. When the curve begins to plateau, any higher dose is medically unjustifiable.

An important precedent for compliance-related Food and Drug Administration labeling with regard to efficacy can be found in the package insert directions for cholestyramine (Questran). Although this labeling gives an average figure of 19% for the reduction in the combined rate of coronary death and nonfatal myocardial infarction for the entire experimental population during a 7-year period, there is also an admirably detailed breakdown by estimated average dosage intake for reduction of both serum cholesterol and coronary heart disease risk (see Table 31–1).

The cholestyramine labeling provides four determinations of dose–response values: an average value and one at each of three dosing levels. the full compliance effectiveness has been shown to be approximately twice the average compliance effectiveness. Crude as the estimates of compliance probably were (based on counts of returned unused packets of the medicine), they show an unmistakable dose–response relation for both end point variables and give a much clearer picture to prescriber and patient of what can be achieved with different intakes of the medicine.

The Helsinki trial of gemfibrozil (Lopid) has taken the same approach to the analysis of drug effectiveness. Patients in this 5-year clinical trial were divided into four quartile groups on the basis of average capsule counts. The boundaries between the four quartiles were 69%, 85%, and 93% of the recommended dose. Lipid responses to gemfibrozil rose with increasing quartile of compliance for total, nonhigh-density lipoprotein, low-density lipoprotein, and high-density lipoprotein cholesterol and for triglycerides. The quartile with the highest rate of compliance achieved substantially

---

[1]In such an analysis, patients are treated as if they took the treatment to which they were assigned, regardless of whether they actually took it.

TABLE 31–1.[a] *Relation between compliance and therapeutic endpoints for cholestyramine*

Packet count	Total cholesterol lowering (%)	Reduction in coronary heart disease risk (%)
0–2	4.4	10.9
2–5	11.5	26.1
5–6	19.0	39.3

[a]From Food and Drug Administration–approved labeling for package insert.

greater lipid-lowering effects than the average of all the subjects in the trial (see Table 31–2).

As with the cholestyramine study, the gemfibrozil study demonstrated the impact of variable compliance and the value of patient-specific compliance data in determining drug effectiveness.

Reliance on the assumption of uniform compliance with directions for use of prescription medicines during a clinical trial might be defended on the grounds that approximately the same rate of noncompliance can be assumed to occur with therapeutic use after regulatory approval as with clinical investigation before regulatory approval. This argument is not persuasive, however, both because it rests on an unproven hypothesis and because it ignores the enormous variation among individual patients.

The patient in a placebo-controlled trial is informed that there is a 50% chance of not receiving the test medicine. In contrast, the patient in everyday medical practice knows that the medicine prescribed has been proved effective. This difference is likely to result in differences in compliance. In addition, an experimental population is chosen by use of informed consent, has been screened to exclude extremes of age and comorbid states, avoids the use of concomitant medication, and is closely followed, often by expert physicians. In everyday medical practice, medicines are given to patients of all ages, some with multiple diseases and on multiple medicines, by physicians of varying competence. Some of these differences might increase com-

TABLE 31–2.[a] *Compliance-dependent effects of gemfibrozil on plasma lipids in the Helsinki heart study*[ab]

	Gemfibrozil				Placebo			
	Q1	Q2	Q3	Q4	Q1	Q2	Q3	Q4
Cholesterol								
Total	−4.4	−7.7	−11.3	−12.7	+2.0	+0.8	+1.4	+1.2
High-density lipoprotein	+6.5	+8.1	+10.2	+12.0	−1.0	−1.0	−2.3	−1.0
Non–high-density lipoprotein	−7.1	−11.1	−16.0	−18.0	+2.4	+1.0	+2.0	+1.8
Low-density lipoprotein	−3.6	−6.8	−10.3	−12.1	+2.5	+1.5	+2.8	+3.0
Triglycerides	−22.9	−32.6	−42.7	−42.0	+0.3	−2.0	−0.6	−1.9

[a]Data from V. Manninen, et al. *Lipid alterations and the decline in the incidence of coronary heart disease in the Helsinki study. JAMA* 1988; 260:641–651.
[b]Q1, compliance <69% by pill count; Q2, compliance 69 to 84% by pill count; Q3, compliance 85 to 93% by pill count; Q4, compliance >93% by pill count.

pliance in practice; others diminish it. It is not surprising that routine medical experience cannot be equated with investigative use.

Moreover, even if the average rate of compliance during clinical trials was shown to approximate the average compliance during routine medical use, the assumption of uniform compliance ignores the documented variation among individual patients. This in turn distorts the medicine's effectiveness data.

On occasion, compliance data can serve to distinguish between a therapeutic failure and an adverse reaction. Consider, for example, a patient with cardiac rhythm disturbances in an antiarrhythmic drug trial who suddenly experiences an arrhythmia. Two possible explanations are drug toxicity or therapeutic failure. If monitoring shows an overdosing during the period immediately before the event, drug toxicity would seem likely. But an event occurring after 3 days without intake of any medicine suggests not therapeutic failure (as might be a reasonable conclusion if compliance had been good to perfect), but the result of lack of the medicine in the body.

This correlation is of particular importance in three types of situations. First, there are some situations in which effectiveness is difficult to demonstrate. Averaging noncomplying patients with complying patients may well influence the results so that effectiveness cannot be demonstrated at a statistically significant level. Second, the Food and Drug Administration and other regulatory authorities will at times require the use of active controls in addition to or in lieu of placebo controls. Where two equally effective medicines in a clinical trial have different rates of patient compliance, the difference in effectiveness shown between the two medicines could be statistically significant and clinically impressive, even though it resulted solely from a disparity in regimen compliance. Third, a significant number of nonresponders in a clinical trial can itself throw substantial doubt on the practical effectiveness of a medicine. This may occur even if the average rate of effectiveness, based on all patients, is statistically better than that of the placebo. The more marginal the demonstrated effectiveness, the more difficult it will be to obtain regulatory approval or to establish a market for the product if it is approved.

Thus, the current approach to determining drug effectiveness in clinical trials, by using the average rate of effectiveness, has a number of unintended results. First, it may reduce the likelihood that in a clinical trial, an effective medicine will, in fact, be shown to be effective. Second, in compensating for this deficiency, it forces the investigators to increase the dose to compensate for undercompliance. Third, this dose increase in turn inevitably results in a larger incidence of and more severe adverse reactions, which will be discussed below.

During the past decade, Food and Drug Administration has increasingly been concerned about the need to conduct clinical "titration" trials to determine the precise dose level of a new medicine that achieves optimum effectiveness and safety. The purpose of this approach is to reduce the prescribed dose to the lowest effective level to reduce both the incidence and the severity of adverse reactions. This is a laudable objective that serves a genuine public health purpose. As long as the current approach of determining average effectiveness prevails in clinical trials, however, the objective of determining the lowest effective dose cannot be achieved because of the distortion created by widespread noncompliance. Under the current approach, the lowest average effective dose can be determined, but a true dose–response relation cannot be generated. Even worse, the current approach forces compliant patients to overdose.

In contrast with this current approach, accurate monitoring of compliance allows the development of a true dose–response relation from a single trial using a specific recommended dose level, because it also takes into account the actual dose taken by each individual patient. The difference between the two approaches (i.e., monitoring compliance versus assuming compliance) can readily be seen in the following example. Assume that Drug A is effective at a daily dose of 10 mg, is no more effective at a dose of 15 mg, and is ineffective at a dose of 5 mg. In a clinical trial, 50% of the patients take the specified dose of 10 mg, 25% take an overdose of 15 mg, and 25% take an underdose of 5 mg. Under the current approach of determining average effectiveness, the results would show that the medicine was effective in 75% of the patients and ineffective in 25% of the patients at a dose level of 10 mg. With accurate monitoring, however, the results of the trial would show that 10 mg is 100% effective, 15 mg is no more effective, and 5 mg is ineffective. The difference in the results between these two approaches is thus extraordinarily important.

Recently, the Food and Drug Administration indicated its willingness to consider approval of a new life-saving medicine after a phase II clinical trial that clearly demonstrates effectiveness. The type of dose–response relation that could be obtained through use of sophisticated monitoring of compliance would seem to be a critical element for any such definitive phase II study in the future.

Although the Food and Drug Administration does not have the legal authority to base its drug evaluations on the net social benefit of a new medicine, other governmental and private organizations do take a cost-benefit analysis into account in establishing formularies, determining reimbursable cost, and making other related technology assessments. A relatively low average rate of effectiveness for a medicine can thus place the product at a serious marketing disadvantage. Accurate correlation of dose with effectiveness and the consequent correlation of cost with benefit should provide a more favorable profile for a medicine.

IMPACT OF NONCOMPLIANCE ON REGULATORY DETERMINATION OF DRUG SAFETY

It is axiomatic that as the dose of a medicine increases, the likelihood of adverse reactions increases. Just as ignoring variable compliance in a clinical trial results in an underestimate of the medicine's effectiveness, it also results in an underestimate of the medicine's adverse reaction profile.

No medicine approved by the Food and Drug Administration as safe and effective since 1962 has subsequently been removed from the market because of new information demonstrating a lack of effectiveness. There have been numerous well-publicized instances, however, in which clearly effective medicines have been removed, because at the dosage recommended or under the conditions of use specified, an unacceptable level of adverse reactions has occurred. Frequently, these effective medicines have been withdrawn from the market by their manufacturers even though the Food and Drug Administration has urged that they remain available for a relatively small number of patients for whom the benefit–risk ratio would remain favorable.

Thus, it is essential to establish the lowest dose that provides an acceptable clinical benefit and to target the medicine to those patients who need it and are expected to respond. To determine this optimal dosing level, more precise clinical trials and more accurate dosing information are critically needed.

IMPACT OF NONCOMPLIANCE ON REGULATORY REQUIREMENTS FOR DRUG LABELING

From the discussion above relating to the determination of the effectiveness and safety of the medicine during clinical trials, the impact on the package insert is clear. Under the current approach of determining average drug effectiveness, it is likely that the recommended dose will be higher than the actual minimum effective or optimal dose to compensate for the dilution effect of the patients in the clinical trials who did not comply with the recommended dose. Using the dose–response information obtained from accurate monitoring, however, a true dose–response relation can be described in the package insert. In effect, a dose–response relation stratifies the dosing schedule to be set forth in the approved labeling.

Virtually all prescription drug labeling today is technically misleading because it does not show the effects of taking the medicine in complete compliance with directions for use. By providing physicians with the results of clinical trials that measure only average drug effectiveness and that do not determine a dose–response relation, and by failing to state that the recommended dosage was set without consideration of patient compliance with directions for use, the labeling provides physicians with dosing information that is inherently erroneous, even if well-intentioned.

With the availability of a true dose–response relation for a new medicine, drug labeling will become more accurate. The correlation of dose with effectiveness can be spelled out with clarity, perhaps in a table such as that used for cholestyramine (Questran). Both physicians and patients will have available the expected beneficial effect to be obtained from full compliance, average compliance, and low compliance.

This has important implications for drug therapy as well as for avoiding adverse reactions. In the past, physicians have assumed that the lack of therapeutic response in a patient was the result of therapeutic failure. Knowing the dose–response relation, however, the attending physician will have therapeutic information that could lead to more effective professional intervention. Rather than assuming therapeutic failure of the medicine, the physician can be led to more careful questioning of compliance by the patient and to modification in dosage if necessary. The types of professional intervention designed to increase compliance would be given greater impetus. Knowledge of the likely individual patient-specific response to an identified dose of the medicine will, in short, provide incentive to the physician to investigate the true cause of the lack of therapeutic response in the patient.

In some instances, information on the effect of even minor patient noncompliance may lead to new packaging and labeling strategies designed to reduce this problem.

Development of patient-specific dose–response data for a generic medicine could also have important promotional implications. Under the Drug Price Competition and Patent Term Restoration Act of 1984, a company that obtains clinical evidence required by the Food and Drug Administration to support a new claim for a medicine obtains a 3-year period of market exclusivity before generic medicines can make the same claim. By developing specific dose–response data, a company can potentially redefine the optimal dose, in terms either of the level or the frequency and other conditions of use. This exclusive labeling could provide an important marketing advantage.

IMPORTANCE OF ACCURATE MONITORING OF PRESCRIPTION DRUG USE DURING MARKETING AFTER REGULATORY APPROVAL

The need for correlation between drug use and clinical end points in individual patients does not end when the investigational trials are completed and a regulatory authority has approved the medicine's submission. Equally important decisions depend on this information after marketing of the medicine begins.

To the extent that a valid dose–response relation is available before marketing, the recommended dosage and the information contained in the package insert will maximize the potential for safe and effective use of the medicine. Nonetheless, prescription drug labeling cannot prevent individual patient noncompliance, through overuse or underuse of the medicine. Thus, a reliable monitoring device has additional uses after regulatory approval of a submission. First, it can assist in controlling patient compliance with the directions for use of a medicine. Second, it can pinpoint the cause of unexpected problems with either the effectiveness or the safety of a medicine.

In daily medical practice, the clinical signs observed by a physician in any specific patient may wax and wane, without apparent correlation with the dose that is being administered. The physician has insufficient information to titrate the dose to the individual patient's medical needs because actual dosage information is inaccurate or unavailable.

For some medicines, strict control of dosing is absolutely essential for effectiveness. An excellent example of this relation is the oral contraceptive. Failure to comply with the daily dosing schedule destroys the medicine's effectiveness. For that reason, the familiar calendar pack was developed and is standard throughout the industry. The precise percentage claims of effectiveness for oral contraceptives are possible only because noncompliance is either reduced to a minimum or documented and taken into account in analyzing data on effectiveness.

Just knowing that a monitoring device is a silent but ever-present diagnostic observer of the patient will, in itself, perform a valuable compliance function. People tend to behave more reliably when they know that they are under observation and thus accountable for their action. They tend to speed when no policeman is visible and to slow down when they believe a policeman is in the vicinity. Simply knowing that a device will reliably report drug compliance is likely to result in a higher rate of compliance than would otherwise occur. Yet it is clear that some patients will still be noncompliant, and in diseases as different as melancholia, epilepsy, and glaucoma, monitoring of data allows clinicians to explain therapeutic failure and to take appropriate action to a degree not achievable through the use of other clinical data.

Compliance information on marketed medicines is of enormous regulatory importance. Unexpected therapeutic failure or adverse reactions must be reported by the manufacturer to regulatory authorities. Not infrequently, these problems will eventually be reflected in revised labeling. Without the availability of patient-specific compliance information, all therapeutic failures and adverse reactions will be deemed by regulatory authorities to have resulted from use of the medicine at the dosage recommended in the package insert that was approved. Thus, labeling changes will be seriously considered. Only with the availability of patient-specific compliance information can this presumption be overcome.

As noted above, in a number of recent well-publicized incidents, effective medicines have been removed from the market (e.g., zomepirac, benoxaprofen, nomifensine, suprofen, ticrynafen) because of an unacceptable rate of adverse reactions. Although it is impossible to determine precisely what would have happened if a dose–response relation had been available before marketing and patient-specific compliance information had been available after marketing, it is conceivable that some of those medicines could have avoided the regulatory nightmare that occurred.

The availability of patient-specific compliance data has other important ramifications as well. Exposure to malpractice and product liability litigation, for example, should be significantly reduced where specific data document an actual erroneous dosing regimen used by the patient.

CONCLUSION

Compliance with prescribing directions is often poor and has serious implications for drug regulation, research, and medical care. New, improved techniques for quantifying noncompliance are capable of providing important advances in our approach to drug treatment. The development of interventions to enhance compliance with medication regimens will improve patient safety.

Subject Index